——— The ———

Chronic Bronchitis and Emphysema Handbook

The
Chronic Bronchitis and Emphysema Handbook

REVISED AND EXPANDED EDITION

Dr. François Haas

Dr. Sheila Sperber Haas

with Illustrations by Kenneth Axen

John Wiley & Sons, Inc.

New York • Chichester • Weinheim • Brisbane • Singapore • Toronto

This book is printed on acid-free paper. ♾

Copyright © 2000 by François Haas and Sheila Sperber Haas. All rights reserved

Published by John Wiley & Sons, Inc.
Published simultaneously in Canada

This publication is designed to provide accurate and authoritative information in regard to the subject matter covered. It is sold with the understanding that the publisher is not engaged in rendering professional services. If professional advice or other expert assistance is required, the services of a competent professional person should be sought.

Library of Congress Cataloging-in-Publication Data:

Haas, François.
    The chronic bronchitis and emphysema handbook / François Haas, Sheila Sperber Haas.—Rev. and expanded ed.
        p. cm.
    Includes bibliographical references and index.
    ISBN 0-471-23995-X
    1. Lungs—Diseases, Obstructive—Handbooks, manuals, etc. 2. Lungs—Diseases, Obstructive—Popular works. I. Haas, Sheila Sperber. II. Title.

RC776.O3 H33 2000
616.2'4—dc21   00-023916

Printed in the United States of America

10 9 8 7 6 5 4 3 2 1

This book is dedicated to people everywhere who are struggling to reclaim their lives from COPD, to the family and friends who support them in this battle, to the health care professionals who really *listen* to them and give them the best edge possible in this fight, and to patient advocates who fight for better weapons and a more fair advantage in this lifelong struggle.

Contents

Preface

It has been nearly 10 years since the publication of our initial handbook for patients with COPD—chronic bronchitis and emphysema. Until recently we saw no significant changes in treatment or outlook for COPD patients—and thus no reason for doing a second edition. In the last two years, however, three important issues have emerged.

First is the development of lung reduction surgery. Second is the dramatic increase in awareness of complementary—or alternative—therapies, along with progress in understanding what they can accomplish and greater acceptance by mainstream medicine. Third is the even greater need for patient advocacy. Since we wrote the first edition, we are more convinced than ever that changing health care management is increasingly forcing COPD patients to go to bat for themselves. And this book now includes more of the tools and ammunition that you'll need.

COPD can be an exhausting and overwhelming burden to live with. Patients who constantly fear running out of air, who watch their capacities dwindle prematurely, struggle with a grossly heightened sense of their fragility. They and those close to them are usually frightened, depressed, and angry. Doctors treating COPD patients do the best they know how to do. The problem is that so many were taught only to treat the medical aspects of COPD—and many have never learned since to appreciate the importance of rehabilitating these patients.

The word *rehabilitate* comes from the Latin *rehabilitare*, which means to restore. Restoration to a happier, healthier lifestyle should be the goal of any treatment program—and it is certainly our aim in educating you. This book's guiding principle regards *rehabilitation* as synonymous with *comprehensive care*—rehabilitation in its broadest and truest sense. It should not be merely an adjunct to the treatment of COPD, but ideally encompasses medical management and is itself the treatment. It is the means for reversing the downward spiral that begins with impaired pulmonary function and ends in near-total impairment of the patient and, all too frequently, his or her family.

The most basic premise of all rehabilitation—including pulmonary—is that positive change can be achieved under even the most dreadful circumstances imaginable, and thus no effect of illness, save for death, is absolute. The concept of pulmonary rehabilitation actually first emerged after World War I. Then in 1942, during World War II, the Council on Rehabilitation stated that, "rehabilitation is the restoration of the individual to the fullest medical, mental, emotional, social and vocational potential for which he/she is capable."

The Council added that in addressing both the physical and mental aspects of any chronic illness, rehabilitation must be tailored to maximize improvement and minimize the impact of illness or progressive deterioration for both patient and family. The next decade—the 1950s—saw the pioneers of pulmonary rehabilitation establish successful techniques for meeting these goals, techniques that now allow COPD patients to resume useful and satisfying lives.

Although the medical literature is filled with reports verifying the solid benefits of comprehensive pulmonary rehabilitation, the medical establishment still views it with at best benign neglect, and at worst—outright hostility. They brand it a waste of time and money rehabilitating patients with a disease that can only get worse. Skepticism and a lack of enthusiasm persist among many physicians, *including* pulmonologists. The reasons for this skepticism are not surprising.

1. Many programs that call themselves comprehensive in truth provide only fragmented care, and thus produce only fragmented benefits.

2. Because most programs fail to incorporate follow-up in their design, alleged benefits remain anecdotal.

3. Many programs use physiological parameters—such as pulmonary function tests and arterial blood gases—as measures of overall success. However, these are neither sensitive nor appropriate measures of benefit.

4. A great many programs fail to recognize the dynamic link between the various components of impairment. Failure to address one or more of these components may greatly diminish the benefit of treatments directed to others. For example, failure to recognize and treat depression and/or anxiety may result in noncompliance with medication or

an exercise program and, in turn, failure of the rehabilitation effort. The resulting—and erroneous—conclusion is that pulmonary rehabilitation doesn't work.

5. Because the absolute necessity for a team approach continues to be unappreciated by most physicians, they fail to acknowledge that not even the most skilled, caring, and conscientious physician can meet all the needs of the patient with chronic lung disease.

6. There is a failure to appreciate that rehabilitation is not accomplished in 3 weeks or 3 months, but is a lifetime process.

Although the situation is improving—with many medical facilities now offering some degree of pulmonary rehabilitation—it is doing so at a frustrating pace. So the great majority of COPD patients—and many of the doctors who care for them—are still convinced COPD means a fearful, breathless life of increasing inactivity and helplessness, drugs to quiet intense anxiety and depression, more and more frequent hospital stays, and a decidedly premature death.

But COPD patients with the good fortune to have learned—from their doctor or elsewhere—of a comprehensive rehabilitation program know this doesn't have to be so. They work, they walk, they travel, they garden, they exercise, they make love, they laugh, they socialize. Their COPD symptoms are far less intrusive, their disease has slowed its pace, and their hospital stays are shorter and much less frequent.

Doing what they want may take a lot of planning and effort, and may happen at a much slower pace than it used to. But, because these patients no longer have to turn their backs on the things important to them, the quality of their lives has immeasurably improved and they feel in control once again.

Forty-five years ago, Dr. Albert Haas began the pioneering pulmonary rehabilitation program here in the Rusk Institute at the New York University Medical Centers. Since that time, we have been helping patients with emphysema and chronic bronchitis live longer and dramatically better lives.

We help them learn to: breathe more effectively, get into good physical condition, get rid of excess phlegm, use less energy to do things, return to work, resume favorite leisure activities, put intense anxiety and depression in the past, get their marriages back on track, like themselves again. The less advanced their disease and/or the more they participate in their own care, the greater their progress.

Education is your key: education about your disease, and the variety of things you can do to cope with it. The problem until now for COPD patients was that the needed information wasn't easy to come by. This lack of public information about the disease has been a crippling problem for most COPD patients, because it was precisely this information that would have helped them cope with their illness and achieve the best their life still has to offer them.

That is why we wrote *The Chronic Bronchitis and Emphysema Handbook*. It is a comprehensive guide for COPD patients *and their families*, because we clearly realize the enormous impact of COPD on family as well as patient.

Aiming to produce as complete a book as possible, we had several goals in mind. First of all, that this book *not* be a substitute for a well-trained physician and physical therapist; our aim is to educate COPD patients, not treat them. Second, that the book be clearly written, enjoyable to read, and a pleasure to look at. Third, that the book should go beyond the medical aspects of COPD to include everything relevant to handling the disease. (A glance at the table of contents indicates the range of topics we consider relevant.)

Our first aim reflects one of our biggest objections to most popular medical books, their strong implication that "Follow these rules and you will be cured." Some books actually give treatment rules, telling readers what drugs and doses to take. Once an ill person is diagnosed, however, he or she needs to be treated by a competent professional who knows his or her particular case. Each patient is an individual, and no two individuals should be treated exactly alike just because they have the same disease. The need for any element of COPD treatment must be determined in the context of the whole person. This requires a qualified (meaning competent and *educated*) doctor.

A second important consequence of *educating* patients properly is that it allows them to participate actively—and therefore effectively—in their own treatment. Educating the patient's family means enabling them to participate too, to the patient's benefit and their own. For any illness, we believe that achieving the most effective treatment requires participation by doctor *and patient and family*.

And because treating COPD effectively involves a broad range of medical and rehabilitation services, patient and family do best when they are well-prepared for active involvement with the entire group of highly skilled professionals they will be working with: doctor, physical therapist, respiratory therapist (sometimes), vocational counselor, psychological counselor, social worker (sometimes).

Our second goal was to write a book that is easy and enjoyable to read. Making information accessible involves more than just putting it all together in one place. Readers may notice some repetition in defining certain technical terms. There are two reasons for this. One is that people differ in their capacity to retain relatively technical information. Readers who do not easily retain such facts will not have to hunt around for definitions when technical words and concepts reappear after a while. The second reason is that some readers prefer to skip around instead of reading a book by chapter order. We do not want information to be incomprehensible because a reader has not yet read preceding sections.

The illustrations in this book are unique, and a pleasure to look at. For this success we thank our friend and colleague of many years, Kenneth Axen, Ph.D., who shares our conviction that illustrations should combine clearly presented information with visual interest. And because he is a scientist who studies breathing, he was able to develop these illustrations on his own, freeing us to concentrate on the research and writing.

Two elements of our writing style deserve some comment. The different subjects presented in the book require two different ways of addressing the reader. When presenting background or technical information, we address the reader impersonally. In talking about experiences that most or all readers have—or will have—we address you personally. You will also notice that we sometimes use the pronouns *he* and *him*. This does not reflect any sexist bias, but simply our strong distaste for the awkward *he/she, him/her*, etc., which substantially breaks up the flow of a sentence. Constantly alternating between *he* and *she* also makes for bumpy reading. So when you read these masculine pronouns, please picture male and female doctors and patients.

One last thought concerns our qualifications for producing this book. We each have a Ph.D. (François in biophysics and heart-lung physiology, Sheila in psychology). François's father, Dr. Albert Haas, was one of the first architects of pulmonary rehabilitation. So the content and value of pulmonary rehabilitation have been part of the air he has breathed since he was a young child. François directed the Cardiopulmonary Laboratory at the New York University Medical Centers, which carries out lung testing and diagnosis, for close to twenty years. His research studies on how the lungs work have included ways to make cardiopulmonary rehabilitation even more effective. François now devotes himself full-time to pulmonary research, with a prominent focus on rehabilitation issues. Sheila is a medical and science writer with a passion for making the complex appear simple.

Last but not least, we owe special thanks to the army of patients, physicians, nurses, and other health care professionals for the insight, compassion, and conviction with which they daily put theory into practice.

To whatever degree *The Chronic Bronchitis and Emphysema Handbook* helps COPD patients and their families achieve the kind of realistic perspective about their disease that allows them to live confidently and reasonably calmly with it, and so remove needless limitations from their lives—to this degree our goals will be realized.

François Haas
Sheila Sperber Haas

The
Chronic Bronchitis
and Emphysema
Handbook

1

You and COPD: An Introduction

What Is COPD?

COPD means Chronic Obstructive Pulmonary Disease. It is an umbrella name covering *pulmonary emphysema* and *chronic bronchitis.* These are both chronic lung diseases that damage the air passageways, interfering with the lungs' capacity to breathe enough air in and out. These two diseases typically occur together, although one or the other often predominates.

Other general terms for these two diseases, all of which point to their chronic nature and their interference with getting air in and out of the lungs, include: Chronic Obstructive Airway Disease (COAD); Chronic Obstructive Lung Disease (COLD); Chronic Airflow—or Airway—Obstruction (CAO); and Chronic Airflow Limitation (CAL).

How to Use This Guide

If you have picked up this book to read, you know or you suspect that you or someone close to you is suffering from emphysema or chronic bronchitis. Perhaps a doctor has told you. Or perhaps changes you've noticed—like breathlessness when walking up stairs, a heavy cough that won't go away, or a lot of mucus from your lungs that doesn't clear up—have aroused your suspicions. (If you haven't mentioned these to your doctor, take a look at the questionnaire at the end of this chapter. Your answers will indicate whether you should see your doctor.)

Before you read further, you should know what you can—and cannot—expect from this guidebook. You cannot substitute it for a doctor. But you can use it to help find the best possible medical treatment. The book gives you an accurate and complete COPD education to help you: learn how to find the right specialists to diagnose and treat you; understand your disease so you can recognize appropriate treatment; know the variety of medical and rehabilitation techniques that will control your symptoms, improve your health, and better the quality of your life.

Why is it necessary to know all this? Successful treatment of COPD combines a broad variety of specialized techniques from pulmonary and rehabilitation specialists. Common sense alone cannot tell you what's right for you. And it's very difficult to learn it all from your doctor. It's a fact of life today that few doctors have the time or staff to educate their patients—and patients' families—in any depth. And many have little practice in translating medical jargon into normal speech.

In addition, many doctors remain unaware of the profound benefits to be gained from lung rehabilitation programs. They mistakenly assume that anyone with a disease that's eventually going to get worse can't benefit very much from rehabilitation efforts.

So patients often have to go to bat for themselves. This book gives you the tools and ammunition you'll need. It combines everything you need to know about controlling your disease and improving your life, in language you will understand.

Turning Your Life Around

Here are a few concrete examples of what COPD patients can gain from education and rehabilitation.

Rosa M. had suffered with a mix of emphysema and chronic bronchitis for years. Her family doctor prescribed medication and encouraged her to be increasingly inactive, convinced he was helping her. Whenever one of her frequent respiratory infections became life-threatening, he hospitalized her promptly and gave her the best care. Rosa gradually grew breathless more and more easily. By the time she entered the N.Y.U. Medical Centers' Pulmonary Rehabilitation program, she was a pulmonary cripple who could no longer do any of the things she loved: travel, visit museums or art galleries, attend concerts, take leisurely walks, give dinner parties. At home, she had become frustratingly dependent on her husband.

An evaluation determined that Rosa's pulmonary resources were seriously limited, but not enough to justify the crippled life she was leading. This crucial knowledge guided the rehabilitation program we designed for her.

After conditioning her muscles, learning how to breathe more effectively and how to use her energy economically, Rosa gradually resumed her favorite activities and her participation in life at home. Learning how to avoid major lung infections made hospital stays a rarity. Rosa and her husband—both no longer frightened and depressed—now live with renewed pleasure, vigor, and hope.

Harry D. entered the Pulmonary Rehabilitation program with very moderate COPD that had wrecked his life. He was a 55-year-old skilled furniture refinisher who loved his work and enjoyed the comfortable income it had provided. But the various chemicals his work required, and the dust raised by sanding, were so irritating to his lungs that—even with a protective mask—he could no longer work.

Harry sat around at home, afraid of everything that made him breathless—and angry at the world. His ego was crumbling. The emotional consequences of unemployment accompanied by the pressures of a dramatically lowered income were also destroying Harry's marriage. Harry's doctor suggested he enter the N.Y.U. Medical Centers' Pulmonary Rehabilitation program.

In addition to a program like Rosa's, Harry was also scheduled for vocational and psychological counseling, and both Harry and his wife joined a support group. Harry discovered he has excellent accounting skills, loves the work, and can do it at home if he prefers. He and his wife have achieved a positive adjustment—including satisfying sex—to the unavoidable changes COPD brings. Harry's zesty optimism has returned, his wife's basic emotional strength is flourishing, and their marriage is now responding resiliently to the challenges of his disease.

Leon L. was participating in an experimental pulmonary rehabilitation program in our laboratory. Our initial evaluation of his lungs indicated moderately severe COPD. Several months into the program he was offered a very desirable job in Kingston, Jamaica. Medically, Leon was fully capable of handling the work. Yet he was going to turn down the opportunity because he was, in his own words, "afraid to let go of my safety net." Fortunately, we finally convinced him that his fears were out of line. When he returned to New York City after three and one-half productive years in Kingston, our evaluation showed that his pulmonary status had remained stable.

(You can read Leon's story in much greater detail—and in his own words—at the end of Chapter 13: how his disease developed, how frightening and incapacitating it became, how he learned to take care of himself, and how that turned his life around.)

The Downward Spiral

These examples stand out from among the typical COPD stories because of their happy endings. Sadly, the breathlessness—technically called *dyspnea*—that becomes one of COPD's hallmark symptoms leads a great many patients to fear a wide range of jobs and satisfying, health-promoting leisure activities—exercise, outings, trips, etc.—that are still within their physical capacity.

When dyspnea first begins, it initiates a downward spiral (see Figure 1.1). Patients so fear becoming breathless that they withdraw from activities they can still pursue. Then they start to lose shape—partly from their disease, *and partly from their reduced level of physical activity*! They are "deconditioning" themselves.

What happens when your physical conditioning starts to slide? Formerly easy activities become difficult. They leave you winded. But COPD patients are convinced it is only their disease making these activities dif-

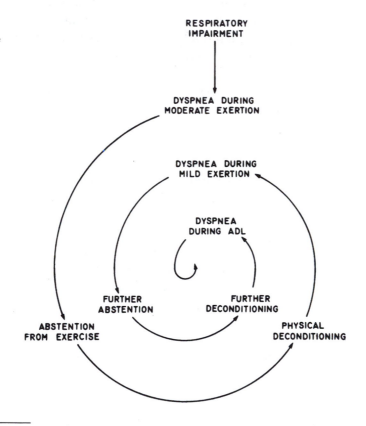

Figure 1.1 In chronic pulmonary disease, dyspnea from energetic activities can eventually result in such severe physical deconditioning that daily household and self-care tasks assume a difficulty out of proportion to what the patient's heart and lungs are actually capable of undertaking.

ficult. Because they are terrified of feeling breathless, they drop those activities from their shrinking repertory, become more deconditioned, experience breathlessness with even lighter physical demands, give them up too, and so on. They react to everything through a filter of fatigue and anxiety. They see their lung disease as an inescapable prison, not realizing that they have helped to build it and lock themselves in.

These needless limitations prematurely turn COPD from a serious disease into a crippling one, significantly diminishing quality of like for the patient and his family. But the harm appears to go beyond emotional impoverishment. The growing view is that these needless limitations may also speed up the actual physical progress of the disease.

Minimizing the Limitations

You should clearly understand that COPD ranges from mild, perhaps unnoticed, forms to severe, debilitating conditions. Whatever the stage of your COPD when it was first diagnosed, the essential goals are the same: (1) to gain a fundamental understanding of what has happened to your lungs, and (2) to determine what can be done to minimize the consequent problems.

These goals are reached via two paths taken simultaneously. One is appropriate medical treatment, which includes far more than pulmonary evaluation and medication. It must incorporate an extensive rehabilitation program involving social, psychological, and vocational counseling as well as physical measures. The other avenue is education. You must make every attempt to educate yourself about your disease. *With proper medical intervention and education, the progression of the disease can be significantly slowed.* Although existing damage cannot be undone, some of the negative effects may be reversible.

The information in this book is specifically intended to help educate COPD patients and their families. We hope that providing solid, comprehensive, understandable information and a realistic perspective about COPD will help our readers remove needless limitations from their lives. You can live calmly and confidently—and much more fully—with your condition.

Some COPD Facts

Emphysema and Chronic Bronchitis in a Nutshell

Our airways are structured like a many-branching, upside-down tree. The trunk (our *trachea*) receives air from our mouth and nose. It divides into the main branches entering the lungs' five lobes. With each successive branching, these airways become more numerous and narrower. Each branched pathway finally ends in a cluster of *air sacs*. This is where the oxygen in fresh air passes into our blood while carbon dioxide passes from our blood into our lungs (to be exhaled).

In *emphysema*, overstretched and torn air sacs cannot hold much fresh air and cannot fully release their stale, carbon dioxide-containing air for expiration. In *chronic bronchitis*, chronic airway inflammation leaves them permanently swollen, which narrows them. The airway irritant causing the inflammation also makes them produce great quantities of mucus—which blocks them. Both types of damage limit the amount of fresh air coming in, and stale air going out.

Doctors refer to these two related lung conditions with the same term because of outstanding similarities. They are both typically (although not always) caused by smoking. They usually appear together in the same person (although the degree of each will vary). Most of the symptoms—and their treatment—are similar. And with both diseases, decades usually intervene between the start of damage and the point at which it progresses far enough to be noticed.

The net effects of these obstructive lung diseases include a chronic cough, often with heavy mucus production. In addition, the breathing effort needed to pull air in and push it out through narrowed airways requires a great deal more energy. This is experienced as shortness of breath. Eventually, the lungs' ability to transfer oxygen into the bloodstream and remove carbon dioxide from the blood is damaged. Within this general picture, differences emerge that depend on which disease predominates. (See Chapter 3 for a more detailed look at these differences.)

How Long Have We Known About COPD?

Emphysema was the first of these two chronic lung diseases to be formally recognized. The earliest medical descriptions appeared in the late 1600s. One example is the eminent British physician of that era, Sir John Floyer, describing his examination of the lungs of a "broken-winded mare":

In the thorax, the Lungs appear'd very much swelled or puffed up, and appear'd much bigger in the Broken-winded mare than usual. . . . I blew up some Lobes of the Lungs and found the Air would not come out again, nor the Lungs subside by themselves; by which it was plain, that the Bladders of the Lungs had been extended or broken . . . that caused a continual Inflation of the whole Lungs . . . which causes a continual Dyspnoea [breathlessness], in which the external Air can't pass freely thro' the Trachea and its Branches in Inspiration and Expiration; and this difficulty occasions the great Labour and Nisus [physical effort] of the Respiratory Muscles.

But roughly 150 years passed before emphysema was fully described and defined. Laennec, the great French physician—and inventor of the stethoscope—achieved this in the 1820s. Anatomists of his day first pinpointed the lungs' damaged air sacs and the air that becomes trapped inside them as the typical physical evidence of emphysematous lungs. Laennec mistakenly thought that persistent cough and breathlessness recurring during the winter months—the primary symptoms of chronic bronchitis—were also due to emphysema's structural damage. Now we know that it is a separate, although related, lung disease. So although the symptoms of chronic bronchitis have been recognized as an irreversible lung disease since antiquity, an accurate understanding of the pathology underlying them is quite recent. No medical writings, however, indicate when Laennec's mistaken view was revised.

How Common Is COPD?

The frequency of chronic bronchitis and emphysema has risen so dramatically during the past 50 years that they now constitute a major health problem in industrialized countries—and the rate is still increasing. In the seventeen years from 1979 to 1996, the estimated number of Americans with chronic bronchitis and/or emphysema increased from 9.5 million to over 16 million (from roughly 4.0% to 6.0% of the country's population).

But these figures probably underestimate the actual total. It is suspected that a significant number of COPD patients do not report their condition in national health surveys.

Who Gets COPD?

Because COPD develops slowly—usually requiring 20 to 30 years of smoking before symptoms prompt a person to seek medical help—most patients are in their 60s or older. The typical COPD patient is, or has been, a long-term cigarette smoker.

Because smoking is far and away the single most important risk factor for COPD, the social pressures determining who smokes also influence who is most likely to develop COPD. One factor is sex. For many decades, smoking was far more acceptable for men. So today's COPD patients are predominantly male. But the social acceptance of women smokers that developed after World War II is beginning to erase this extreme imbalance.

The other factor is socioeconomic class, which influences how much smokers typically smoke, and how strong these cigarettes are. Blue-collar workers, for example, tend to smoke stronger cigarettes and more frequently than white-collar workers do. That explains why in England and Wales over the last 50 years, the bronchitis-related mortality rate for the lowest socioeconomic class has been six times higher than for the highest; and why in the United States, the COPD-related mortality rate among unskilled and semiskilled laborers is twice as high as among professionals.

Socioeconomic class also influences how a COPD patient does once his disease develops. Families with lower incomes can usually afford only a small—often overcrowded—house or apartment. Overcrowding makes respiratory infection more frequent, as well as encouraging a premature return to work after illness. Both situations speed up lung damage in COPD. The poorest families also tend to live in more polluted neighborhoods, providing an additional constant and inescapable respiratory irritant. And adding insult to injury—patients in this lower income bracket frequently do not have access to the best medical care.

Family Clustering   In both high-risk groups, COPD tends to cluster in families. This means that the vulnerability to COPD is inherited. Heredity—the genetic element—was first considered important in COPD's development back in the 19th century. Recent research confirms that genetic factors predispose people in certain families to the development of chronic obstructive lung diseases when the causes are present.

We now know that: (1) relatives of bronchitis patients (compared to relatives of other types of patients) have a much greater likelihood of developing bronchitis; (2) siblings of bronchitis patients, compared to their husbands or wives are also more likely to have bronchitis; (3) airflow measurements are much more alike between siblings (who share genetic material) than between their parents (who do not), although they all live in the same environment; (4) identical twins (who share the same genetic material) are much more likely both to have COPD than are fraternal twins (who are like non-twin siblings in terms of shared genetic material).

But these research results only tell us that heredity usually determines who will develop COPD given the right circumstances. In most cases we don't yet know what physical differences create this predisposition.

The one clear-cut family scenario involves a known inherited enzyme deficiency. Men and women lacking enough of this enzyme are predisposed to the rapid, early development form of emphysema, which hits them in the decades before their 50s. (In this form of emphysema, the enzyme—*alpha₁-antitrypsin (AAT)* or *alpha₁-antiprotease (AAP)*—that normally prevents loss of the lungs' elastic fibers is not produced in sufficient amount.) Yet even this inherited condition interacts with the harmful effects of smoking. In one study of COPD patients suffering from AAT deficiency, the average age at which shortness of breath was first noticed was 44 years for nonsmokers and 35 years for smokers.

Not everyone with this deficiency, however, develops COPD. Also, emphysema can occur, although rarely, in nonsmoking families with normal *alpha₁-antitrypsin* production. Obviously, other as yet unidentified hereditary factors must also increase risk for COPD.

How Serious Is COPD?

The seriousness of any disease must be gauged from the answers to three separate questions: Is it life-threatening? What is the economic impact on the family and/or society? How does it interfere with your ability to live your life as you would like? A disease can be considered serious in regard to one aspect, even though it is negligible as far as others are concerned.

Threat to Life

COPD causes 4.7% of all deaths in the United States, making it the fifth most common cause of death here. In 1997, for example, this meant that at least 110,000 deaths were caused directly by COPD and its related medical problems. That year COPD also made another 160,000 Americans too weak to survive other, unrelated medical conditions. So 270,000 COPD-related deaths in 1997 is a far more realistic figure.

From 1970 to 2000, the likelihood of COPD's, being a direct or contributing cause of death has tripled. This increasing likelihood of dying from COPD is even more pronounced for women than for men. In 1970, COPD killed 4.3 men for each woman. By 1983 this ratio had decreased dramatically to 2.4 men for each woman, reflecting the post-World War II upsurge in women smokers. By 1997 it had fallen even farther, down to 1.5.

Economic Impact

The proportion of COPD patients whose disease limits their activities is the highest of all major disease categories! Over 50% report some degree of limitation. More than one-half of this group is confined to bed at least part of the time.

In 1990, the estimated total annual economic drain produced by COPD was a staggering $15 billion. Only a small fraction of this was spent on actual medical costs. It overwhelmingly reflects disability payments and the premature loss of earnings. Thousands of COPD patients each year reach a degree of impairment that forces them to leave work and rely on disability payments. In 1983 and 1984 alone, more than 16,000 each year were awarded first-time disability benefits. During the 1980s, both health care costs and the number of COPD patients escalated, dramatically deepening the annual economic drain. By 1990, COPD was the cause of 16.2 million doctor's visits and 1.9 million hospital days. This translates to an estimated annual cost of $7.6 billion spent on COPD patient care along with $8.6 billion lost from reduced productivity due to disability and premature death.

Effect on Lifestyle

Although there are no statistics describing COPD's impact on the ways in which patients shape their professional lives and leisure time, the many anecdotal reports from patients illustrate the potentially serious impact of these diseases even in their milder states. The three COPD portraits we sketched earlier in this chapter give a sense of the destructive impact COPD typically has on the lives of patients and their families. Jobs, favorite leisure activities, and independence are forfeited. Income is suddenly limited. Close relationships are undermined. Fear, anxiety, loss of self-esteem, depression, and anger replace the anticipated satisfactions of one's later years.

Minimizing This Impact

But COPD's impact in terms of lives diminished and then lost can be substantially lessened. Even though this disease is usually quite advanced by the time patients become aware of a serious health problem, it does not have to be such a frequent killer. Patients with COPD are *not* inevitably fated to deteriorate and die from this disease.

With the kind of medical help stressed in this guide, many patients are able to slow their disease enough and cope with their symptoms so effectively that they live longer and fuller lives. Their eventual death is from an unrelated cause.

QUESTIONNAIRE

	Yes	No
1. Do you get winded more easily during exertion than you did one year ago?	☐	☐
2. Do you worry about your shortness of breath?	☐	☐
3. Have you been bothered for the past several years by a cough that takes about three months to shake?	☐	☐
4. Do you have roughly a three-month period each year when your lungs produce a lot of phlegm (also called "sputum" and "mucus") that you bring up?	☐	☐
5. If you are bringing up phlegm now, is it colored (milky white, gray, yellow, green)?	☐	☐
6. Do you regularly find blood in your phlegm?	☐	☐
7. Does your breathing sound noisy?	☐	☐
8. Do you snore at night and feel tired in the morning?	☐	☐
9. Do you need more pillows than you used to sleep comfortably?	☐	☐
10. Does it feel easier to breathe if you bend forward and lean on your arms?	☐	☐
11. Do you tend to purse your lips when you breathe out?	☐	☐
12. Have you recently developed a bluish tinge in your lips and/or under your fingernails?	☐	☐
13. Have you been smoking for about 20 years, and have never seen a doctor?	☐	☐
14. Do your ankles swell fairly regularly?	☐	☐
15. Did either of your parents die from pulmonary disease before age 60?	☐	☐

If you answered "Yes" to any of these questions, we suggest you see your doctor and tell him what you have been experiencing. Although in your case it may be nothing to worry about, these symptoms can indicate the presence of significant respiratory disease.

2

The Respiratory System: What It Is, How It Works, and What Goes Wrong in COPD

The business of the respiratory system is twofold. It supplies the body's tissues with oxygen, the gas needed for burning the food we eat to produce energy. It also rids the body of excess carbon dioxide, the gaseous waste product from energy production. This combined process is called "metabolism."

Respiration involves all the processes that contribute to getting and using oxygen and eliminating carbon dioxide. It can be examined at two levels, one small and one large. Processes involving the individual cell concern the microscopic machinery that uses oxygen to transform the food we eat into energy, producing carbon dioxide as the waste product. Large-level processes occur at the organ level. They involve the basic machinery—the lungs, airways, rib cage, respiratory muscles, heart, and blood vessels—bringing about this exchange of gases. This is the process called breathing.

If our respiratory system becomes obstructed, we're in trouble. Not enough oxygen coming in means not enough energy. The result at less severe levels is feeling tired and breathless from moderate activity. At lower levels, it means not enough energy to get out of bed without help of some kind. Dropping oxygen levels eventually affect the heart, which overworks itself trying to make up for this lack. And not enough carbon dioxide going out means—at less severe levels—that we're tired and don't feel well. If increasing buildup reaches toxic levels, it means eventual coma.

Why Is This Chapter Important to You?

You can't really understand your disease until you know how and why COPD's damage stresses your respiratory system, and perhaps your heart—and the consequences of this stress. Without this understanding, your doctor's examinations, and any lung tests you undergo, won't make much sense to you. You won't understand the medications you are, or will be, taking—not what they do, nor why you need them. You won't realize what your medical and physical therapies are working to accomplish. This will make it very difficult to sustain your motivation and cooperation in your treatment.

To sum this up in one phrase: *Education is your key to coping successfully with COPD.* The more you know, the greater the resources you are placing at your disposal *and* the more competent and responsible you can be in utilizing them. The results—concrete and substantial—are a longer lifespan, and a more satisfying one!

What This Chapter Covers

First, we draw a picture of the healthy respiratory system—its large parts, how they work to supply you with enough oxygen and remove enough carbon dioxide, and the power supplied by your respiratory muscles and the lungs' elastic character. Then you'll see how COPD impairs your lungs' ability to take in fresh air and get rid of stale air, and why you now have to work so hard to breathe. (Chapter 3 will draw together all the COPD bits and pieces for a comprehensive portrait of each disease, including how each one evolves over time.)

You can't get a working understanding with generalities and part of the picture. So this chapter contains a fair amount of detailed information on respiratory structures and how they work. We have done our best to make this information clear and readable without omitting important pieces of the puzzle. And since you will be reading about yourself, that should add a great deal of interest.

Our Breathing Machinery

Nose Job

We usually inhale through our nose. But the nose is not just a simple passageway to our airways. The interior of the nose is far more expansive than it appears to the uneducated eye. Within the skull it becomes an extensive labyrinth of passageways that funnels into the throat. The inner walls of the nose are covered with a sticky layer of mucus. They also are richly supplied with heat-radiating blood vessels.

When we breathe in (inspire), three things happen as fresh air is bounced around in this complex array of nasal passages: virtually all of the dust particles it normally contains are trapped in the mucus (which then travels to the throat to be swallowed), the air is warmed by the blood

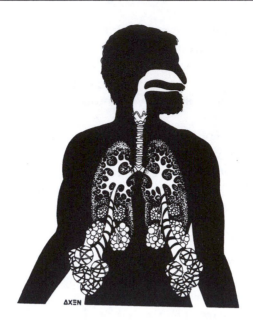

Figure 2.1   Anatomy of the respiratory system.

vessels, and it picks up moisture. This "treated" air passes through the throat, through the voice box (which holds the vocal cords), and into the trachea. (The throat divides into the *trachea*, which is the windpipe, and the *esophagus*, the tube leading to the stomach.)

Airways

The airways form a many-branching structure that starts with the trachea (Figure 2.1). First the trachea divides into the two wide branches (called *bronchi*) entering the lungs. Each of these divides into two, then these four branches each divide into two, and so on. In all, the airways divide 23 times—becoming narrower and narrower—as we follow them from the trachea to the 300 million tiny air sacs, or *alveoli*, where oxygen and carbon dioxide are exchanged. We call the larger airways *bronchi*, and the narrower ones *bronchioles*.

The basic respiratory unit is the structure combining the two final branchings (the tiniest bronchioles) with the alveoli they serve. Its formal name is the *acinus*. We will discuss the acinus more actively later in this chapter, when we describe the tissue damage emphysema causes.

Air Sacs

The air sacs are where oxygen and carbon dioxide are actually exchanged. The blood circulating in the membranous walls around the individual alveoli picks up oxygen while it gives up excess carbon dioxide (Figure 2.2). This excess leaves the body in the next exhaled breath (expiration). (Not all the carbon dioxide is disposed of, because a certain level must be maintained in the blood.)

Lungs and Ribs

Healthy lungs are made up of five pink, spongy lobes. Three are on the right side of the chest cavity and two on the left side, with the heart between them (Figure 2.3). Air sacs, airways, and blood vessels are the lungs' primary structural elements (see Figures 2.4 and 2.5). These spongy organs are protectively enclosed in a bony, yet flexible, airtight "cage" made up of part of the backbone (called the *thoracic*—meaning "chest"—vertebrae), the collarbones, the breastbone, and the ribs. (Look at Figures 2.3 and 2.6.) The ribs are attached to the thoracic vertebrae in a way that allows them to move up and down to change the size of the chest cavity.

Inspiratory Muscles

The main muscle of inspiration is the *diaphragm* (Figure 2.6), the thin, dome-shaped muscle separating the chest and abdominal areas. Because

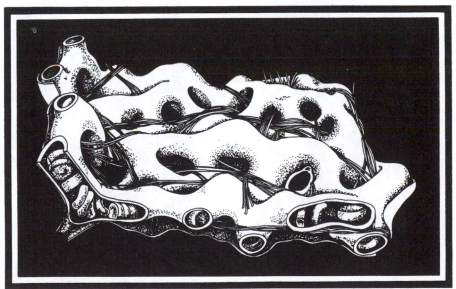

AXEN

Figure 2.2   The alveolus wall shows the red blood cells flowing between it and the capillary wall. Interwoven in the wall is a network of elastic fibers.
Source: Redrawn with permission from E. R. Weibel, *The Pathway for Oxygen: Structure and Function in the Mammalian Respiratory System* (Cambridge: Harvard University Press, 1984), p. 314.

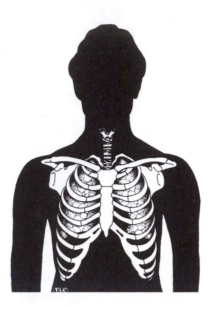

Figure 2.3   Anatomy of the chest cavity. The heart is the shadowed structure by the base of the breastbone (*right*). Two of the lungs' lobes are also on that side. The opposite side contains the other three lobes. These organs are protected by the ribs, breastbone, and collarbones.

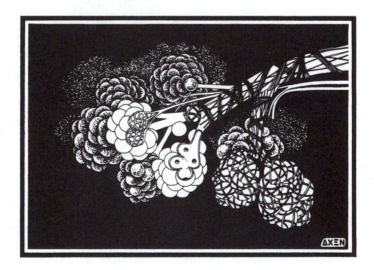

Figure 2.4   The pulmonary lobule. The long, slender portion is a small preterminal airway surrounded by airway muscle cells. Each of its tiny branches ends in an acinus—a group of related alveoli. Blood vessels run parallel to the airway and branch into the capillary bed surrounding these alveoli.

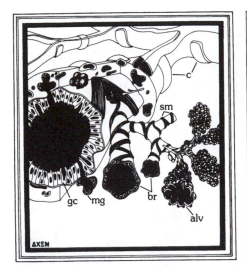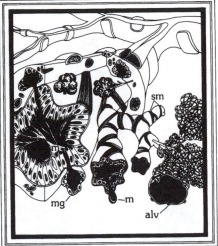

Figure 2.5   Low-magnification view comparing healthy (*left*) and chronic bronchitic (*right*) airways and their surrounding tissues.

Labels: gc = goblet cells; c = cartilage; br = bronchi; mg = mucous gland; m = mucus; sm = smooth muscle; alv = alveoli.

Source: Redrawn with permission from T. Des Jardins, *Clinical Manifestations of Respiratory Disease* (Chicago: Year Book Medical Publishers, 1984), pp. 2, 106.

the diaphragm lowers as it contracts, it increases the size of the chest cavity by making it longer. The ribs are attached to each other by the two sets of *intercostal muscles*, which also change the size of the chest cavity.

The *external intercostal muscles* contract during inspiration, pulling the ribs outward to help the diaphragm enlarge the chest cavity. The expanding chest cavity pulls the lungs along with it. As the lungs' airways and air sacs expand, they cause air to be sucked in through the nose (or mouth) and trachea.

What makes this happen is the creation of a vacuum as air pressure in your lungs drops. You see, a little air always remains in your lungs when you breathe out. As your lungs begin to expand again, this remaining air suddenly has more room. So it spreads out, and its pressure drops. This rapid pressure drop creates a vacuum. And the vacuum sucks air from the outside down into the air sacs. (Think of a vacuum cleaner!)

Expiratory Muscles

Return of the chest cavity to its original—or resting—size as the lungs empty of air usually occurs passively, meaning without muscle power. It

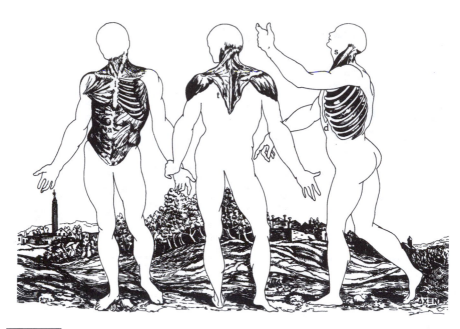

Figure 2.6   The respiratory muscles. *Right:* The major muscle of inspiration—the diaphragm (d)—seen through the rib cage, and the major accessory muscles of inspiration—the sternocleidomastoid (s)—in the neck. *Middle:* The major respiratory accessory muscle in the back—the trapezius (t). The part of the muscle above the shoulders is inspiratory, increasing the size of the chest cavity by raising the shoulders. The section along the back is expiratory, reducing chest cavity size by lowering the shoulders. *Left:* The major expiratory muscles in the abdominal wall (a), and the inspiratory external intercostals (i). (The expiratory internal intercostals are hidden.)

happens in much the same way that an inflated balloon or a stretched rubber band spring back to their original size. Then, just as air pressure in the lungs drops when they expand, it increases again as the deflating lungs compress the air back into a smaller space. And this growing air pressure in the air sacs pushes air back out of the lungs and through the nose or mouth. (As the lungs spring back, they pull the chest wall in too.)

But expiration must become active during strenuous activity. Then it is helped by contraction both of the *internal intercostals* and of the large muscles of the *abdominal wall* (Figure 2.6). We will see why this is necessary shortly.

In addition to these major respiratory muscles that enlarge and decrease the bony cage surrounding the lungs, a secondary group of muscles—appropriately called the *accessory respiratory muscles*—joins the work during activities that make extremely heavy demands on the respiratory system. These accessory muscles are in the neck, shoulders, and back (see Figure 2.6). They help primarily during inspiration.

What Controls Your Respiratory Muscles?

The respiratory muscles are controlled by the respiratory center located in the most primitive part of our brain, called the brain stem. This control is automatic and continuous. We do not have to be conscious of our breathing for it to work. (But this control can be influenced by the more sophisticated parts of our brain involved in our emotions, in talking, and in thinking.)

The brain-stem respiratory center tells the respiratory muscles when to contract, how strongly to contract, and how much the chest cavity must expand. But how does your respiratory center "know" all of this?

It is from the amount of carbon dioxide in the freshly oxygenated blood (called *arterial* blood) your heart pumps through your body. Rising carbon dioxide levels in your arterial blood (when, for example, your body burns more fuel for exercise) immediately excite the respiratory center. It then strengthens the signal it continuously sends along the nerves that link it with the respiratory muscles. Responding to this stronger signal, these muscles make your breathing faster and deeper. Because this increases ventilation, the body gets rid of carbon dioxide at a much faster rate. This way, the level of carbon dioxide in arterial blood is maintained at the same level that exists during normal breathing.

Sometimes the regulatory center is no longer sensitive enough to respond to carbon dioxide changes. If this happens, there is a back-up system. Then respiration is regulated via the amount of oxygen in arterial blood, and/or by the amount of acids in the blood. One kind of acid (carbonic acid) is formed when carbon dioxide encounters blood plasma, and the other (lactic acid) is a byproduct of exercising muscle.

But whatever the effective regulatory signal, if the respiratory muscles cannot respond to the brain center's stronger message and carbon dioxide production remains higher than normal, the system has broken down. Respiration has failed.

Then the amount of carbon dioxide in arterial blood will continue rising. The initial increases in carbon dioxide cause a sense of fatigue. But once it goes beyond a certain level, carbon dioxide becomes toxic. It disrupts normal metabolism, causes confusion, and—if it goes high enough—eventually results in coma.

Microscopic Anatomy: The Acinus and Emphysema

Following any of your lungs' airways along its narrowing and branching length, we eventually reach the next-to-the-last, or *terminal*, bronchiole. Each terminal bronchiole ends in an acinus—the lungs' most elementary respiratory unit (Figure 2.4). Within the acinus, the terminal bronchiole branches one final time. Each endpoint branch is a *respiratory bronchiole*.

What makes the terminal and respiratory bronchioles different from all other airways are their direct connections with the alveoli. Both of these tiny bronchioles have isolated alveoli opening directly into them along their length. Each respiratory bronchiole also ends in a cluster of up to seven alveoli. The cluster of "acini" branching off from an individual preterminal airway is termed a *lobule*. (Viewed under the microscope, each lobule resembles a bunch of grapes, as shown in Figure 2.4.)

Emphysema Attacks the Alveoli

Because emphysema destroys elastic fibers in the membranous walls surrounding individual air sacs (how this happens is described in the next section), these alveoli lose their ability to recoil to their original size during expiration. Then, as an alveolus remains stretched, the rest of the membrane fibers eventually break. The wall is destroyed, merging the air sac with its neighbor. As this process continues, alveoli become larger and fewer. It is somewhat like tearing down the interior walls in a building of multi-room apartments until each apartment is only one large room (Figure 2.7).

The Problem

The alveoli's membrane walls—which are richly supplied with capillaries, the circulatory system's tiniest vessels—are the actual gas exchange sites. Progressively reducing this wall space increasingly limits the amount of oxygen that can enter the blood flowing through the lungs in two ways. Most important is that shrinking this gas exchange membrane seriously limits the amount of gas exchange that can occur. (For greater detail, see the "Gas Exchange" section at the end of this chapter.)

Second is that blood is now sent rushing through the lungs in less time than the complete oxygen uptake process requires. The heart pumps the same amount of blood through the lungs each minute, regardless of any changes in the lungs. If there are suddenly less blood vessels for this blood to travel through, then it must move through the remaining vessels more quickly than before. In emphysema, this speed eventually goes beyond

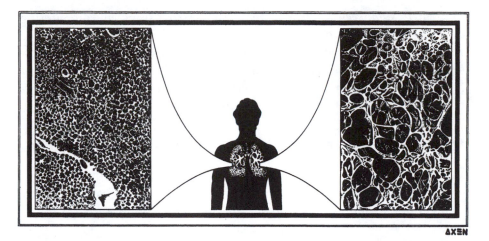

Figure 2.7   *Left:* We see under the microscope the tight, sponge-like appearance of healthy lung tissue. *Right:* The microscope shows us the emphysematous lungs' typical large air spaces resulting from destruction of the alveolar walls.

the time needed for the oxygen-carrying blood cells to take on a full load of oxygen. During nondemanding activities, this oxygen deficit is fairly minimal. But during activities that increase heart rate—sending the blood even faster through the lungs—any drop in arterial blood's oxygen content is very apparent to patients with severe emphysema.

Hypoxia is the technical term describing the condition of inadequate oxygen.

Two Types of Emphysema

The two types of emphysema refer to where in the acinus alveoli are dying. It is most common to have one or the other. Some patients develop both kinds.

Panlobular (panacinar) emphysema involves weakening and enlargement of the air sacs clustered at the end of respiratory bronchioles. Destruction may be so severe that the entire visible structure of an affected acinus disappears. The disappearance of many neighboring acini creates a "spider web" appearance on a lung X-ray. The lungs look like they are full of holes. As a natural part of aging, this type of emphysema in mild form is common among the elderly. When panacinar emphysema appears in younger people, it is caused by the body's inadequate production of the elastic fiber-preserving alpha$_1$-antitrypsin enzyme. These cases are more virulent and debilitating.

Centrilobular (centriacinar) emphysema destroys single alveoli entering directly into the walls of terminal and respiratory bronchioles. Then these airway walls enlarge, and the alveoli disappear. Because the alveoli clustered at the end of the acinus are unaffected, the bulk of the acinus is not destroyed. This form of emphysema, the most common of the two, is often associated with chronic bronchitis.

Physical Properties of the Respiratory System

When the respiratory muscles work to expand the chest cavity, they must overcome the two characteristics of the respiratory system that oppose any changes in its volume. These are its *elastance* and *resistance*.

Elastance

Elastance, or *elasticity*, is easy to understand. We've all experienced it first-hand with rubber bands and balloons. They are elastic structures. After stretching a rubber band or blowing up a balloon, they spring back—*recoil*—to their original shape when you let go.

The lungs and chest wall are both elastic structures, too. If they were removed from the bony confines of our chest, the lungs would instantly spring back to a much smaller volume while the chest wall would spring outward to a larger volume. But because the lungs and chest wall are a tightly coupled system, each continuously pulls against the other. When the inward pull of the lungs and the outward pull of the chest wall are equal—the balance point—the system stops moving. This is what happens when you reach the end of a normal—meaning "nonstrenuous"—expiration. The lung volume (the amount of air still in your lungs) at this equilibrium point is called the *resting end-expiratory volume*.

Because inspiration must enlarge the lungs' volume beyond this balance point, muscle power is needed to work against their inward pull. It is supplied by the inspiratory muscles. Then, when these inspiratory muscles relax, the elastic respiratory system spontaneously springs back to its resting volume. (The built-in elastic recoil means muscle power is not usually needed to accomplish expiration, so it is a passive process.) This fully describes the healthy respiratory cycle during quiet breathing, and even during mild exercise.

As exercise demands increase, however, so must breath size. It increases in two directions—inspirations get larger, and expirations are now pushed beyond their usual stopping point. The more the lungs are stretched during inspiration, the stronger and stronger is the inward pull back to equilibrium. So the inspiratory muscles must work harder and harder to continue increasing breath size. The accessory muscles also pitch in. Pushing expiration beyond the resting point means it is no longer a passive process. The muscle power needed to overcome the outward pull of the chest wall is supplied by the expiratory muscles.

What Makes the Lungs Elastic?

About one-half of the lungs' elastic recoil force comes from *surface tension,* a process of attraction between water molecules that goes on within each alveolus. The other half comes from the elastic nature of certain *fibers* throughout the lungs' structure. Emphysema seriously weakens both these forces, because it destroys many elastic fibers and interferes with surface tension. First we will describe each source, then how emphysema's damage occurs.

Surface Tension   During inspiration, surface tension is the force that develops among the water molecules in the liquid film covering the inner walls of the alveoli. Fluid (salty water) bathes all of the body's cells and surfaces. In the lungs this fluid also contains *surfactant,* a chemical manufactured by the body that interferes with water's natural tendency to form a spherical drop with a strong pull into its center.

Why Is Surfactant Important?   In the alveolus, this unopposed force would draw the tiny air sac closed and prevent it from reopening. But surfactant—with its ability to disturb the magnet-like attraction water molecules have for each other—changes the story.

After an expiration, when the lungs are relatively empty of air, surfactant molecules squeeze water molecules away from the surface of the forming bubble. This weakens the bubble's inward pull, thereby allowing inspiration to start. But as the lungs—and the alveoli—inflate, the surfactant is diluted as it spreads over an increasingly larger area. Dilution weakens its ability to interfere with the attraction between water molecules. So as the alveoli stretch, the attraction—or surface tension—between water molecules grows. As soon as the inspiratory muscles relax, this inward force then helps pull the lungs back to their original size.

Elastic Fibers   The other half of the lungs' elastic force comes primarily from specialized fibers in the lungs' fibroelastic skeleton—the tissue that gives shape to the lungs. These fibers are found in the alveolar walls (Figure 2.2), and in the elastic connective tissue embracing the airways and air sacs. The most important of these fibers contain the protein *elastin*. They behave like rubber bands. They stretch several times their length during inspiration, and during expiration they spontaneously return to their normal length.

The amount of elastin in the lungs' fibroelastic tissue—which depends on how much old elastin is destroyed and how much new elastin is synthesized—determines its behavior. (Continuous, simultaneous cell destruction and renewal occurs throughout the body. It is not unique to the lungs.) Healthy lungs maintain the proper balance between destruction and renewal. A change in either upsets the balance, interfering with respiration. If too little elastin is destroyed, the lungs become very difficult to expand. If too much is destroyed, the lungs hyperexpand and can't recoil effectively.

The process of elastin destruction and renewal involves complex regulation. Certain specialized lung cells produce new elastin. Others produce *elastase*, the enzyme that destroys aging elastin. The liver produces *alpha*$_1$-*antitrypsin*, the enzyme controlling the amount of elastase so too much elastin isn't digested. In emphysema, these checks and balances have stopped working. Too much elastin is destroyed because elastase is no longer adequately controlled, apparently because alpha$_1$-antitrypsin production has dropped to a trickle.

The loss of elastin (and thus elasticity) means both that the lungs expand beyond the normal during inspiration, and can no longer resume their normal—or resting—size during expiration. As a consequence, alveoli overinflate and eventually rupture. In a vicious cycle, this reduces elasticity still further because each lost air sac further impairs surface tension's contribution to the lungs' recoil ability.

Resistance

Resistance is the friction-like force opposing the actual flow of air in and out of the lungs' airways. It is created as air moves past the airway walls. (Friction, occurring when two surfaces slide over each other, is the force opposing this movement.)

The amount of resistance depends on both how wide the airway is and how fast air is traveling through it. If an airway's opening becomes twice as narrow, for example, resistance increases 16 times. Then the respiratory muscles have to work much harder to continue breathing the same amount of air at the same speed.

To get a feel for this, breathe through a drinking straw while it is fully open, and then after you pinch it partially closed. Repeat this experiment while you breathe more quickly.

During relaxed inspiration, the inspiratory muscles easily supply the force that overcomes resistance. During passive expiration, resistance is overcome by the same energy (from surface tension and elastin fibers) that causes the inflated lungs to return to their normal size. But during exercise (because breathing is more rapid), or in COPD (because the airways are narrowed), this may not be enough. When that happens, the expiratory muscles must help overcome resistance.

COPD and Resistance   Whether emphysema or chronic bronchitis predominates, airway narrowing in COPD always disturbs expiration more than inspiration. There are two reasons for this: (1) Even in healthy lungs, resistance in all but the smallest airways is greater during expiration. They expand during inspiration (lessening resistance) and recoil to their resting width during expiration (increasing resistance). So COPD's airway narrowing is added to this normal expiratory increase in resistance. (2) In the smallest airways, emphysema reverses the normal situation. As we learned in discussing surface tension in healthy alveoli, resistance in the respiratory and terminal bronchioles normally lessens during expiration. But elasticity loss in emphysematous air sacs means that their recoil is no longer present to pull these tiny airways open as inspiration ends and expiration begins.

Patients with chronic bronchitis predominating also experience some increase in inspiratory resistance, too. Why? Airway narrowing is much more pronounced. Long-term airway irritation chronically inflames the airway walls, causing them to swell. This swelling reduces their internal diameter. Long-term irritation also results in excessive mucus production, which plugs these airways and narrows them further.

Breathing Is Work, Especially in COPD

Healthy Lungs, Normal Work

To summarize: The normal work of breathing is the work needed to expand the respiratory system from its resting position, plus the work needed to overcome friction created by air moving against the airway walls. Overcoming both elastance and resistance combines the efforts of the inspiratory and expiratory muscles. And as we just described, taking larger breaths and breathing faster both make the respiratory muscles work harder.

COPD Lungs, Hard Work

Higher Resistance   Because COPD permanently narrows the airways, the air flowing through them meets greater resistance—sometimes more than 25 times normal. So the respiratory muscles often have to work harder—especially during expiration—even under nonstrenuous circumstances. Since resistance is affected by breathing speed as well as airway width, a problem with one can often be compensated for by changing the other. When moderate COPD has narrowed your airways, breathing out more slowly than normal does away with a lot of the added resistance. But this compensation eventually fails if airway obstruction continues to worsen.

Then airflow resistance continues increasing, and the compensatory time needed for breathing out becomes longer and longer. Simultaneously, the lungs are continuing to lose elasticity. Finally, the loss of elasticity becomes so widespread that elastic recoil is too weak to push air out of the lungs effectively. Then each expiration requires so much time—from the combined inroads of high resistance and low elastance—that it cannot be completed before the next inspiration must start. Air now remains trapped in the lungs.

Hyperinflation   The expiratory muscles jump in to help expiration, but this effort increases pressure around the airways, narrowing them further and trapping more air. The COPD lungs—which for some time have already been somewhat hyperinflated at rest—now become grossly hyperinflated.

Because such hyperinflated lungs cannot return to their normal resting position, they interfere with the inspiratory muscles. The diaphragm—our main source of inspiratory power—can no longer contract effectively. Normally it is dome-shaped, pulling the dome down as it contracts. But hyperinflated lungs press down on the dome to such a degree that the diaphragm is always in a contracted position. And the other inspiratory muscles can no longer return to their full—that is, optimal—resting length before contracting again.

The more any muscle approaches its optimal length between contractions, then the more it can contract, the stronger it is, and the more it can do. In advanced COPD, the inspiratory muscles have, in effect, been shortened. So the biggest breath they can help achieve is a lot smaller than it once was.

Overload   Working against increasingly greater airflow resistance and the stress of hyperinflation can eventually exhaust the respiratory muscles.

If this happens, respiration fails. And as we have already mentioned, failure permits the amount of carbon dioxide in the blood to rise to potentially fatal levels.

What Controls the Airway Opening?

We need to present two final pieces of the puzzle before moving on to Chapter 3's detailed description of what actually happens in COPD. The first of these is a more detailed knowledge of our airway structure, and the forces that normally control their width (so important in determining the amount of airflow resistance our respiratory muscles must work against). Then we can fully appreciate what goes wrong in COPD. Figure 2.5, which graphically illustrates this information, will be very helpful to refer to as you read.

Our airway walls are made up of cartilage, smooth muscle (one of the three muscle types), mucus-producing glands, connective tissue, and epithelium (the type of tissue that covers all outer and inner body surfaces, including the lining of vessels and other small cavities). Because the relative amounts of these components change—in healthy lungs—as you move into the lungs along the airway branches, the large, medium, and small airways are distinctive in composition as well as in size. (See Figure 2.5.)

Mucus

Connective tissue (the fibroelastic framework) kind of holds the overall structure together. Mucus—the layer of sticky fluid covering the lining of epithelial cells—is made up of water, large molecules of sugar and protein, and salts. It is technically called *sputum*. Mucus is produced by goblet cells in the lining of medium and large airways, and by mucous glands deep in the airway wall. (In a healthy nonsmoker, the proportion of goblet cells greatly decreases as the airways become smaller.) The mucus-producing goblet cells are interspersed among other epithelial cells with moving, hair-like projections called cilia (Figure 2.8). These two types of cells form a protective alliance that keeps the airways sterile. Mucus traps foreign particles—including bacteria—that enter the airways, then the cilia push both mucus and particles up to the mouth to be swallowed or coughed out.

Excessive amounts of mucus—such as the lungs produce during respiratory infections—are an irritant once they reach the larger airways. Its presence there stimulates the cough reflex, which expels it. (When a cough is stimulated, the respiratory muscles contract forcefully while the

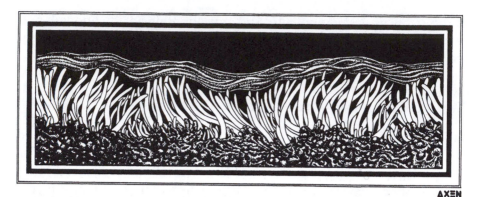

AXEN

Figure 2.8   Drawing of scanning electron microscope micrograph of cilia from human bronchial epithelium. Cells, microscopic inhaled particles, and bacteria are trapped in the thin layer of mucus. The beating cilia move these particles toward the mouth, where they are either swallowed or coughed out.

vocal cords stay tightly shut, building up very high pressure in the lungs. Then the vocal cords fly open and air blasts out of the lungs, sometimes as fast as 70 mph.)

Chronic bronchitis overwhelms the cough reflex in several ways. To begin with, it paralyzes the cilia. As they stop working, mucus starts accumulating in smaller and smaller airways (Figure 2.5). It combines with the inflamed airway lining to increase expiratory airflow resistance substantially. This high resistance prevents air from blasting out of the lungs at high speeds. The cough is still stimulated appropriately, but it has become too weak to dislodge the mucus filling the upper airways.

Muscle

Cartilage—which helps support all but the smallest airways—forms unclosed rings around them. Its presence decreases substantially in each airway generation until it disappears in the smaller airways. A layer of smooth muscle lies between the epithelium and cartilage, forming a continuous muscular ring encircling the airways (Figure 2.5). In healthy lungs, how much it contracts basically determines the size of the airway opening.

As we shall see in a few paragraphs, COPD adds further influences. To minimize these influences, it becomes important to use medication that alters the airway muscle's behavior. We want it to open as wide as it can. (Understanding this section will help a lot when you get to Chapter 7 on medications.)

How this airway muscle behaves results primarily from the balance between the *autonomic nervous system*'s two opposing parts. (This balance also controls the mucus-producing glands.) The autonomic nervous system continuously controls our automatic bodily functions, constantly adjusting them to maintain our interior environment with a minimum of fluctuation. Its two divisions—the *sympathetic* and the *parasympathetic*—usually work in opposite directions.

The nervous system acts via *mediators*, chemicals that it produces and releases. Mediators "talk" to muscles via *receptors*, specialized areas that all muscles have on their surface. Each type of mediator has its own type of receptor. That receptor can't be activated by any other mediator. Because muscles have more than one type of receptor, they can respond to more than one kind of mediator.

When airway muscle receptors sense the presence of the specific chemical mediators they respond to, the machinery that contracts the muscle is either started or turned off, depending on the mediator. Two types of airway muscle receptors cause the muscle to contract. One is activated by acetylcholine (*cholinergic receptors*) released by the parasympathetic nervous system. The other type recognizes adrenaline (*adrenergic alpha-receptors*) released primarily by the adrenal glands (part of the sympathetic nervous system). Receptors that turn off the contraction machinery, allowing the airway muscle to relax, also recognize adrenaline but are called *adrenergic beta-receptors*. Adrenaline's relaxing (or bronchodilating) effect predominates because there are many more beta-receptors than alpha-receptors.

So when the healthy respiratory system is at rest—meaning the absence of conditions (such as exercise) temporarily increasing the body's demands on it—the opening size of each airway is the end result of the balance between the cholinergic and adrenergic alpha-receptors on one side, and the adrenergic beta-receptors on the other.

But when the respiratory system is affected by COPD, pathological factors further influence the airway opening. In emphysema, the smallest airways shut down during expiration. In chronic bronchitis, the mucus glands can more than quadruple in size, substantially narrowing medium and large airways with their sticky secretions. And goblet cells begin appearing in even the smallest airways. Because of their small size, these airways are very vulnerable to complete blockage by mucus. Once that blockage occurs, air in the surrounding alveoli remains trapped there. These air sacs become distended, and the walls eventually rupture. *This is why chronic bronchitis and emphysema are typically found together. If emphysema has not already developed separately from the chronic bronchitis, it will eventually be produced by it.*

Treating COPD must include ways to normalize the airway openings as much as possible. As we will see in Chapter 9 on bronchodilator medication, this is based in part on finding drugs that stimulate the airway muscle beta-receptors to promote muscle relaxation and prevent the cholinergic and alpha-receptors from initiating muscle contraction.

Gas Exchange

Remember that gas exchange is what breathing is all about. It's also what COPD disrupts. Let's end this chapter with a brief description of where and how successful gas exchange takes place. (In the next chapter, we get to the problems.)

At rest, healthy people move about a half-liter (close to a half-quart) of air in and out of their lungs with each breath. They do this about 12 to 14 times a minute. (This adds up to eight liters, almost eight quarts, every minute.) As the lungs inflate, some of this air fills the larger airways. The majority fills the smaller airways and air sacs. Here in the alveoli, some of the oxygen in this fresh air and all of the excess carbon dioxide brought to the lungs by the blood are exchanged.

At rest, the right side of the heart pumps about five liters (almost five quarts) of blood through the lungs every minute. Then the blood is returned to the left side of the heart, where it is pumped throughout the body. Blood going from the heart to the lungs is called *venous blood*; once it leaves the lungs to return to the heart it is called *arterial blood*. Venous blood is oxygen poor, but rich in carbon dioxide. As venous blood passes through the lungs, oxygen is replaced and carbon dioxide removed. Then the blood loses oxygen and picks up carbon dioxide as it flows through the body's tissues, returning to the right side of the heart to be pumped through the lungs again (Figure 2.9).

Not all of the freshly inhaled air participates in this exchange of gases. Air that does not is called *dead space*, which includes all of the air filling the larger airways and those alveoli that aren't, for the moment, receiving any blood, and most of the air entering alveoli that temporarily have relatively little blood circulating around them. In addition, a tiny amount of blood normally does not participate effectively in this gas exchange, because it has gone to inadequately filled air sacs or has somehow bypassed the air sacs completely.

Despite this, the amount of blood passing through the lungs each minute so closely matches the amount of air reaching the alveoli each minute that a healthy person's blood—even during exercise—carries close

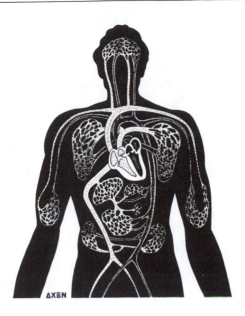

AXEN

Figure 2.9 The circulatory system. Densely stippled areas indicate a high concentration of oxygen (air, the heart's left side, arterial blood). The lightly stippled areas indicate blood from which oxygen has been removed (in the veins and the heart's right side). Blood gains oxygen as it passes through the lungs, then gives up oxygen as it passes through the tissues.

to the maximum amount of oxygen it can, and successfully gets rid of all the excess carbon dioxide it has picked up.

This gas exchange process is so efficient because of the incredible expanse actually covered by the thin, blood vessel-filled membrane that forms the walls of the lungs' 300 million air sacs. It is this membrane through which gas exchange occurs. If this membrane could be stretched out flat, it would cover a tennis court!

Obstructed Airways Hurt

But seriously obstructed airways disrupt this matchup. Air entering the lungs of a chronic bronchitis patient—one who has a substantial number of airways plugged with mucus—is very unevenly distributed. Much of it goes to the unobstructed areas of the lungs. But the blood coming from the heart to pick up oxygen and shed carbon dioxide is not redistributed to anywhere near the same degree. Too much of it goes to obstructed areas of the lungs, the areas that cannot fully oxygenate it or adequately remove the carbon dioxide it carries (Figure 2.10). The result is a *ventilation-blood flow imbalance.*

The patient becomes chronically hypoxic—that is, the level of oxygen in his blood regularly falls below what it should be. Then his body's muscles—including his respiratory muscles—cannot get the amount of oxygen they need to function effectively. The level of carbon dioxide in his blood rises above what it should be, adding to his sense of fatigue.

Loss of Gas Exchange Membrane Hurts

Lungs that have lost a substantial part of the gas exchange membrane—which is the basis of emphysema—can no longer accept anywhere near eight liters of air and five liters of blood each minute. Gas exchange can no longer occur fast enough to satisfy the body's needs.

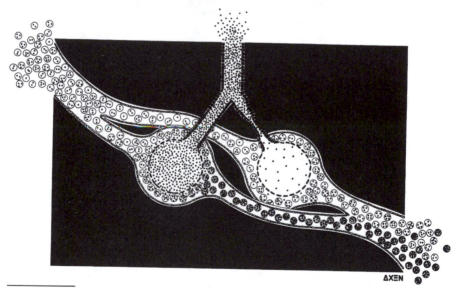

Figure 2.10   How airway obstruction affects the amount of oxygen in arterial blood. In this schematic illustration of ventilation-blood flow imbalance, each dot represents an oxygen molecule. Because the obstructed alveolus gets less air than the other one, fewer oxygen molecules are available for the blood circulating around it. The net effect of the obstruction depends on how much of the lungs are involved. With only a small part obstructed, the lack of oxygen from that area is negligible when it mixes with well-oxygenated blood from the substantial healthy areas of the lungs. As more and more of the lungs' airways become obstructed, the shrinking healthy areas compensate less and less. Eventually, as in severe chronic bronchitis, the blood can no longer meet the body's oxygen demands.

3

COPD: The Damage, the Symptoms, the Progression

Now you have a general idea of the elements that make up your respiratory system and how they normally work together. You've also seen where and how emphysema and chronic bronchitis create problems. Here we focus on the diseases themselves and tie all the pieces together. What does each disease look like? How and why are emphysema and chronic bronchitis so closely related? How does COPD progress over time?

NOTE: As you read through these descriptions, try to keep in mind that these two diseases—each in its own way obstructing the flow of air in and out of the lungs—usually occur together. We describe their mechanisms separately for ease of presentation and understanding. But in the real world, the two sets of processes usually work hand in hand.

The Evils of Tobacco

Cigarette smoking is the overwhelmingly most important cause of COPD. It causes two major kinds of damage to the lungs—the air sac damage we call emphysema, and the airway/air sac damage we call chronic bronchitis. Realizing that smoking injures our lungs isn't a modern notion. Over 300 years ago, the seventeenth-century physician Tobias Venner published the first warning against smoking and lung damage in his book *Via Recta and Vitam Longam* (*The Long and Healthy Life*): "Tobacco . . . disturbeth the humors and spirits, corrupteth the breath . . . exisaccateth the windpipe, lungs, and liver."

Table 3.1 illustrates the four variables—age, number of cigarettes smoked per day, recent or planned change in that number, and existing airway obstruction (measured by FEV_1)—that, combined, best predict the chance of developing COPD within the next ten years. ("COPD" means some combination of emphysema and chronic bronchitis.)

Table 3.1 Risk Factor Points: Your Chances of Getting COPD

Age	Points	Cigarettes/Day	Points	FEV$_1$ % Predicted	Points	Change in Cigarettes/Day	Points	Total Points	Risk* (Cases/100)
				Men					
25	0	0	0	121	−14	−60	−9	<7	Low Risk
27	1	10	2	118	−12	−50	−7	8–14	1
29	2	20	5	115	−10	−40	−6	8–17	2
31	3	30	7	112	−8	−30	−4	8–19	3
33	4	40	9	109	−6	−20	−3	20	4
35	5	50	11	106	−4	−10	−1	21	5
37	6	60	13	103	−2	0	0	22	6
39	7			100	0	10	1	23	7
41	8			97	2	20	3	24	8
43	9			94	4	30	4	25	9
45	10			91	6	40	6	26	11
47	11			88	8	50	7	27	13
49	12			85	10	60	9	28	15
51	13			82	12			29	18
53	14			79	14			30	20
55	15			76	16			31	23
57	16			73	18			>32	High Risk
59	17			70	20				
61	18								
63	19								
65	20								

Women

Age	Points			FEV₁ %	Women Points			Total	Risk
25	0	0	0	121	−16	−60	−17	<10	Low Risk
27	1	10	4	118	−14	−50	−14	11–17	1
29	2	20	9	115	−11	−40	−11	18–20	2
31	3	30	13	112	−9	−30	−8	21–23	3
33	4	40	18	109	−7	−20	−6	24	4
35	5	50	22	106	−5	−10	−3	25	5
37	6	60	27	103	−2	0	0	26	5
39	7			100	0	10	3	27	6
41	8			97	2	20	6	28	7
43	9			94	5	30	8	29	8
45	10			91	7	40	11	30	10
47	11			88	9	50	14	31	11
49	12			85	11	60	17	32	13
51	13			82	14			33	14
53	14			79	16			34	17
55	15			76	18			35	19
57	16			73	21			36	21
59	17			70	23			>37	High Risk
61	18								
63	19								
65	20								

*This table gives your risk for getting emphysema and/or chronic bronchitis in the next ten years. Add up your points for the risk factors: age, smoking, percentage of predicted FEV₁ (get this from your doctor), and any recent or planned change in your smoking habit. Look up your probability in the last column.

Source: Table reproduced from T. T. Higgins, "Epidemiology of Bronchitis and Emphysema." In *Pulmonary Diseases and Disorders*, 2nd ed., A. P. Fishman, ed. New York: McGraw-Hill, 1988.

For example, a 45-year-old man smoking two packs daily, with no plans to change his smoking habit and mild airway obstruction (FEV_1 = 82% of predicted) scores 31 points. This translates to a 23% chance that he will develop COPD by age 55. (A "23% chance" means that, of 100 people with his age, smoking habit, and airway obstruction, 23 of them will develop COPD by the time they reach 55.) But if he stops smoking, his risk falls to 9%.

And compared to nonsmokers, cigarette smokers are ten times more likely to die from COPD, cigar smokers three times more likely, and pipe smokers one and one-half times more likely.

The next question: How does cigarette smoking cause lung damage that impairs their ability to work, and gets worse as time goes by?

Emphysema

Emphysema's immediate cause depends on whether it is the first or second of the COPD diseases to appear. When it develops first, its cause is a presently incurable enzyme imbalance in the lungs that allows destruction of too many elastic fibers in the lungs' framework and air sac walls. A tiny number of these patients inherit this enzyme imbalance. The vast majority develop it from smoking cigarettes for many years.

When chronic bronchitis—typically caused by smoking—is the first to develop, it eventually hyperinflates the lungs because mucus obstructing the smallest bronchioles prevents air sacs from fully emptying. Then elastin in these overstretched alveoli walls breaks down. The route is different, but the same point is reached. (This route will be described more fully in the section on Chronic Bronchitis.)

Enzyme Imbalance

What medical researchers have learned from studying people who have inherited this imbalance permits us to understand the mechanism behind this problem, regardless of its cause.

An important element in the body's repair system are enzymes that destroy proteins—the basic building blocks of all tissue. They get rid of aging cells to make way for new ones, and help in other ways to fight disease. To prevent these enzymes from digesting too much protein, our body also produces regulatory enzymes that continuously circulate throughout our body in our plasma—the fluid in which our blood cells travel.

Alpha₁-antitrypsin is the most abundant of these regulatory enzymes. It is manufactured in the liver, then released into the plasma for transport.

Its primary role is inhibiting the enzyme *elastase,* which is manufactured by a type of white blood cell and released into the plasma surrounding them. Elastase—as its name implies—digests *elastin.*

Elastin is the basic construction material in the lungs, providing the bulk of the framework and the alveoli walls. Elastase digests aging elastin cells so they can be replaced by new ones. Normally, alpha$_1$-antitrypsin adequately controls the amount of elastase in the lungs so it doesn't destroy healthy tissue too. But with too little alpha$_1$-antitrypsin, elastase proliferates. It destroys healthy elastic cells. This is the beginning of emphysema—when it precedes chronic bronchitis.

Clinical scientists have gathered two kinds of proof linking this abnormal relationship to emphysema. In animal experiments, higher elastase levels clearly produce emphysema. In humans, inadequate alpha$_1$-antitrypsin is the single factor *always* associated with COPD.

Inherited Alpha$_1$-Antitrypsin Deficiency   (For patients who want an in-depth discussion, Chapter 4 is devoted to this form of emphysema.) Our 31 chromosomes contain about 100,000 genes—the blueprints for all our inherited characteristics. We have two sets of chromosomes, one from each of our parents. A gene on chromosome 14 determines how much alpha$_1$-antitrypsin our liver produces. Depending on what each parent passed on to them, some people have two normal alpha$_1$-antitrypsin genes, some have two defective genes, and some have one of each.

When a gene pair has one defective member, the consequence generally depends on the trait. For traits needing only one active gene, the defective one is not called into service. But for traits that rely on both genes—and alpha$_1$-antitrypsin is one of these—even one defective gene can cause trouble. And a pair of defective genes can wreak havoc.

With just one defective alpha$_1$-antitrypsin gene, a person's liver still produces roughly 75% of what it should. The subtle problems this can cause do not involve emphysema. But the person with two defective genes produces only 15% of this critical regulatory enzyme—too little to control the destruction of elastin. Most of these people eventually develop emphysema (and are also susceptible to chronic liver disease). The emphysema symptoms are usually obvious by age 35 if they smoke, and by age 45 if they don't. (This deficiency is more common in some countries than others. It affects 1 of every 6,000 people in the United States, for example, but 1 of every 1,000 in Sweden.)

Self-Made Alpha$_1$-Antitrypsin Deficiency   Uncontrolled destruction of the lungs' elastin by the elastase enzyme is also how smokers develop emphysema. In fact, cigarette smoke packs a triple whammy when it comes to injuring the lungs' elastic network, by (1) inactivating alpha$_1$-antitrypsin; (2) causing pulmonary inflammation, which brings still more elastase (via elastase-containing neutrophils) into the lungs; and (3) slowing production of new elastic cells.

Emphysema Develops   By whichever route, destruction of too many elastic fibers in the lungs' framework and air sac walls is the first step in emphysema. This loss of elasticity results in hyperinflated air sacs, and impairs the lungs' ability to recoil effectively during expiration. The hyperinflated air sacs become permanently enlarged. Eventually the walls of these overstretched air sacs break down, merging neighboring alveoli into one large air sac (look back at Figure 2.9). At the same time, the disease invades the walls of previously healthy alveoli.

Destruction of capillary-rich air sac walls means that much of the lungs' capillary network—which is responsible for taking oxygen into the body and discarding carbon dioxide—is gradually lost. This continually reduces the amount of gas exchange that can occur. The inspiratory muscles start working harder to take air in.

Since the enlarged alveoli can no longer provide the force that normally keeps the smallest airways fully open during expiration, expiratory resistance increases considerably. In compensation, expiration becomes slower and longer, and often is eventually aided by the expiratory muscles even during nonstrenuous activities. But the increased force exerted by the expiratory muscles' compensatory behavior compresses the small airways even further. Their collapse during expiration traps air in the attached alveoli. This process begins limiting the amount of stale air that can be breathed out, and therefore the amount of fresh air that is breathed in.

Expiratory resistance can eventually become so high that it actually prevents expiration from finishing before the next inspiration must begin. This increases air trapping, and limits even more the amount of air that can be moved in and out of the lungs.

Substantial air trapping—when more air than normal remains in the lungs at the end of each expiration—means the lungs can no longer return to their normal resting position. Because they must remain partially expanded, the inspiratory muscles cannot relax—stretch out to full length—in between breaths. A shorter muscle is less effective, and so must work harder. At some point, the accessory inspiratory muscles start to help out on a full-time basis.

An irony of this disease is that each new development increases the workload on the respiratory muscles, while at the same time diminishing further the amount of oxygen available to produce the energy this work requires.

So emphysema patients are characterized by hyperinflated lungs and by chronically diminished airflow—especially during expiration. Gas exchange is moderately disrupted. The consequences of these lung changes are most noticeable during activities requiring physical effort. Patients find themselves breathless doing things that once gave them no difficulty.

Chronic Bronchitis

When the lungs' airways are regularly assaulted by a troublesome irritant over a long time, as in cigarette smoking, they eventually respond in two ways (look again at Figure 2.5). They become permanently inflamed, with fluid swelling the tissue that lines the airways. Since this narrows the airways, airflow resistance increases. The lungs also radically increase mucus production in a powerhouse attempt to clean out this irritant. In a two-pronged effort, the mucus glands grow several times their normal size and the goblet cells both become far more numerous and spread out to populate even the smallest airways.

In this early stage of chronic bronchitis, the excessive sputum does not yet block the patient's airways because the cough is still strong enough to move a great deal of it out of the lungs. Because this mucus is not permitted to stagnate in the airways, it has not yet become a hospitable site for bacterial growth. The impressive sputum reservoir that the lungs produce is still *nonpurulent,* a medical term meaning "without bacterial content." The airways are still sterile.

But gradual paralysis of the cilia—the tiny hair-like structures responsible for moving mucus up and out of the airways—permits mucus to accumulate in smaller airways. Then air can no longer rush out of these airways fast enough to create a powerful cough. Eventually, the patient's cough becomes too weak to propel enough mucus out of his larger airways. Loss of the body's airway-clearing mechanism lets prodigious amounts of mucus stagnate in his lungs. This warm, dark, damp, and sticky environment is ideal for bacterial growth.

In the next stage of chronic bronchitis, then, bacteria colonize the airways. In this respect the airways now resemble the digestive tract, where bacteria are normally in permanent residence. But what is normal for the intestines is not so for the lungs. Once bacteria populate the airways, pulmonary infections become frequent. (Professionals in the field feel that continuous bacterial presence in the airways may actually perpetuate and worsen the mucus secretions. A vicious circle has developed.)

With each pulmonary infection, the dramatic increase in airway mucus production that would normally occur is added to an already huge mucus pool. Eventually, the peak excesses of mucus associated with respiratory infections begin to creep into the smallest airways, those crucial links to the air sacs. Little or no gas exchange occurs in these alveoli until the mucus recedes. As this periodic obstruction of the terminal and respiratory bronchioles becomes more widespread and slower to recede, air becomes trapped in the surrounding alveoli. *These air sacs become permanently hyperinflated.*

Deterioration of the elastic fibers in these air sac walls is given a big assist by the neutrophil-produced elastase increase that has been part of the inflammatory response for however many years the patient has been smoking. In the face of these combined forces, the progression of emphysema is inevitable. One chronic obstructive lung disease has now led to another.

This periodic obstruction gradually becomes permanent in more and more of the smallest airways. Then air can no longer reach the capillary blood in these air sac walls to deliver oxygen and remove carbon dioxide. A ventilation-blood flow imbalance has been created. This imbalance significantly reduces oxygen and raises carbon dioxide in the blood. In technical terms, the patient is now chronically *hypoxic* (low oxygen) and *hypercapnic* (high carbon dioxide).

COPD's Natural History

The "natural history" of COPD—by which we mean the progression of physical damage and its impact on the patient—depends on whether bronchitis or emphysema predominates.

Chronic Bronchitis Predominating

The typical patient with chronic bronchitis predominating first visits his doctor because he has been unable to shake a bad cold that has "settled in my chest." It is the first or second time that he has been steadily coughing up large quantities of mucus for several months after getting a cold. He is usually between 40 and 55 years old and a heavy smoker, and more often male than female (although these odds are changing).

Although the patient has just become aware of his symptoms, the disease has been silently progressing for several decades. During this time his airways have been continuously assaulted by the harmful substances inhaled in his cigarette smoke. These substances have inflamed his air-ways, gradually increased mucus production throughout his airways, and eventually damaged the ability of his ciliated epithelial cells to move mucus out of his smaller airways. His cough—still moderately effective—now has to work hard to keep up with the pace of mucus production in his larger airways. In addition to inhaled cigarette smoke, any other air pollutants in his environment start adding to the insult.

The airway-narrowing effects of mucus accumulating in smaller air-ways, plus the preexisting inflammation, continue to increase expiratory airflow resistance. The patient's cough eventually becomes too weak to dislodge mucus in his upper airways. The mucus accumulating through-out becomes permanent host to bacteria, predisposing the individual to respiratory infections. As his condition progresses, the patient periodically complains of disabling shortness of breath (medically termed *dyspnea*). Blood tests at these times reveal too little oxygen and too much carbon dioxide in his blood. These worsenings, or exacerbations, tend to occur during air pollution peaks and at the start of a cold or flu. Such condi-tions particularly increase the production and retention of mucus, which in turn increase airway obstruction.

But aside from these occasional bouts of hypoxia and hypercapnia, coughing and heavy sputum production are the patient's only prominent symptoms in what is still an early stage of his disease. His lungs are still managing to function adequately at nonstrenuous activity levels, and oxygen and carbon dioxide levels remain within normal limits.

Without energetic therapeutic intervention, however, the patient inevitably gets worse—although just what precipitates transition to the second stage is not fully clear. It is thought that continued smoking and recurrent infections cause more and more obstruction in the small air-ways. Some eventually remain fully blocked for so long that the airway segment below the blockage actually amputates from lack of oxygen. The affected air sacs disappear as their membranous walls die and become absorbed. The remaining airway fragments are useless scar tissue.

The larger airways, too, are gradually narrowed by mucus as enlarged mucous glands dominate both large and small airways and goblet cells proliferate. Peeking in the airways with a microscope from time to time would show us increasing hypersecretion of mucus everywhere. Routine pulmonary function tests now reflect airway obstruction because it is severe enough to increase resistance measurably. This noticeable resistance to airflow can make breathing more difficult. Yet despite the abnormali-ties at this stage, the large amount of reserve capacity in our lungs still allows most patient to maintain acceptable levels of oxygen and carbon dioxide in their blood when they are between pulmonary infections and/or pollution peaks.

The third stage of this disease, though, is characterized by continuous, progressive disturbance in the ventilation-blood flow relationship. There is no longer a workable matchup between the availability of oxygen and the presence of blood-filled capillaries to absorb it. This results from the ever-increasing degree of smallest airway obstruction, plus the development of emphysema. Most patients with chronic bronchitis have developed centrilobular emphysema by now, affecting isolated alveoli higher up in the acinar. But in some, more widespread air sac destruction has resulted in panlobular emphysema. (In any case, as a patient grows older, age-related changes in the lungs hasten this loss of elastic recoil, adding to the likelihood of infection and airway obstruction.)

In these more advanced stages, the difficulty in maintaining an adequate oxygen level in his blood sometimes gives a bluish-gray tinge to the patient's skin. Progressive withdrawal from physical activity over the years has turned the majority of these patients flabby and overweight. Their typical skin color and physique have led to the descriptive term *blue bloaters* (Figure 3.1).

Eventually, the lung pathology in chronic bronchitis damages the patient's heart. Part of his problem stems from the loss of air sac capillaries through "amputation" and emphysematous changes. The other part comes from his worsening ventilation-blood flow imbalance. With continued low oxygen, the muscles encircling the small blood vessels leading to the remaining capillaries contract permanently, narrowing these vessels. Constant contraction eventually overdevelops these vascular muscles, which thickens the walls—and narrows them still more. And we know from discussing the airways that when a tube narrows, what flows through it meets with greater resistance. So with the vascular pathways far less numerous and much narrower, pushing blood through the lungs now takes a lot more work than it used to.

(Ironically, this damage results from a blood-flow response that is actually helpful in healthy lungs. In that case, when a tiny area is temporarily oxygen-deprived, the vessels feeding the capillaries there temporarily narrow to divert the flow of blood to well-oxygenated areas. But in COPD, poor oxygenation becomes both widespread and chronic. So *all* the blood vessels feeding pulmonary capillaries constrict, and *remain* that way.)

Matters worsen when some COPD patients with advanced chronic bronchitis (and a small number with severe emphysema) develop a condition that intensifies this effort further. The condition is called *polycythemia*,

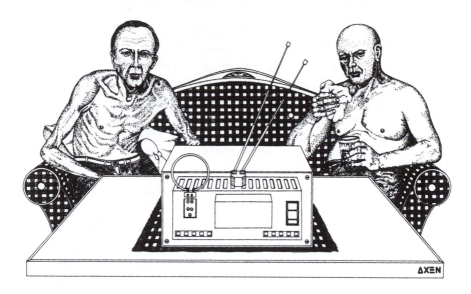

Figure 3.1 The person on the *left* has the typical appearance of a patient with emphysema predominating—a pink puffer. Although he has good color, he appears distressed. He uses the muscles of his neck (accessory muscles) while breathing in. He sits forward in his chair bracing his arm on the arm rest, and he naturally adopts pursed-lip breathing (see Chapter 13, pages 183–186). In contrast, the person on the *right* has chronic bronchitis predominating—a blue bloater. He is typically overweight, and his color is dusky gray. His lips and fingernail beds may be distinctly blue (cyanosis). He coughs frequently, but the cough may not be effective in bringing up sputum.

which translates from Latin to mean "too many red blood cells." Here is another example of a normally adaptive response to lowered oxygen becoming destructive when it is stimulated by chronic pathology.

When a healthy person who normally lives close to sea level travels up to the mountains, his body compensates for the lower amount of oxygen in high altitude air by increasing its production of red blood cells. Although each red cell now carries less oxygen than at sea level, having more red blood cells available to carry oxygen can maintain the blood's oxygen level.

For a relatively small number of COPD patients, this adaptation goes too far. Red blood cells increase so rapidly that they actually thicken the blood. Pushing thickened blood through the lungs' damaged vascular network stresses the heart still more.

The segment of the heart that pumps blood through the lungs—called the *right ventricle*—is responsible for this exhausting work. The right ventricle gets larger to help it summon up this extra effort on a daily basis. Eventually, however, the heart can no longer maintain this nonstop additional effort. The demands it must meet are overwhelming. It begins to fail.

This condition is called *cor pulmonale*. (The direct translation from Latin is "lung heart.") The patient can still get up out of bed every day, but his condition is now fragile and unstable. He is constantly on the verge of heart and respiratory failure.

Emphysema Predominating

The patient with emphysema predominating is from 50 to 75 years old (and most often male) when he first feels the need to see his doctor. He complains of pronounced breathlessness that has suddenly begun bothering him regularly during active pursuits (like playing with grandchildren). Unlike his chronic bronchitic counterparts, the emphysema patient does relatively little coughing, his sputum production is scanty, and upper respiratory infections are only occasional. He tends to be thin—often to the point of emaciation—and anxious.

The degree of airflow obstruction in nonsmoking emphysema patients is normally mild. More pronounced airflow obstruction is usually due to an accompanying chronic bronchitis. If this chronic bronchitis component is small, the emphysema patient can remain essentially symptom-free for life aside from his intense breathlessness during mild activity—termed *exertional dyspnea*. In the more advanced stages of emphysema, the patient exhales audibly with his lips pursed and uses his accessory respiratory muscles prominently. But because there is no severe large airway obstruction to disrupt gas exchange, oxygen and carbon dioxide levels remain normal and his complexion is rosy. From their pursed-lip breathing and healthy color, these patients are described as *pink puffers* (Figure 3.1).

As long as any coexisting chronic bronchitis remains minor, this patient's oxygen level will fall only temporarily—at the start of an upper respiratory infection. In this "benign" state of affairs, he is much less likely than his chronic bronchitis counterpart to develop *cor pulmonale*. His chances will rise dramatically, however, if the coexisting chronic bronchitis becomes more widespread and severe. Then he will become chronically hypoxic, resulting in constant and substantial added work for the heart that eventually wears it out.

The natural history of patients with emphysema predominating, compared to predominantly chronic bronchitis, holds many more gradations in severity. It ranges from increasing shortness of breath during exertion over a potentially long lifetime with perhaps an occasional respiratory crisis in later years, to progressively incapacitating breathlessness and fatigue at rest as more and more of the lungs disappear from the combined destruction of emphysema and widespread chronic bronchitis.

Modifying This Natural History

Although these chronic, progressive lung diseases cannot yet be cured, they can be treated. We use a variety of therapeutic measures to slow their progress significantly, and substantially reduce the degree and impact of their symptoms. As we shall see in later chapters, the management of both these diseases involves:

☐ Making changes to prevent the inhalation of harmful substances (such as cigarette smoke, polluted air), to slow your disease's progress and increase the effectiveness of all other treatment measures.

☐ Preventing pulmonary infections, to slow your disease's progress and reduce stress on your lungs and heart.

☐ Reducing airway obstruction—via appropriate medication, more effective breathing techniques, and postural drainage to expel mucus—to slow your disease's progress, improve your ventilation-blood flow balance, and lessen airway resistance. This lightens the workload for both your respiratory muscles and heart, and gives you a lot more energy.

☐ Improving your muscle conditioning (which makes your muscles simultaneously capable of greater effort and less needy of oxygen) and learning alternative ways of moving and working that use less muscle power (and therefore less oxygen), to improve the oxygen level in your blood. This expands the amount and variety of activities available to you, as well as reducing stress on your respiratory muscles and heart.

☐ Providing supplemental oxygen, if necessary, to maintain a normal oxygen level in your blood. This improves your energy, mood, concentration, and mental functioning.

4

Inherited Emphysema: Alpha₁-Antitrypsin Deficiency

Elastin is the lungs' basic structural material, providing the bulk of the overall elastic framework and the alveoli walls. *Elastase* is an essential enzyme for maintaining healthy lungs because it digests ineffective, aging elastin fibers so they can be replaced by new ones. (It is called a *protease* enzyme because it digests a protein.) *Alpha₁-antitrypsin* (*AAT* for short)—another enzyme normally abundant in the lungs—digests excess elastase, which otherwise would start eating into healthy elastic tissue. (A more detailed view of these enzymes is in Chapter 2.) If for some reason there is not enough AAT to keep the amount of elastase under control, it starts destroying healthy elastic tissue faster than it can be replaced. This is the beginning of emphysema.

Although with most emphysema patients the culprit is cigarettes, a small percentage develop this chronic lung disease because they inherited one or two defective genes for producing the AAT enzyme. People with two defective genes produce almost none at all. People with one defective and one healthy gene produce this regulatory enzyme, but either in very small amounts, or in an altered form that functions poorly. The American Lung Association reports that approximately 1 in every 2,500 people in the United States has some form of AAT deficiency. Based on the total U.S. population, this amounts to 100,000 people. The Alpha1 Association—the national support and advocacy organization—is in the same ballpark. They estimate that 80,000 to 100,000 men, women, and children are affected by AAT deficiency, and they point out that only a fraction of them have been diagnosed. The Alpha1 Association nicknames the disease *A1AD*, and patients often refer to themselves as *alphas*.

The Dynamics of Disease

Our 31 chromosomes together contain about 100,000 genes—the blueprints for all our inherited characteristics and physiologic functions. We have two sets of 31 chromosomes, one from each parent. The AAT gene resides on chromosome 14. It is nicknamed the *PI* gene—short for *protease inhibitor*—and designated *14q32.1*. (Since there are still many genes with unidentified functions, we give every gene an "address" that pinpoints its location, and we also give names to those whose function we already know.) AAT—the most important member of the family of protease enzymes—is produced primarily in the liver. The rest of it is produced by certain white blood cells, and by cells in the intestines and kidney. Everyone has two AAT genes—one on the chromosome 14 passed on from the mother, and one on the father's chromosome 14. Most people have two normal genes, some have two defective genes, and some have one of each. Defects are the result of mutations that affect a gene's ability to function properly. Although at least 90 different harmful mutations have been identified in this gene, the "Z" type is overwhelmingly the most common.

As a general rule, for any important function—like AAT production—a pair of defective genes wreaks havoc. When just one gene in the pair is defective, the consequence varies. Some functions require only one healthy gene—with the second acting as back-up just in case something goes wrong with its partner—and then a defective gene simply remains silent. But for functions requiring two healthy genes—and AAT is one of these—even one defective gene causes trouble. The enzyme is produced, but either in an inadequate amount or as a malfunctioning enzyme.

The majority (95%) of patients with the most severe deficiency have inherited the Z variant from each parent. The remaining 5% of these patients represent about 20 other mutation types, and include a few people with one normal gene. The person with two defective genes produces almost none of this critical regulatory enzyme—far too little to control the destruction of elastin. Most of these people eventually develop emphysema. (They are also at risk of developing chronic liver disease, especially children and adults older than 50. Liver pathology develops in about 10% of these children and 25% of these older adults.) With one defective gene, a person's liver typically still produces roughly 75% of the normal amount. So the subtle problems this may cause don't often emerge as definable symptoms. According to both the World Health Organization and the Alpha1 Association, only a small proportion of the number of people estimated to have this deficiency—both severe and less severe—have been diagnosed.

Cigarette smoke both seriously speeds up the destruction of lung tissue and transforms a single-gene defect into a far more significant health problem. Because smoking irritates the lungs, white blood cells are attracted to the site to repair the damage. As they happen to be the same white blood cells that produce elastase, this substantially adds to the excessive amount of elastase already bathing the interior of the lungs. Adding insult to injury, oxidants in the smoke itself inactivate much or all of the AAT that might still be present. In A1AD people who smoke, emphysema symptoms are usually obvious by age 35. Not smoking gives them another 10 years before reaching this point.

Although little is known yet about the harm caused by environmental air pollution to A1AD people, it is likely that such oxidants as ozone, sulfur dioxide, and nitrogen oxides also speed up the progression of emphysema in these cases. Similarly, the existence of respiratory infections in early childhood also seems to be a risk factor for early development of emphysema in these people.

Screening

Because the overwhelming majority of emphysema patients are *not* AAT-deficient, screening for this condition is prohibitively expensive. What little large-scale screening does take place is in the service of research. Groups of blood donors have been screened in an attempt to determine the percentage of people in the general population who are walking around with undiagnosed A1AD. About 300,000 newborns have also been screened. This is another way to try to estimate the percentage of people born with this condition. And in addition, following infants long-term who are found to have this deficiency will gradually provide important information about the natural history of this disease.

Screening all siblings of a diagnosed A1AD patient is important, because approximately 25% of them also carry the defective gene. Once identified, currently "silent" carriers can be counseled to stop smoking— if they are smokers—and evaluated as candidates for the early initiation of *augmentation therapy* (see below), which is thought might slow the disease's course. The AAT Deficiency Detection Center in Salt Lake City, Utah, offers free screenings to people with a higher-than-average risk. Between 1991 and 1996, the nearly 17,000 samples they screened identified 514 PI-ZZ individuals. These 514 translate to about 15% of A1AD patients diagnosed with a severe deficiency during those 5 years in the United States. Free screening is also available through the Alpha1 Association.

Treatment

Treatment for A1AD patients is of two types. The modalities used for *all* COPD patients—including lung volume reduction surgery—are appropriate. These therapies are fully discussed in the relevant chapters elsewhere in this book. In addition, you now have access to *augmentation therapy*. This is directed at treating your primary defect—minimal or ineffective AAT—by giving you significant doses of the healthy human enzyme.

Augmentation therapy was not an existing option until the late 1980s, when purified human AAT was approved by the U.S. Food and Drug Administration (FDA) as an orphan drug. It had not yet been proven effective, but it was safe. Although preliminary studies since then have shown a modest improvement in lung function, a conclusive clinical trial is highly unlikely. Because it would have to be randomized—meaning that some patients would be blindly assigned to receive the real treatment and others to receive a fake (placebo)—it will probably be impossible to find patients who would consent to possibly not receiving the real treatment. If the treatment turns out to be highly effective, volunteers assigned to the placebo will have jeopardized their lives. There is also the ethical question: Do we have the right to ask people to risk sacrificing their lives for the possible future benefit of others?

Instead, the natural history of this disease and the effect of intravenous enzyme delivery in patients with a severe deficiency are being studied through several large multicenter registries (a coordinated listing—covering a large area or entire country—of patients with a particular disease). One is the registry maintained by the United States National Heart, Lung, and Blood Institute, one is the Danish-Dutch registry, and the other is the German registry. The Spanish registry of PI-ZZ patients (begun in 1993) is also collecting data. Unfortunately, each study has been designed differently, which will probably make it impossible to add these observations together or even compare them. Two other factors make clear conclusions even more unlikely: each registry involves a relatively small number of patients, and this disease progresses relatively slowly. It is an irony that even if this treatment actually significantly slows the loss of lung function, it may be impossible to carry out the kind of experiment that can demonstrate this in a scientifically and medically meaningful way.

About 2,000 people worldwide are using commercial enzyme augmentation products. Because their half-life in the body is five days at the most, intravenous infusions have to be given weekly to maintain protective effects. Side effects—although few and minor—include headache and a variety of muscle and joint aches and pains.

Because the therapeutic benefit of augmentation therapy is uncertain and this therapy is costly, the criteria for selecting patients is controversial. The American Thoracic Society recommends that only patients with seriously inadequate AAT levels—*and* who do not smoke or have stopped smoking—should be treated. Although it is common sense that therapy be started before irreparable lung damage has developed, there are no data yet supporting this judgment.

Because intravenous dosing is inconvenient and adds significantly to this therapy's cost, aerosol delivery of human AAT is currently being evaluated to see if it increases the amount of enzyme in the fluid that bathes the airway tissues. Not only would this permit patients to use this treatment at home, but smaller doses would be needed because the protein is administered directly to the lungs. The hope for the relatively near future is gene therapy. Instead of adding the actual enzyme, the gene responsible for making it would be delivered to the respiratory tract. In this way, enough of the protein would be continuously manufactured in the airways and alveoli to raise levels high enough to prevent deterioration of pulmonary function.

Prognosis

The official prognosis for A1AD people is still poor. Only 16% of those with the PI-ZZ variant survive to age 60. This compares to 85% of the healthy population. The actual picture, though, is probably better than this statistic. The beneficial effects of both AAT augmentation and new surgical procedures have come about too recently to have affected a large enough percentage of patients to make a significant dent in these figures. In actual fact, it is likely that both longevity and quality of life for A1AD people have been improving—and will continue to improve—as newer therapies come into regular use.

Resources

AAT-deficient patients benefit from one of the most active, productive support organizations around: the Alpha1 Association. They are the main source of information for new developments and local support groups, provide an interactive multimedia educational program for newly diagnosed patients (*Alpha to Alpha*), and offer a great deal of basic disease-related information—as well as assistance and a variety of resources—on their terrific website. Their two publications for members are the *Alpha₁ Quarterly Review Journal,* which reprints informative medical articles, and the newsletter *Alpha₁ News.* The new Family and Peer Support Program matches a peer counselor to newly diagnosed patients and their families. On their website, *Alpha2Alpha* provides access to live chats with other Alpha₁ patients. And for patients without access to a local support group, an e-mail support network will keep letters arriving regularly. You can contact the Alpha1 Association at:

8120 Penn Ave. S., Suite 549
Minneapolis, MN 55431-1326
800-521-3025 *or* 612-703-9979; *fax* 612-703-9977
A1NA@alpha1.org; www.alpha1.org

The American Lung Association's website provides introductory information on this disease and its treatment: *www.lungusa.org/diseases/luna1ad.html.* They can be reached by phone at 800-LUNG-USA.

The AAT Deficiency Detection Center in Utah can be reached at 800-288-8371 for information and instruction sheets.

5

Seeking Help

A family member or close friend, rather than the patient himself, is usually the first to recognize the alarming persistence of COPD's major early symptoms—chronic bronchitis's coughing and excessive mucus production, and emphysema's shortness of breath from mild exertion. The patient typically attributes them to a lingering cold or flu, or to the unavoidable consequences of getting older. Even though pulmonary damage has been gradually progressing over many years, the majority of people we meet recount a story in which the incapacitating aspects of their disease appeared to materialize overnight. This sudden discovery brought them to the doctor's office.

Yet the ideal time to begin medical treatment for COPD is: *the sooner the better*. The earlier intervention begins, the more it can accomplish. So help should be sought as soon as the persistence of symptoms, no matter how mild, is noticed. Do not think you are making a big deal out of nothing. Many serious diseases, including COPD, begin with symptoms so mild that it is usually impossible for a nonmedical person to realize what is underlying them. So it is your responsibility to see your doctor when your body has not been functioning as it should. Your doctor's job is determining if this change is natural or not, temporary or not, and helping you handle it appropriately.

Finding the Right Doctor

What Kind of Doctor?

Two medical specialties overlap for treating COPD: the family physician and the pulmonary internist. Most COPD patients begin with one of these. Then as their disease progresses, other specialists—such as a cardiologist—often join the treatment team.

The Family Physician   The family doctor (also known as a general practitioner or GP, a primary care physician, or an internist) is usually the first
doctor most people consult. In rural areas, this is often the only doctor a
COPD patient ever sees. Starting at this point has a major advantage
(unless you are new in town or have recently changed doctors): your family doctor knows your history and your general state of health. The main
disadvantage is that general practitioners must keep up with changes in so
many areas of medicine that without a specific interest in pulmonary disease, they may be less aware of treatment advances until these changes
eventually filter down throughout the medical community. *Despite this,
the family physician can adequately manage most cases.* The occasional complicated case should usually be referred to the appropriate specialist.

Pulmonary Internist   In areas where a wealth of medical choices exist,
people tend to bypass the family doctor and go directly to a specialist.
Someone with a respiratory problem would choose a *pulmonologist.* These
physicians first specialize in internal medicine, then spend further years
studying pulmonary medicine, and then must pass an examination to
become "board certified" in this subspecialty. Because of a focus on pulmonary disease, the pulmonologist is well informed on the latest treatment advances for COPD.

Where to Look

Unless limited medical resources in your area mean that you have no
choice, finding the right doctor can be difficult. A good way to begin is
seeking recommendations, either from friends or acquaintances (particularly someone with a pulmonary problem), or from another physician.
Keep in mind, though, that nonmedical people are likely to recommend
doctors whose bedside manner is particularly pleasing. Another doctor
will recommend a colleague he went to school with, or whose medical
competence has particularly impressed him. (A medical student we know
has decided to seek friends' recommendations for nonsurgical problems,
but would get another doctor's advice if she needs a surgeon.)

Obtaining a personal recommendation is not the only way. Most large
communities have a Lung Association that can recommend physicians or
clinics. The American Lung Association—headquartered in New York
City at 1740 Broadway, New York, NY 10019; 212-245-8000—can also
advise you on locating a physician or clinic. (Other organizations that
might be helpful in this regard are listed in the Appendix.)

Another approach would be to call the appropriate departmental office
(Family Practice or Pulmonary Medicine) of the nearest large medical

center. This can be particularly helpful if your symptoms become aggravated while traveling and you need nonemergency medical help.

The National Jewish Medical and Research Center (in Denver, Colorado) is, as the name implies, one of the foremost centers for treatment and research in pulmonary diseases. The Center provides a trained staff of registered nurses to answer general questions over the telephone about lung diseases. The caller can also request the names of appropriate hospitals and specialists in his area. This free Lung-Line is manned Monday through Friday from 8:00 A.M. to 5:00 P.M. Mountain time. Messages are taken at other times, and these calls are returned as soon as the Lung-Line reopens. The toll-free number if calling from outside Colorado is 800-222-LUNG, and from within the state is 303-398-1477.

One source to avoid is a magazine's "Best Doctors" type of list. These evaluations are subjective, and are sometimes little more than a popularity rating.

Making the Right Choice

For those of you who have the luxury of choosing among two or more medically competent physicians, it is critical to select one whose personality works well with yours. As with other long-term relationships, the effectiveness of the patient-physician duo depends much on good chemistry, and the trust and communication that this helps promote. A physician whose attitude is "I'm the doctor and you do as I say," for example, will work poorly with patients who find it important to know what is being done, what effects can be expected, and why.

Three complaints arise most frequently when we ask patients who changed physicians why they did so. Their former doctor: (1) did not explain things sufficiently; (2) was unwilling to try lowering medication dosage; or (3) was hesitant to try new approaches and treatment. Yet most felt satisfied with their current doctor. The first complaint, as we indicated, is basically a matter of personality. Most physicians' approach to medication and new treatments depends much on the attitudes they developed during their medical studies.

The two opposite points of view regarding medication use are "minimal-to-none" vs. "aggressive therapy." The aversion to medication that many patients and some physicians hold stems from the desire to avoid possible side effects of drug therapy as much as possible. Most physicians fall somewhere in between these two extreme viewpoints.

As to nontraditional or not-yet-traditional treatments, physicians are trained to be conservative. "Conservative" in this case means not abandoning treatments of proven benefit until something of greater proven benefit comes along. Doctors are rightly skeptical about new treatments that have not yet passed the rigors of modern investigational criteria. Although some of the physicians we have spoken with adhere only to a traditional treatment plan, the great majority will accept a new form of therapy once they are convinced that: (1) it cannot harm the patient, and (2) the patient will still continue traditional treatment along with it.

Although these different philosophies have no effect on a physician's competency in treating the person, they do affect the doctor-patient relationship. Finding a doctor whose attitudes are in step with your own point of view greatly facilitates good communication. It helps to get an idea of a particular physician's personality and philosophy as early on as possible.

When we were looking for a pediatrician for our soon-to-be-born first child, we interviewed several who came highly recommended to us and then chose the one with whom we felt most comfortable. Although we don't know of any medical group other than pediatricians who often allow such interviews, it doesn't hurt to ask

Unfortunately, though, you will probably have to commit yourself to a first appointment in order to gather this important information. Our advice—assuming you can afford to lose the initial fee—is not to settle for the first physician you see unless you feel strongly that this is someone you can work well with. And if a relationship that begins well does not continue to meet your needs as a patient, then it is time to look for a doctor who does.

The severely ill patient who needs frequent hospitalization has an additional factor to consider in choosing a doctor. Since hospitals vary in their standards of patient care, the hospital affiliations of the doctors you are considering become important.

Patients belonging to an HMO may be limited to the participating specialists. It is still essential to meet these physicians and make your choice among them. But if even the best of them leaves you dissatisfied, then if it is feasible we suggest that you contact the closest teaching hospital and locate a specialist there who meets your standards. He can function as a consultant and guide your HMO team.

Who Is Responsible for What?

So you have found a doctor whose personality and attitudes you feel will permit a productive relationship based on mutual respect, confidence, and cooperation. What should you be prepared to expect from each other as this relationship begins?

Your Doctor's Responsibilities

You, the patient, are entitled to certain things from your doctor: (1) an accurate diagnosis of your disease and, if possible, identification of factors that make your condition worse; (2) attentiveness to your "story" and honest answers to your questions about symptoms, treatment, and the future; (3) a treatment plan that will permit you to live as normal a life as possible; (4) an education that will teach you both about your disease and the proper use of medications and other therapeutic techniques; (5) adequately close contact—meaning that your doctor is reachable and returns telephone calls within a reasonable amount of time—so that appropriate intervention, when needed, can be done quickly enough to avoid a hospital stay if this is possible; (6) prompt hospitalization when it is needed.

If you become a patient in the clinic of a large city hospital, these responsibilities—except for (1), (3), and (6) usually do not apply. Although the clinical aspects of your disease will be competently treated, the reduced staff and funds of the typical city hospital leave their physicians without the time needed to pursue the other aspects, even though they are necessary for optimum treatment.

An Added Responsibility Toward the Smoking Patient

Because the doctor treating COPD cannot make any substantial impact on the disease when a smoking patient continues this highly destructive habit, the doctor should then assume a strongly supportive role in helping these patients stop. The American College of Physicians' Health and Public Policy Committee emphasizes the importance of this active role as antismoking counselor. We know that many cigarette smokers can quit, and that their doctor's help and support are tremendously important to their success. Studies show that such encouragement is especially important for smokers trying to quit without involvement in a stop-smoking group.

There are several ways in which doctors can help support their smoking patients' efforts to stop smoking. Some involve motivating these patients. Others require doctors to educate themselves in the techniques found effective by stop-smoking groups. Throughout, doctors must consistently urge their smoking patients to stop. An effective doctor is able to personalize for patients both the risks of smoking and the values of stopping. And it goes without saying that doctors treating COPD patients should be appropriate role models (that is, nonsmokers themselves).

Once smoking COPD patients have made the commitment to give up cigarettes, it becomes very important to express faith in their ability to stay off them. In addition, the doctor should guide these patients in self-control techniques; prepare them for the withdrawal symptoms they may experience; provide educational materials; and refer those patients who need it to an effective group or individual who specializes in helping smokers stop and/or stay stopped.

Your Responsibilities

Your doctor is entitled to expect certain things from you.

1. He needs your honesty in answering all of his questions, as hiding anything (the recreational use of drugs, for example) diminishes his ability to treat you effectively and seriously weakens the relationship's underpinning of mutual trust.
2. He needs to know that you are committed to getting better—that you are a full partner in whatever treatment plan is developed. (If you don't follow this treatment regimen, you are wasting both his time and yours.)
3. You should be gaining insight into your condition. This includes acceptance of your disease as a chronic condition, and an awareness of what improves or worsens your symptoms.
4. You will call him whenever your symptoms or the effect of your medication changes.
5. You will not abuse his responsiveness by calling him for inappropriate reasons. You will gradually learn when it is—and is not—important to talk with your doctor.

For this last point, our pediatrician again provides an excellent example. We asked at our interview with him how to decide whether a particular situation required us to call him. He refused to give us any criteria for making that kind of decision because he preferred—*at the beginning*—to be called to the phone about unimportant matters rather than risk missing an emergency. He added that we would learn when it was important to call him as we gained experience in being parents and got to know our particular child. So as you gain experience in dealing with your COPD, you will come to know very clearly when you need to call your doctor.

Another pediatric story gives an example of abusing your doctor's sense of responsibility. A woman called her pediatrician to discuss what she knew was a minor matter. But because she did not feel like waiting around 15 to 20 minutes for his return call, she claimed that her son was in the midst of a medical emergency. She got the doctor on the phone instantly, but once he realized that the "emergency" was the result of her impatience, he told her to find another pediatrician immediately!

6. Remember that doctors are human beings. And all human beings have both good and bad days. So don't be offended when your doctor is occasionally somewhat curt or preoccupied during a visit or

telephone call. Give him some understanding when he is having an off day. And do him the justice of bringing up the problem for discussion if it persists.

7. If you are a smoker, do your utmost to give it up! (Much more on this in Chapter 8.)

6

How Do I Know
I Have COPD?

The three most common chronic obstructive pulmonary diseases—emphysema, chronic bronchitis, and asthma—all present a confusingly similar symptom picture. Dyspnea, difficulty in moving air through the airways, chest tightness, and wheezing are common with all three. Coughing is a basic symptom of chronic bronchitis, and frequent with the other two. The airway hyperreactivity of asthma often appears when chronic bronchitis temporarily worsens.

These similarities muddied the diagnostic waters for a very long time. Back in 1794, the distinguished 18th-century Edinburgh physician William Cullen complained that: "The term asthma has been commonly applied . . . , even by many . . . [specialists], to every case of difficult breathing. . . . By not distinguishing it with sufficient accuracy from other cases of Dyspnea, they have introduced a great deal of confusion into their treatises on this subject." The road leading to accurate diagnosis of the COPD entities opened up when the French physician Laennec developed the stethoscope early in the nineteenth century.

The principles of treatment for each COPD entity are also very similar. Therapy is aimed primarily at decreasing or reversing the airflow obstruction created by abundant mucus secretion, and/or hyperinflation, and/or airway muscle contraction, and/or other inflammatory processes.

If the goal of therapy is the same regardless of the diagnosis, then why is there any real need to distinguish between these three respiratory diseases? Because current and future plans for coping with the disease's overall impact on your life are very different depending on which disease you have. This will become very apparent in the chapters concerning the various aspects of treatment and their effects.

How does a physician distinguish between these diseases? Evaluation follows a logical, orderly course that combines an accurate patient history, physical findings, and objective measurements from lung function tests and other laboratory studies. We learn if significant airway obstruction exists, how severe it is, and whether it is primarily in the smaller airways or more widespread. We find out if the impact is substantial in both phases of the breathing cycle, or primarily in expiration. We see to what degree basic respiratory function—by which we mean supplying the blood with adequate oxygen and sufficiently removing excess carbon dioxide—has been harmed. We also learn whether or not the respiratory pathology has affected the heart's health. We also can identify some helpful treatment measures.

History Taking

The history's overall purpose is to establish the nature and time frame of your current symptoms. Most physicians also find that taking a careful medical history is an invaluable diagnostic aid and helps evaluate your disease's severity and its impact on your life. And just from talking, information about factors that aggravate your symptoms may well come to light. A clear understanding of symptoms can also disclose a disability or discomfort that may require rehabilitation therapy. Finally, the conversational give-and-take of the history-taking process provides an excellent opportunity for you and your physician to establish a mutually trusting relationship.

There are five traditional categories of questions that your doctor asks. They concern: social history, family history, past medical history, present complaints, and a review of the different organ systems (neurological, digestive, etc.). Each category begins with general questions and proceeds to more specific ones. *Above all, be honest in your answers.* (You won't help yourself by hiding, for example, the recreational use of drugs.) When all questions have been asked, if you think that your doctor has missed possibly important information it is your responsibility to tell him. (Before your appointment, you might consider writing down everything that you see as relevant to your symptoms.)

General Questions

First, your doctor will ask you about your past. Did you have asthma as a child? Have you had pneumonia several times? Do you have recurrent sinusitis? The doctor will also want to know your smoking history: do/did you, how much, and for how long. There will be questions about your occupation and whether it might be exposing you to respiratory irritants. Your doctor will also inquire about your family's relevant history. Do/did any family members have emphysema, asthma, or chronic bronchitis, or a vulnerability to sinusitis or pneumonia?

Specific Questions

If answers to his general questions suggest COPD, your doctor's remaining questions will help clarify his understanding of where you stand in relation to the three major symptoms of respiratory disease: cough, sputum production, and dyspnea.

Although a persistent *cough* is the most easily noticeable of these symptoms, it is usually people other than patients who are aware of it. Patients themselves often deny anything unusual, chalking it up to "smoker's cough" or "a lingering cold," and so haven't thought much about it. Yet any persistent cough indicates something abnormal, and its characteristics can help characterize the disease causing it.

A long-term "productive" cough—one that regularly brings up mucus—is the primary early symptom of chronic bronchitis. In fact, one of the criteria defining chronic bronchitis is the presence of a productive morning cough for three consecutive months of the year, two years in a row.

The typical chronic bronchitic's cough is a paroxysm. The uncontrollable response is caused by anything (laughter, exercise, excitement, etc.) that makes him breathe more deeply. Some patients even faint during particularly violent coughing fits. The cough is often worse in the morning because mucus accumulates in the airways during sleep (although these patients are rarely awakened at night by coughing). When the patient coughs, people in earshot often hear prodigious amounts of mucus rumbling in his airways. Yet these coughing fits do not always bring much up. Patients typically complain that their cough does a poor job of clearing congestion.

Regular coughing—especially a productive cough—is not a hallmark of the patient suffering primarily from emphysema. Some of these patients do cough regularly, some just occasionally, and some cough only if their condition worsens substantially—and when a cough exists, it is usually a dry one.

Noticeable *mucus production* is also abnormal. Healthy people produce no more than two teaspoons worth of sputum each day, and swallow most of it unawares. Patients with chronic bronchitis predominating produce substantially more, although the amount varies with the patient: a large soup spoon of mucus at the small end of the continuum, with a cupful at the other.

Equally important to diagnosis are how your mucus looks and feels. Is it thin and watery ("serous") and therefore easy to bring up, or is it thick and slippery ("mucoid")? Patients with especially thick mucus may need special treatment to help them clear their airways. Is it clear (which is normal), or shaded white to gray from particulate matter, for example, dust or air pollution residues? Mucus that is yellow or green reflects an inflammation of some sort—most likely a respiratory infection or an allergic response. A putrid odor—which indicates infection—is another diagnostic aid. In addition, your doctor will ask if your mucus has recently changed color. Any recent appearance of blood in your sputum should also be mentioned. This usually indicates either an infection or particularly violent coughing fits. But it can also be a symptom of more serious lung diseases.

Dyspnea is the uncomfortable, sometimes frightening, sensation that "I am not getting enough air to breathe." This highly subjective experience cannot be measured, and exactly what causes it remains a mystery. Neurological, muscular, biochemical, and physical processes all combine to control our breathing. How each of these factors does—or doesn't—contribute to creating the sense of breathlessness is still unsolved. We do know that the symptom of dyspnea is not limited to respiratory diseases. So for each patient complaining of dyspnea, the physician needs to determine whether the cause is respiratory or nonrespiratory.

Although dyspnea may be an important symptom even in the early phases of emphysema, the patient usually remains unaware of it for quite some time. Its onset is insidious, progressing slowly and ever so gradually, happening with less and less—the decreases almost unnoticeable—exertion. When chronic bronchitis is the primary disease, shortness of breath is usually not a problem until the disease is in its advanced stages. Then it becomes severe.

The Physical Examination

When the question-and-answer period is over, your doctor will examine you. First he listens to your chest with his stethoscope to hear how air passes in and out of your lungs. With healthy lungs, he hears a soft, low rushing sound. With obstructed airways, the sound the air makes depends on the nature of the obstruction.

Airway obstruction—present in chronic bronchitis—produces wheezing, the sound of turbulence caused as air is forced around mucus and through narrowed airways. Although for a long time wheezing was thought to happen only during expiration, recent evidence indicates that it occurs during inspiration too. Wheezes differ in tone and loudness depending on when they are listened to (during inspiration or expiration, during a temporary worsening or not), and exactly where in the lungs. A *rale* (pronounced *rahl*) is another abnormal sound heard in COPD patients. This is the noise air makes as it bubbles through accumulated mucus. In patients with advanced emphysema, the large number of grossly hyperinflated air sacs filled with trapped air make all breath sounds faint and distant. But the most severe cases of COPD often produce no breath sounds at all. The obstruction is so great that air cannot be pushed through the airways with enough force to produce the amount of turbulence needed to make a detectable sound.

We know what the different sounds mean. The problem is agreeing on what to call them. Laennec was, understandably, the first to describe abnormal breath sounds. But his clarity has been lost. In his initial treatise, Laennec called all abnormal lung sounds *rales* from the French word for *rattle*, and qualified each rale with the proper adjective (e.g., *gurgling rales* were due to air passing through fluids). But the popular association of *rattle* with "death rattle" led Laennec to abandon it for *rhonchi* (from the Greek work for "snore"). Things got scrambled when Laennec's work was translated into English. *Rales* and *rhonchi* were suddenly used to describe different types of sounds.

Three broad categories of breathing sounds, each with subtypes, soon developed in the United States: (1) *rales* (*crepitations* and *crackles*), describing delicate sounds from the smaller airways; (2) *rhonchi*, the coarser gurgling sounds of air passing through mucus in the larger airways; and (3) *wheezes*, the continuous musical sounds associated with air passing through narrowed, obstructed airways. Recently, both the American Thoracic Society and the American College of Chest Physicians suggested a different categorization system: *crackles* for discontinuous sounds, and *wheezes* for high-pitched musical sounds.

What else will you doctor look for when he examines you? He will observe the way you breathe, the muscles you use, the shape of your chest, and your sitting posture to get a sense of how severely your breathing is obstructed.

The patient with more severe obstruction gives the appearance of intense inspiratory activity, forcefully inspiring and then expiring slowly against pursed lips. Because his seriously hyperinflated lungs have pushed out his ribcage and flattened the diaphragm sitting beneath them, he is barrel-chested and his neck muscles bulge. (Because the patient's flattened diaphragm—along with shortened inspiratory intercostal muscles—don't provide adequate inspiratory power, he now regularly uses his accessory inspiratory muscles, located in his neck, which has overdeveloped them.)

The patient sits forward in a chair with his arms or hands braced against his knees or the table in front of him (look back at Figure 3.1), a position that naturally makes these muscles more effective.

The physical examination can also indicate the general adequacy of gas exchange. In chronic bronchitis, the patient with bluish lips and fingernail beds (a condition called *cyanosis*) does not have enough oxygen in his blood. If there is also excess carbon dioxide retention, the veins become visibly engorged.

Heart function in the earlier stages of COPD is normal. But in more advanced cases, especially where chronic bronchitis predominates, cardiac complications are frequent. The observable physical signs are: extensive cyanosis; swollen ankles (called *peripheral edema*); engorged jugular vein (the large blood vessel in the neck); enlarged liver.

So you have abnormal breath sounds and you use your inspiratory muscles excessively. Perhaps you also cough up a lot of mucus, or your lips are tinged with blue, or you have become barrel-chested. All of this clearly confirms that your problem involves obstructed airways. The physical examination's purpose—substantiating the existence of airway obstruction suggested by your history—has been fulfilled.

At this point, an array of objective tests will help your doctor decide which of the three obstructive respiratory diseases—chronic bronchitis, emphysema, or asthma—is your problem and how severe it is, and provide some idea of your prognosis. (Deciding which of the different possibilities is the actual problem is the "differential diagnosis.")

Laboratory Studies

Pulmonary Function Tests

There are three basic types of pulmonary function tests. Lung volume measurements—done quietly—measure the volume of air in your lungs at different points during breathing. Ventilation measurements—done under relatively dynamic conditions—are concerned with the air flowing into and out of your lungs. Gas exchange measurements determine how the alveoli are functioning. (Although there are many more tests than the ones described below, we discuss only those that have proved over time to be the most informative.)

Most of these pulmonary function tests provide more detailed evidence for the presence or absence of airway obstruction, and document the severity if obstruction exists. One of these pulmonary function tests also provides definitive diagnostic information for asthma. Asthma is confirmed if this test shows dramatic reversibility of airway obstruction when bronchodilator medication is used. If test results exclude asthma, then the finger points to emphysema and/or chronic bronchitis. And if bronchodilator medication improves airflow to some small degree, then we know that a small component of that patient's airway obstruction is reversible.

Your performance on each of these tests will be compared to the *predicted values* appropriate for you. These are average measurements form large groups of healthy people. Each group combines people of the same race, sex, age, and height. Your measurements will most likely be considered normal if they fall within the range from 80 to 120% of the average for your particular group. But predicted values are guidelines, not rigid judgments, and final interpretation of the pulmonary function tests is undertaken in the context of information gained from your history, physical exam, and chest X-ray.

Lung Volume Measurements   Figure 6.1 illustrates the different portions of the total lung volume usually measured during a pulmonary function test and how they are traced by the spirometer (the test instrument). In all these tests you breathe through a mouthpiece—much like those on snorkels and scuba tanks—attached to the spirometer. You wear a nose clip to make sure that all the air moving in and out of your lungs goes through your mouth.

You will be asked to breathe quietly for a few breaths, and then be told to squeeze as much air out of your lungs as you possibly can. The amount of additional air squeezed out after quiet expiration would have ended is your *expiratory reserve volume.* After this maximum expiration, you will be asked to fill your lungs slowly with as much air as they can hold, and then again squeeze out as much as you can. The amount of air breathed out in going from you maximum inspiration to your maximum expiration is your *vital capacity.* Next you will be told to take another maximum inspiration, then just breathe out quietly. The amount of air breathed out as you go from your maximum inspiration to the end of a quiet expiration is your *inspiratory capacity.*

Some air always remains in the lungs after even a maximum expiration, an amount called the *residual volume.* Since it can never be breathed out, this residual amount—and therefore the two lung volumes that include it in their total—must be determined indirectly with the spirometer. These other two volumes are the *functional residual capacity* (the amount of air remaining in the lungs at the end of a quiet expiration, that is, the residual volume + the expiratory reserve volume), and the *total lung*

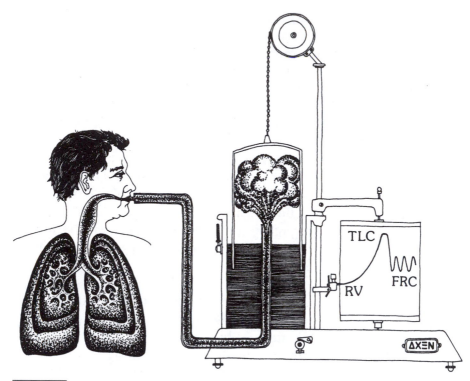

Figure 6.1 Evaluation of lung function using classical spirometry. The upper-most point on the chart is *total lung capacity* (TLC), the lowest is *residual volume* (RV), and the difference between the two is the *vital capacity* (VC). When normal expiration ends, the remaining volume is the *functional residual capacity* (FRC). The repeating small breaths on the right of the tracing are the *tidal volume.*

capacity (the total amount of air contained in the lungs after a maximum inspiration—that is, summing all of the individual volumes).

With one indirect technique, you breathe in a specific amount of helium gas and its concentration in your lungs is measured. Then the amount of air that has to be in your lungs to produce that concentration can be calculated. The other indirect technique measures the amount of oxygen that it takes to wash all of the nitrogen gas out of your lungs. (The air we breathe contains about 80% nitrogen.) For either method, all that you must do is breathe quietly until the recording equipment indicates either that (1) the helium being breathed in is not being diluted any further, or (2) all of your lungs' nitrogen has been expelled.

These static lung volumes document the presence and severity of air-way obstruction rather than identifying its cause. When the airways are obstructed, all of the volumes measured directly (expiratory reserve volume, inspiratory capacity, vital capacity) tend to be smaller than normal. How much smaller is usually related to the severity of the obstruction. The volumes that must be determined indirectly (residual volume, functional residual capacity, total lung capacity) are larger than normal. All of these changes occur because of hyperinflation and air trapping, as we described in Chapters 2 and 3.

Ventilation Measurements These dynamic pulmonary function tests measure two things. One is the *resistance* that inspired and expired air meet in your airways. (Remember that airway obstruction increases resistance.) The other is *airflow*—the amount of air entering or leaving your lungs in a particular time period—which is partially determined by resistance.

Resistance must be measured in a plethysmograph (which can also be used for the indirect determination of residual volume, functional residual capacity, and total lung capacity). The plethysmograph is a five-foot-high box, two and one-half feet in both width and depth, with one or more clear sides (see Figure 6.2). You sit inside this box, wearing a nose

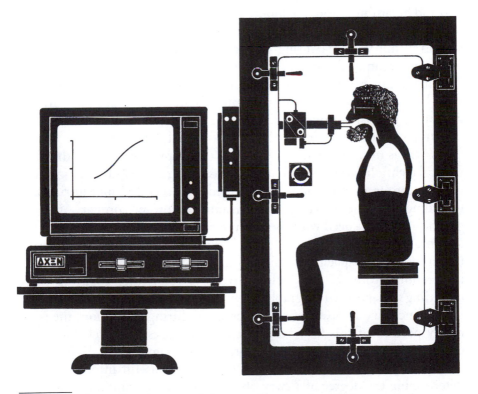

Figure 6.2 Lung function test of airway resistance using plethysmography.

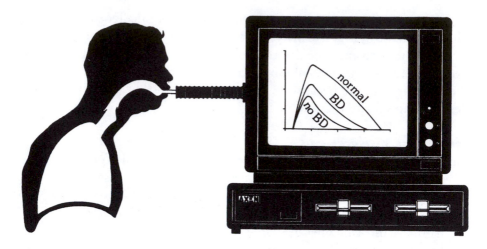

Figure 6.3   Lung function test of expiratory airflow using flow-volume curves. *Bottom curve:* Typical of COPD. *Middle curve:* Obstruction somewhat reversed by bronchodilator. *Top curve:* Normal pattern included for comparison.

clip and breathing through a mouthpiece. The basic maneuver is repeated several times. First you breathe quietly, then pant gently about once per second. While you are panting, a shutter will close off the mouthpiece for just a few seconds. As soon as it reopens, you breathe quietly again. The information gained from this test is the speed with which air flows out of your lungs and the effort your respiratory system is making (its "driving pressure") to push air out at this speed. Then airway resistance and various lung volumes are calculated from this initial data.

Airflow is measured with a technique that is probably one of the most fruitful technological developments for assessing airway obstruction. You breathe through a mouthpiece connected to specialized monitoring and recording equipment that gives an instant-by-instant comparison (on a graph) of airflow speed with the volume of air already in the lungs at that instant. This is recorded on the graph during one maximum expiration (from total lung capacity to residual volume) followed by one maximum inspiration (from residual volume back to total lung capacity). The recording's shape on the graph is curved, and is called a *flow-volume curve.* Since airway obstruction is magnified during expiration, the expiratory portion of this flow-volume curve produces a very characteristic picture when airway obstruction is present (see Figure 6.3).

The flow-volume curve contains particularly useful information for determining the degree of airway obstruction: (1) the amount of air that can be pushed out of the lungs in one second (called *FEV$_1$* for "forced expiratory volume in one second"); (2) the highest airflow rate achieved during this one second (called *PEFR* for "peak expiratory flow rate"); and either (3) the average airflow for the middle 50% of the expiratory curve (called $FEF_{25-75\%}$ for "forced expiratory flow for the mid-50%"); or (4) the airflow occurring when exactly one-half of the vital capacity has been expired (called V_{50} for "expiratory airflow at 50% of vital capacity." When the airways are obstructed, these airflow measurements usually decrease.

Assessing the Reversibility of Obstruction Traditionally, the airway obstruction produced in COPD was considered irreversible. Happily, current wisdom finds that it is actually partially reversible in many COPD patients. To see if you fall into this category and, if you do, to determine the degree of reversibility, two sets of pulmonary function tests will be done, one right after the other. Between the two sets, you will be given a spray bronchodilator medication (and instructed how to use it). If your second set of tests shows significantly improved airflow, your airway obstruction can be improved by this medication.

Failure to respond to the bronchodilator on the first try does not automatically mean that this medication cannot improve your airflow. A retest should be done, because there are several possible reasons for an initial failure to respond. What are these reasons? Unfamiliarity with the proper technique for taking a bronchodilator often prevents enough of the drug from reaching the airways where it is needed. Or, if the primary area of obstruction is in the smaller airways, it can't be reached by an inhaled bronchodilator. Finally, a bronchodilator cannot counteract obstruction caused by mucus plugging, inflammation, or structural changes in the airways.

The only problem with the pulmonary function retest after using the bronchodilator concerns the lack of firm guidelines for establishing whether or not adequate airflow improvement has indeed occurred. Various tentative recommendations are all that currently exist, with most physicians using their own personal criteria. The following recommended criteria for true bronchodilation seem logical to us: post-bronchodilator measurements should be greater than the initial measurements by: 15% in FEV_1, 20% in $FEF_{25-75\%}$, and/or 10% in vital capacity even without any improvement in airflow rates.

Gas Exchange Measurements The ventilation tests tell your doctor to what degree your airways are obstructed and roughly how much of your lung tissue is lost or nonfunctioning. But they do not tell him how well your remaining functional lung tissue is doing at getting oxygen into the blood and carbon dioxide out of it.

To evaluate your lungs' ability to achieve adequate gas exchange, one thing your doctor needs to know is how much oxygen passes into your blood in a specific amount of time. The doctor learns this from a *diffusion test*. He may also want to know exactly how much oxygen and carbon dioxide are in your arterial blood (the blood flowing from your lungs into your heart). This information comes from a *blood gas analysis* (described in the section on Blood Tests later in this chapter).

Measuring the actual transfer of oxygen from your lungs to your blood is difficult. This *diffusion test* would require sampling blood directly from your heart. Happily, there is a much easier way of gaining this information. We dilute a tiny amount of carbon monoxide in the air you breathe. You hold one large breath of this air for ten seconds before breathing out. Comparing the amounts of carbon monoxide in the air you breathed in and the air you breathe out after ten seconds tells us the degree of pressure in your air sacs that is pushing oxygen into your bloodstream.

Chest X-Ray

A chest X-ray provides two kinds of information, depending on whether it is taken in the absence of complications, or during one. Without active complications, it shows only the changes caused by chronic chest hyper-inflation which can occur in all forms of COPD. The normally dome-shaped diaphragm is quite flattened. Some experts find a flattened diaphragm so universal in their emphysema patients that they consider its presence to be unquestionable diagnostic proof. Because emphysema is the one form of COPD involving actual tissue destruction very early on, the X-ray of a patient with emphysematous changes is also highly translucent and the lungs' blood vessels are no longer clearly visible.

When a respiratory complication exists, an X-ray can confirm its nature: pneumonia; local areas of airless lung tissue (called *atelectasis*) due to mucus plugging; the accumulation of air between layers of the thin sheath of tissue covering the lungs (a condition called *bleb*); the collapse of large tissue areas from air seeping in between the lungs and chest wall (called *pneumothorax*); the presence of large air-containing spaces (termed *bullae*) resulting from emphysema's destruction, enlargement, and merging of air sacs.

The X-ray can also show cardiac involvement in the disease process. The heart silhouette is enlarged in chronic bronchitis and in severely advanced emphysema.

Blood Tests

For a patient with pulmonary disease, there are three relevant blood tests: a routine blood analysis, a blood gas analysis, and analysis of alpha$_1$-antitrypsin levels.

The *routine blood analysis* is a screening device designed to assess your general health. It also identifies any as-yet-unidentified disease(s) that could complicate treatment of your respiratory disease. If diabetes is also present, for example, certain airway-relaxing medications must be used with extreme caution.

Blood gas analysis is essential for assessing both the severity of lung disease and effectiveness of the treatment prescribed for it. Arterial blood is required (most other analyses use venous blood.) There are two techniques for obtaining this kind of blood. The first (and most widely used) involves inserting a needle in the easily visible artery on the inside of your wrist. Blood is drawn into sterile tubing attached to the needle. This procedure can be painful even though a small amount of anesthetic is routinely used. The second technique temporarily increases the amount of blood flowing to your fingertip, then samples it. Your hand is dipped in very warm water until the blood vessels are dilated. Then a sterile instrument is used to make a tiny wound about one quarter-inch wide, so that blood can be drawn up into slender glass tubes for analysis.

With either technique, the blood is analyzed for both oxygen and carbon dioxide content. This content is expressed in *mmHg,* a pressure measurement, because gases act in accord to the pressure they exert. (mmHg stands for "millimeters of mercury." Normal atmospheric pressure at sea level is about 760 mmHg. One mmHg equals the pressure exerted by 1/760th atmosphere.) Blood gases can help distinguish between chronic bronchitis or emphysema as the predominant obstructive disease. Both diseases decrease the amount of oxygen the blood carries. Carbon dioxide rises in even moderate chronic bronchitis. In emphysema, though, it remains normal until the disease is severely advanced.

In Chapters 3 and 4, we mentioned a small number of emphysema patients who differ from the stereotype. They are younger than 50, and are not necessarily smokers. Their emphysema is associated with insufficient alpha$_1$-antitrypsin, the enzyme that prevents an oversupply of elastase, the enzyme that normally prevents the lungs' elastic tissue from proliferating. There is now a *blood test that measures the amount of alpha$_1$-antitrypsin.* Normal is approximately 150 mg of enzyme for each 100 ml of blood serum. Patients with this kind of emphysema have less than 60 mg/100 ml of serum. This test is suggested for people whose emphysema symptoms have appeared at a young age, or with a strong family history of emphysema, or with a family member with a proven enzyme deficiency.

Although there is no present cure for this deficiency (several possibilities are being tested), there are still important reasons for knowing if one has it. One is its relevance in genetic counseling. The other is that one can take cautionary measures, either eliminating—or not assuming—those factors (such as smoking) that would greatly increase the likelihood of this deficiency leading to emphysema.

Electrocardiogram

Since many patients with a chronic pulmonary disability are prone to developing cardiac disease (*cor pulmonale*), it is essential to know the cardiac condition of any COPD patient planning to undertake a reconditioning program as part of treatment. (Ideally, this should be all but terminal patients.) This permits patients with an irregular heartbeat and/or signs that their heart is underoxygenated to receive careful cardiac monitoring during their exercise periods, ensuring that this exercise never stresses the heart.

Sputum Analysis

Examining sputum to aid in diagnosis began in classical times with the physicians of Greece and Rome. Galen (A.D. 130–201), the foremost Roman physician during the reign of Marcus Aurelius, described using sputum analysis specifically to diagnose respiratory diseases. Sputum analysis is still an important aid in evaluating patients.

Because abnormal airway secretions tend to collect during sleep, the best time to take a coughed-up sputum specimen is shortly after waking. The ideal preparation is first rinsing your mouth and gargling with an antiseptic to prevent bacteria in your throat and mouth from contaminating your airway secretions. Because mucus cells disintegrate quickly, the specimen should be brought to your doctor—or the laboratory he uses—promptly for examination.

The examination will include sputum color and consistency. In stable bronchitis, mucus is translucent (clear), thick, and sticky. During a respiratory infection, the mucus increases greatly in quantity and becomes opaque and yellow. When color indicates an infection, the bacteria will be cultured and identified so the most effective antibiotic can be prescribed.

Other Tests

Two other tests are sometimes used to assess a COPD patient's condition. One is an exercise test. The other—as far from exercise as you can get—is a sleep study. Let's look at each one in some detail.

Exercise Test   This is commonly called a "stress test." But don't let the name frighten you! A stress test is not designed to overwork or exhaust you, but simply to determine the level of physical activity you can comfortably—and safely—carry out, and how long you can comfortably—and safely—do it. We prefer calling it an "exercise test."

Normally, a person's heart limits the amount of strenuous work he can do and the exercise test identifies this heart-determined limit. COPD has changed that. These patients are limited by their respiratory system. Here, the exercise test is used to identify this limit, and see how it may be safely extended.

First, the exercise test shows us how debilitated new patients are. We can measure exactly how hard they are breathing and how hard their hearts are working at the point they become uncomfortably short of breath. By comparing this with their pulmonary function test results, we know how much of their dyspnea is due to inalterable respiratory limitation, and how much to simply being out of shape. Then we can plan an appropriate reconditioning program (which we discuss in detail in Chapter 13). During this reconditioning program, a repeat exercise test every so often tells us—and the patient—how well he is doing.

We can also see if a patient who has normal blood gases (that is, adequate oxygen and carbon dioxide levels) at rest becomes underoxygenated during exercise. These patients, and those whose oxygen level is always low, return for a second exercise test. Then we see if breathing supplemental oxygen during this test extends their exercise time. (Research shows that oxygen can improve exercise performance and lengthen lifespan in COPD patients with low oxygen in their blood.) If it does, then we know that supplemental oxygen is important in this patient's treatment program.

The test itself is usually done on a treadmill or a bicycle ergometer (Figure 6.4). If you undergo an exercise test, both your heart rate and oxygen saturation (how much of your blood actually contains oxygen, compared to how much should be carrying oxygen) are continuously measured.

Polysomnography   A sleep test (called *polysomnography*) determines whether a patient needs supplemental oxygen at night. Oxygen in arterial

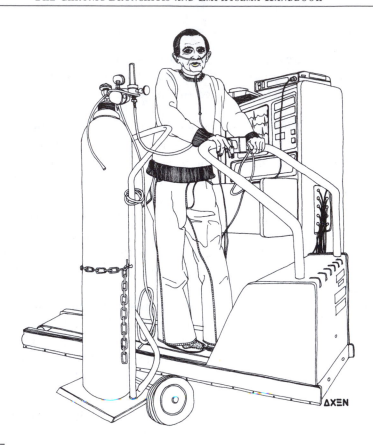

Figure 6.4   The typical stress-testing apparatus combines a treadmill and an electrocardiogram monitor. The patient walks at prescribed speeds and treadmill tilts. Stress tests can even be done with patients who need supplemental oxygen—as shown in the illustration.

blood can drop during sleep. It happens in some presumably healthy people—and it eventually happens in everyone with COPD.

There are two reasons. The greatest drop occurs during sleep's dream stage (called *REM sleep*, for the rapid eye movements that occur during dreams). Intercostal muscle activity normally decreases during this time, and the COPD patient's ineffective diaphragm can't, working alone, maintain adequate ventilation. Another cause is the greater accumulation of airway secretions during sleep because coughing is infrequent then. (Patients who are voluminous mucus producers are particularly vulnerable to small airway obstruction during sleep.) Both these mechanisms decrease sleep oxygenation indirectly as well, because they result in a mismatch of ventilation and blood flow in the air sacs.

The Formal Diagnosis

Arriving at the formal diagnosis of COPD takes all the above kinds of information into account to determine (1) the predominant nature of the patient's airway obstruction, that is, is it primarily chronic bronchitis or emphysema, and (2) its severity, for example, is the obstruction somewhat reversible, and is the heart already involved. Some patients, though, do not fall into a neat category. Then physicians must add the fruits of their experience and intuition to complete the picture.

7

COPD and . . .

When other diseases coexist with COPD, treatment for both becomes much more complex. It is essential that all the doctors treating such a patient be especially knowledgeable about how the drugs that help pulmonary obstruction affect the other disease(s), and how medication used to treat the other condition(s) affect(s) COPD. And each specialist treating the patient *must know exactly which drugs the others have prescribed.*

When more than one chronic condition requires treatment, the rule of thumb is that the most threatening one receives priority in terms of medication chosen. Beyond this, the drugs selected to control the other problem(s) must not aggravate this most critical one. Fortunately, most drugs available for COPD patients offer a variety of safe and effective solutions for the pharmacologic treatment of these complex situations.

We repeat that it is not our intention to dictate the "right" drug combinations, but rather to explain the basic principles that knowledgeable physicians use when they make such treatment decisions.

We can't discuss all complicating conditions that may significantly affect COPD, or this single chapter would become an encyclopedia. We decided to focus on the three most common complicating conditions: cardiovascular disease, diabetes, and surgical procedures. Even if your complicating condition lies elsewhere, this chapter still holds value for you. You will gain an understanding of the kind of knowledge your doctor (or doctors) must have, and the kinds of issues you should be discussing.

Cardiovascular Disease

Because smoking is a risk factor for both COPD and cardiovascular disease, it is no surprise that 50% of COPD patients over 50 suffer from *cardiovascular disease* as well. The term *cardiovascular disease* actually refers to several different problems involving the heart and circulatory system.

□ In *congestive heart failure*, the heart—which is a highly specialized muscle—has become too weak to pump blood adequately. Although both sides of the heart are vulnerable to failure (separately or together), with COPD patients—primarily those with chronic bronchitis predominating—it's usually the right side that fails. This is the side that pumps unoxygenated venous blood through the lungs to gather oxygen and discard carbon dioxide. We call this right side failure *cor pulmonale* (see Chapter 3).

□ In *ischemic heart disease* (also called *coronary insufficiency*), the arteries providing oxygen-rich blood to this specialized muscle have become so narrowed by fatty deposits (called "plaque") that the heart cannot get as much oxygen as it needs. *Arteriosclerosis* and *atherosclerosis* are common terms for this condition. The chest pain that this inadequate oxygen can cause is called *angina pectoris*, or simply *angina*.

□ *Hypertension* is high blood pressure, which refers to the force with which blood pushes through the arteries as it is pumped through the circulatory system. Several different problems can cause hypertension, and sometimes the cause cannot be identified.

□ *Cardiac arrhythmia* concerns malfunction of the heart's electrical activity, with disruption of the electrical signal that coordinates and paces its pumping action. This can make the pumping action of the heart less effective.

When COPD coexists with one of the cardiovascular diseases, COPD therapy must be cautiously administered to meet two additional goals beyond providing effective symptom relief. Most important is that the medication must not aggravate the heart condition. This means avoiding COPD medications that would make the heart work harder or disturb its electrical activity. The second is choosing drugs, when possible, with a direct or side effect that actually helps the heart. An example follows.

A COPD patient with chronic congestive heart failure suddenly becomes wheezy and much shorter of breath than usual. The medication problem is that both symptoms can result from either of these diseases. So before prescribing treatment, the patient's doctor first must determine whether his COPD or his heart failure is the cause. Sometimes the only recourse is trial and error. He might temporarily prescribe a diuretic, which—because it removes water from the body—reduces the heart's work. If the wheezing and dyspnea immediately improve, the patient's heart problem was probably causing them. In this case, a theophylline preparation would be appropriate. In addition to its main effect of bronchodilation, its side effects include diuretic action (making the body get rid of fluid) and making the heart beat more strongly.

How Cardiovascular Drugs Affect COPD

Negative Effects   One treatment of choice for cardiovascular disease is a *beta-adrenergic blocking agent* (for example, *propranolol, nadolol*). Although drugs that block the beta-1 receptors in the heart are good for cardiac problems, they can affect the airways adversely. This is particularly true for those that also block airway beta-2 receptors. Ideally, beta-blockers should not be given to COPD patients because they can constrict the airways. But if they must be used, then it should be one of those more selective for beta-1 receptors (for example, *metorpolol, atenolol*).

Drugs that mimic the effect of *acetylcholine*—the mediator causing bronchoconstriction when the vagus nerve is stimulated—are sometimes given to stop the heart from racing. The problem in COPD is that these drugs sometimes cause bronchospasms. But drugs with the opposite (that is, anticholinergic) effects, such as *disopyramide*—which are given to prevent arrhythmias—can cause bronchial secretions to dry and accumulate. They are best avoided as well.

Positive Effects   Some drugs used to treat cardiovascular disease can also be used to treat COPD, because they cause bronchodilation. *Calcium channel blockers*, which effectively prevent bronchospasm, also help both angina pectoris and high blood pressure.

Nitrates (for example, *nitroglycerin*), which are potent blood vessel dilators, are also used to alleviate angina pain. Although the nitroglycerin doses used in angina do not cause bronchodilation, at least we know that this drug cannot worsen COPD.

How COPD Affects the Heart

COPD stresses the cardiovascular system in several ways, increasing the heart's workload. One stress is increased heart rate, a response to two different situations: the intense anxiety often accompanying COPD, plus limits on the amount of oxygen the lungs can supply. And with severe chronic bronchitis, the heart's right side eventually weakens from contracting too hard for too long to pump blood through the lungs' constricted blood vessels.

COPD is also associated with more frequent *premature ventricular contractions*, often called *PVCs*, meaning that the heart's ventricles—the two large chambers that propel blood to the lungs and to the rest of the body—are contracting out of their normal sequence. In fact, severe COPD with hypoxia often changes the heart's normal electrical pattern even in people with no signs of heart disease.

These cardiovascular stresses can become proportionately more dangerous when the heart's oxygen supply has been reduced by a combination of COPD and ischemic heart disease. It can be hazardous, therefore, to withhold bronchodilator medication, or to use ineffective doses, through the misplaced fear of harmful cardiac side effects.

How COPD Medications Affect the Heart

Beta-receptor Stimulators   Because early bronchodilators—such as *epinephrine* and *ephedrine*—nonselectively stimulate both alpha- and beta-receptors, they constrict blood vessels. This in turn increases blood pressure, heart rate, and the force of the heart's contractions. Because of this substantial increase in the heart's workload, these drugs are contraindicated—meaning "should not be used"—for patients with any kind of cardiovascular problem.

A better choice would be one of the newer beta-2 selective bronchodilators: *terbutaline, salbutamol (albuterol), fenoterol,* and *metaproterenol.* Not only do they add little to the heart's workload, but their vasodilatation side effect lowers blood pressure. This makes them a particularly effective and appropriate choice for the COPD patient with high blood pressure.

Theophyllines   Theophylline and its derivatives are well known both for their potent cardiovascular and central nervous system side effects, and for their narrow therapeutic range (there is little ground between the minimally effective and toxic levels). Both of these characteristics require particular caution if a theophylline preparation must be used to treat a COPD patient who has a cardiovascular problem.

Considerable care must be taken to ensure the lowest dose that is still effective for treatment so that cardiovascular side effects are avoided as much as possible. And because some heart conditions—such as congestive heart failure—can dramatically slow the rate at which theophylline is removed, blood theophylline levels must be monitored even more frequently than usual in these patients. Toxic levels of theophylline are associated with—among other things—rapid heart rate and arrhythmias.

Anticholinergic Agents   Western physicians have used anticholinergic drugs (*atropine* is the most well known) to treat asthma for about 200 years. Recent advances in understanding the effects of acetylcholine on the respiratory system have indicated that anticholinergic drugs can also help COPD patients. This is to the immense benefit of those who also suffer from cardiovascular problems.

The reason? *Ipratropium bromide*—an *atropine-like* drug—is a relatively specific bronchodilator. And it is remarkably free of side effects because it is poorly absorbed across the airways. Beyond this, combining ipratropium bromide along with a beta-2 agonist or theophylline some-times permits reducing the other drug's dosage.

Steroids   Steroids, as we note in Chapter 10, can be important in treat-ing some COPD patients. There is an unavoidable side effect, however, that is potentially dangerous in the presence of cardiovascular disease. Steroids increase the amount of salt retained in the body, causing water retention, which then raises blood pressure and increases the heart's work-load. Of the oral steroids, *methylprednisolone* causes the least salt reten-tion. Still, blood pressure must be regularly monitored, with careful adjustment of both diuretic and blood pressure-reducing medications.

For some patients, an aerosolized bronchodilator plus a steroid can be a reasonable alternative to a theophylline-plus-beta-stimulator combina-tion, as long as blood pressure increases can be prevented.

Summary

When a patient has both COPD and a complicating cardiovascular prob-lem, ipratropium bromide is a helpful bronchodilator and has no negative cardiovascular side effects. It can be augmented by an inhaled beta-2 selective drug such as salbutomol. For the COPD patient whose cardiac problem—such as high blood pressure—does not involve arrhythmias, theophylline can be added to the menu. If theophylline is contraindi-cated, but the other nonsteroid medications cannot open the airways ade-quately, then an oral steroid should be considered. In this case, special monitoring and therapeutic attention must be given to water retention and resulting blood pressure changes.

Regarding cardiac medication, beta-blockers should belong to the beta-1 selective group (*metorpolol, atenolol*) to avoid constricting the air-ways. Or a calcium blocker can be used. Avoid both cholinergic and anti-cholinergic drugs.

Diabetes

When a COPD patient has diabetes as well, the doctor must consider two essential issues when choosing an appropriate bronchodilator medicine. For all such patients, the doctor must know which drugs affect the body's release of stored sugar and its metabolism of sugar in general. For diabet-ics whose disease has affected their autonomic nervous system, the doctor must know what the implications of this are for COPD, and which COPD drugs may worsen this impairment.

Also, diabetics are much more susceptible to all sorts of infections.

The diabetic chronic bronchitic in particular—because his lungs become a fertile breeding ground for infections—needs aggressive surveillance by clinical exam, laboratory tests, and X-rays. Intervention should begin immediately when a beginning infection is indicated.

How COPD Drugs Can Affect Sugar Metabolism

Creating a *glucose* (sugar) imbalance in the diabetic COPD patient is a particular worry when *steroids* must be used to treat the COPD. Glucose is the body's primary energy source. The presence of insulin allows cells to take in the glucose they need. Then the cells use oxygen to burn—or "metabolize"—this sugar to produce their energy. Since the diabetic does not produce the amount of insulin needed to allow his cells to take in enough glucose, he must take supplemental insulin (or a related drug).

One effect of *gluco*corticoids—the group of steroids given COPD patients—is to increase the amount of glucose in the blood while also disrupting the cells' ability to take in sugar. In addition, steroids promote the breakdown of proteins within each cell as a substitute energy fuel. So the blood is flooded with excess sugar, while the cells are burning protein for energy because so little of this sugar is available to them.

When steroids are indicated for a diabetic COPD, these side effects can be somewhat reduced by using large doses of aerosolized steroids instead of smaller oral doses. This, though, produces its own set of problems. Oral yeast infections and loss of voice are frequently troublesome with high inhaled doses. The use of a spacer between canister and mouth, though, can reduce the amount of steroid deposited in the mouth, which may diminish these difficulties. Also helpful are the prophylactic use of antifungal medication (such as oral *nystatin*), plus fastidious oral hygiene. Although inhaled steroids reduce the diabetes-promoting problem somewhat, they by no means make it disappear. So the primary countermeasure may be an increase in antidiabetic medication.

Adrenergic beta-2 selective drugs also increase the amount of glucose in the blood, especially when they are given orally. Even when these drugs are used in aerosolized form, the diabetic must pay greater attention to monitoring his glucose level.

COPD Drugs and Autonomic Dysfunction

The autonomic nervous system in diabetics can develop problems related to heart rate, blood pressure regulation, urination, and male sexual function. In theory, vagal nerve (part of the autonomic nervous system, and a bronchoconstricting pathway) dysfunction should improve COPD symptoms by removing this pathway. In reality, COPD patients with this loss of autonomic control appear to have a greater chance of respiratory failure. Laboratory studies have shown that when their oxygen level falls, they fail to increase their rate and/or depth of breathing to compensate. This becomes a critical concern during an acute episode. That is why diabetic COPD patients with autonomic nervous system impairment—when they develop an infection—usually get supplemental oxygen and have their blood gases monitored without delay.

Both the beta-2 stimulators and the theophyllines improve the ventilatory response of falling oxygen and increasing carbon dioxide. In theory, then, these drugs would appear to be especially appropriate for this subgroup of diabetic COPD patients. We are unaware, though, of any scientific work indicating whether they actually are particularly helpful. It is known that beta-2 stimulators must be given cautiously with these patients to prevent a rapid, uncontrolled drop in blood pressure.

Conclusion

The order of medication preference for the diabetic COPD patient is the same as when COPD coexists with cardiovascular disease. First choice is typically ipratropium bromide, second is inhaled beta-2 stimulators. Next in line are aerosol steroids and—only if they cannot be avoided—oral steroids.

Surgery

It is fairly common for COPD patients to need major surgery at some point. A significant number of them have developed lung cancer, as it shares COPD's and cardiovascular disease's kinship to smoking. A number of other conditions typically associated with advancing age also require surgery.

It used to be that COPD and surgery were a very lethal combination. But light years of progress have been made in the decades since the 1950s and 1960s: improved surgical techniques, commonplace forms of breathing support and cardiac monitoring that weren't even available then, plus pharmacology advances. So surgery itself is far more effective, and pre- and postoperative care of critically ill patients has vastly improved. That is why we find patients with serious pulmonary disease now undergoing surgery much more frequently—and much more safely.

Making the Decision

When a COPD patient develops a condition requiring surgical treatment, his doctor has to weigh the benefits of surgery against the complications it might provoke. In assessing the nature and likelihood of risk, his doctor must consider what is known about the particular procedure's impact on COPD, and try to estimate the chance of pulmonary complications—possibly leading to death—following surgery. But there is often precious little to guide him in this estimation.

Only one surgical procedure permits us—based on a pulmonary function test—to predict reasonably well how a COPD patient will do after surgery. That involves removal of lung tissue, most typically for lung cancer. Other than that, we have to evaluate each patient as he appears to us—and reality can contradict our perceptions. We have learned, for example, that such high-impact procedures as open heart surgery can be survived by severely ill patients who seemed, by all measures, to be very poor risks.

The difficulty in predicting the risk an individual patient actually faces means that doctors who treat advanced COPD patients often face a knotty decision: Should potentially lifesaving surgery be withheld—or not—when the risk of postsurgical pulmonary complications *seems* high enough to cancel the benefits?

A major comfort, when contemplating surgery, is that more and more doctors are learning to avoid—or at least minimize—postoperative complications by recognizing the severity of a patient's COPD, then taking appropriate preventive steps before, during, and after surgery. We note these steps below.

Before Surgery

One of the most important presurgical issues is which hospital to choose. Our advice is to choose one that does a high volume of the procedure you need. It's been shown time and again that the number and severity of complications following a particular surgical procedure go up as the experience of both surgical and nursing staff go down. With more procedures, the postoperative course is substantially smoother and any complications that do arise are far more effectively controlled.

Next is having a good preoperative plan, to minimize your obvious vulnerability to pulmonary complications. The general aim of the plan is maximizing your physical condition. And it helps substantially. Research indicates, for example, that proper preoperative care can reduce the postsurgical occurrence of pneumonia by 60%.

Although the details of your presurgical program would depend on the severity of your lung disease, the basic components apply to any COPD patient.

☐ Stop smoking, if you haven't done it yet. Have your sputum checked, with appropriate antibacterial medication if there is any sign of infection.

☐ Open and clear your airways as much as possible. For starters, fine-tune bronchodilator therapy to optimize airway relaxation and high mucus clearance. A short steroid course to reduce airway inflammation should be considered. Do more frequent chest percussion and postural drainage. Try warm water in aerosol form several times a day to help loosen tenacious sputum for optimal results.

☐ Education. If you haven't yet learned the breathing exercises and how to cough effectively (called *huffing*), learn and practice them now. (See Chapter 13 for the detailed description of these techniques.) Also practice breathing with an incentive spirometer (Figure 7.1) to help deepen your breaths. This will all help prevent your air sacs from collapsing (called *atelectasis*) after surgery.

☐ Learn the simple foot exercises and knee flexion movements that should be done several times an hour after surgery. This is very important in preventing blood clots.

During Surgery

Although the type of surgery usually dictates the kind of anesthesia used, some procedures permit a choice. When a choice exists, the patient should be included in the decision-making process.

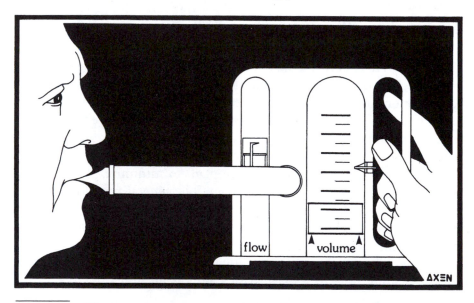

Figure 7.1   The incentive spirometer is designed to give you feedback as you perform your inspiratory breathing exercise. Set the pointer on the right to your prescribed breath-size level. Inhale slowly to raise the flow piston between the arrows until the volume marker reaches your prescribed level. (Illustrated is the *Voldine 5000*®, Sherwood Medical.)

Local anesthesia involves anesthetic agents (such as *xylocain*) that are injected just below the surface of the surgical area, or—as a nerve block—directly into the nerves supplying that area. (This is the kind of anesthetic your dentist injects into your gum.) Nerve blocks can be used in arm and leg surgery. Injecting a local anesthetic into the spinal canal—called *spinal anesthesia*—is used in surgery of the legs and lower abdomen. Because local anesthesia does not usually affect breathing significantly, it is a good choice for COPD patients.

General anesthesia involves loss of consciousness. A muscle relaxant is usually given along with it to relax the muscles at the surgical site. A tube placed down into the trachea during general anesthesia serves two potential purposes: (1) If a patient throws up during surgery, the tube is a barrier preventing vomited stomach acid from being breathed into the lungs. (Inhaled stomach acid would eat away large portions of lung tissue.) (2) If a patient's breathing fails, a respirator can instantly be attached to take over for his respiratory muscles. (In many long operations, it is standard procedure to attach the patient to the respirator throughout.)

General anesthetic agents and muscle relaxants make breathing quite shallow, which reduces ventilation. So the anesthesiologist is especially careful to maintain a high level of oxygen in the air the patient breathes, and to keep the level of anesthesia as shallow as possible to keep interference with ventilation at a minimum.

During prolonged general anesthesia the lungs get stiffer, in part from the shallower breathing. Stiffer lungs means the inspiratory muscles have to work harder, which isn't good for a COPD patient. To minimize this, the anesthesiologist uses mechanical means to inflate the patient's lungs fully every so often during long procedures. The anesthesiologist also ensures that the air mixture the patient breathes is humid enough to keep mucus from thickening and blocking the airways.

After Surgery

If complications occur, it will be in the first few postoperative days. Aggressive—meaning both immediate and vigorous—preventive therapy often avoids, and certainly minimizes, the possibility of serious complications. (This approach isn't meant only for surgical patients with COPD. *Everyone* coming out of surgery benefits from these measures. But they assume heightened importance for patients who are otherwise at significantly greater risk for postoperative problems.)

The key to preventive therapy is to get the patient out of bed and walking as soon as possible. Here is an outline of the major steps involved in ensuring this outcome.

☐ To maintain adequate lung expansion and prevent postoperative atelectasis, conscientiously use the breathing exercises described in Chapter 13, and the incentive spirometer. Both were well practiced before surgery to minimize the impact of postoperative weakness, pain, and fuzziness on doing them properly.

☐ Keep airways as mucus-free as possible to help prevent both infection and atelectasis. This requires an effective cough. The patient who can do so uses the huffing technique, already practiced before surgery. For the patient too weak or fearful to cough on his own, there is *assisted coughing,* in which the physical therapist presses carefully on the patient's abdomen to help explode the air out. Incision pain caused by coughing is minimized by holding a pillow against the wound during the cough.

☐ To aid circulation in the legs to prevent blood clots and maintain range of motion in the joints, the leg and knee exercises taught preoperatively should be done five to ten times each hour.

☐ Deconditioning can occur quite quickly when a person is bedridden. The longer the COPD patient remains deconditioned, the more likely that fatigue and dyspnea will destroy his motivation to resume exercising. To regain exercise tolerance—which means restoring the muscles' efficient use of oxygen—it is extremely important to involve the patient with a reconditioning program as soon as it is medically advisable.

Conclusion

The two most important, and reassuring, facts to emerge from the reported data on surgery in COPD patients are:

1. Patients with severely impaired pulmonary function do relatively well following surgery despite more postoperative complications than patients whose lungs are in better shape.

2. We have a method to minimize the risk of serious complications in all COPD patients—the combination of physical therapy instruction *before* surgery, then physical therapy afterward. Scheduling the initial instruction while the patient is still alert and pain-free is crucial to success. Patients whose first contact with physical therapy procedures is only after surgery certainly do better than patients who have no physical therapy at all. But they don't do nearly as well as those who get a chance to learn and practice the different exercises before surgery occurs.

8

Stop Smoking!

This chapter must precede any discussion of the various medical/rehabilitation treatments for COPD. Why? Because smoking cessation is *the most effective step* in helping patients with chronic bronchitis and/or emphysema. *It is lifesaving.* Although the other long-term therapies can give some symptomatic relief, only giving up cigarettes (and, for some patients with very advanced COPD, the long-term use of oxygen) has been shown to control progression of these diseases (Figure 8.1). Some physicians regard stopping smoking as so critical that they refuse to treat COPD patients who continue to smoke.

One would expect COPD patients—when they learn that continuing smoking guarantees an early death sentence—to be able to give it up. But the unsettling evidence is that only a minority of COPD patients actually stop smoking.

This mirrors the smoking population at large. An American Cancer Society smokers survey shows that nine out of ten want to stop, but are afraid to try. The most common rationalizations for continuing are: "I'm afraid I'll get fat if I stop" and "I need them to relax." The one out of ten who doesn't even want to stop smoking is the basic ostrich with his head deep in the sand: "I don't believe cigarettes are as bad as they say."

"Nicotine is a powerfully addicting drug . . . [that is] six to eight times more addictive than alcohol." So states the American College of Physicians' 1986 position paper put out by their Health and Public Policy Committee. The addiction is both chemical and behavioral. This potent addiction makes smoking cessation programs less effective than they had hoped to be. In fact, they consider themselves successful if only one out of every four clients (25%) stops smoking for one year.

This 25% figure, though, is an average. It masks the variation in success rates regarding both age and sex. Older people are more successful

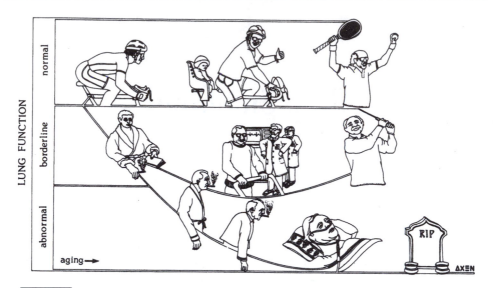

Figure 8.1   Long-term effects of smoking on the lungs. *Top:* Although some lung function is lost as a consequence of aging, the lifelong nonsmoker is able to continue with an active, productive life. *Middle:* Although some lung abnormality is already present, stopping smoking reverses some of the abnormal deterioration. If the person stops early enough and participates in a complete rehabilitation program, some of the lost lung function may return. *Bottom:* Not stopping will result in deterioration of lung function. The person develops COPD symptoms, which for many patients interfere with activities of daily living and lead to premature death.

than younger ones in giving up cigarettes, and men are twice as likely to stop as women.

Many feel that women have more difficulty giving up smoking at least in part because our society's aesthetics label unslender bodies unacceptable. It is a fact that many smokers who stop can expect to gain some weight. (A few pounds result from a slight metabolism slowing, as the nicotine-stimulated increase in metabolic rate disappears. Any further addition is from substituting food for cigarettes.) Some ex-smokers are eventually able to take off this extra weight, some not. From a health standpoint, stopping smoking is infinitely more important than this weight gain. But there is such pressure on women to keep their bodies looking beautiful and healthy that they opt for feeling good about their looks now rather than really feeling good and being healthy in the future.

So how do people give up cigarettes? Substituting a pipe or cigar isn't the answer. The smoker who inhales his cigarette smoke will most likely inhale pipe and cigar smoke, too—which are just as harmful. The only answer is to stop smoking.

The Cigarette Cycle: The Path to Addiction

Smoking cigarette tobacco sets off a self-perpetuating cycle creating a chemical addiction. The new smoker lights up a cigarette, bringing the smoke deep into his lungs with each puff. These deep inhalations lower pressure in his chest and his pulmonary blood vessels, which increases the amount of blood flowing to his heart. Greater blood flow to his heart is experienced as a relaxed feeling. Seconds after this begins, nicotine from the tobacco smoke enters his liver and causes it to release sugar. This sudden shot of sugar in his blood produces a high.

Although it feels good to the smoker, his body's sugar-monitoring system is aroused to correct what it perceives as an imbalance. His pancreas releases insulin to return his blood sugar level to normal. But this drop in blood sugar makes the smoker irritable and hungry, stimulating a desire to smoke and recover that initial relaxed, high feeling.

By now, the nicotine is also stimulating his nervous system to release adrenaline. This speeds up both heart and breathing rates, making the smoker feel even more tense and so sharpening his desire for another cigarette. Lighting this next cigarette perpetuates the cycle. Each additional cigarette entrenches it further.

Superimposed on this physical addiction is the awesome power of habit. The greater number of behaviors linked to the smoking habit, the stronger this habit will be, and the more difficult to break. So giving up smoking involves combating two very different sets of demands, with different time frames. There is physical need, which is conquered in a few weeks at most. And there is the powerful psychological entanglement upon which habits rest, which takes a much longer time to undo.

Giving Up Cigarettes

Breaking the cycle to physical addiction is the first step in giving up cigarettes. Here are two pointers to help control the nicotine urge. First, breathe s-l-o-w-l-y and d-e-e-p-l-y every time you start wanting—or anticipate wanting—a cigarette. This will decrease pressure in your chest and pulmonary blood vessels to give you the same initial feeling of relaxation that inhaling your cigarette smoke has produced. Second, monitor and adjust your food intake to maintain a stable blood sugar level. It is particularly important not to let it drop.

Remember that once your body has gotten used to something, it will not easily give it up. So even following this advice with scrupulous care may not prevent withdrawal symptoms. Don't be alarmed if you experience any of the following—light-headedness, headache, diarrhea, nervousness, and/or insomnia—for anywhere from two days to two weeks. That's how long complete physical withdrawal from nicotine normally takes.

For smokers who can't go cold turkey, or are afraid to try, various types of help exist. We will discuss the four most popular approaches: (1) drug therapy, (2) behavior modification, (3) hypnosis, and (4) acupuncture.

Note: A list of stop-smoking resources in your area is usually available from your local hospital or health center. Also look under "Smoker's Information & Treatment Centers" in your telephone directory.

Before we begin, we want to emphasize that *education* is necessary for success in remaining off cigarettes once you have successfully stopped smoking (by whatever means you choose). The following organizations provide excellent educational materials: the Office on Smoking and Health maintained by the Centers for Disease Control (either use their website—*www.cdc.gov/tobacco/index.html*—or call the public inquiry number—800-311-3435, 404-639-3534—and choose the menu option "other diseases and health risks"); the American Cancer Society (call 800-ACS-2345); the American Heart Association (call 800-242-8721, wait for an operator, and request their smoking packet); and the American Lung Association (call 800-LUNG-USA for the number of your local office).

Drug Therapy

Drugs were the mainstay of many early smoking-cessation attempts. Some were aimed at overcoming the smoking habit by interfering with it or substituting for it. Others were designed to soothe withdrawal symptoms. But they didn't work. Their failure led to the assumption that only nicotine, given in some nontobacco form, could successfully soothe the urge to smoke. The first product approved by the Food and Drug Administration was *Nicorette*, a nicotine-containing gum available since 1985. Now we also have nicotine nasal sprays and nicotine patches that help to satiate the craving for nicotine (Table 8.1). The gum and patches are available without prescription. As the particular formulation that works best for you is an individual issue, you may need to experiment a bit.

If slow, deep breathing and regulating your blood sugar level don't adequately control withdrawal symptoms, Nicorette can decrease them. But the gum itself produces unpleasant side effects in some users (including hiccoughs, nausea, and vomiting). And some users have become dependent on it!

The official advice for using nicotine gum is to combine it with other forms of aid. Merrell Dow, which manufactures Nicorette, recommends that it be used "as a temporary aid . . . while participating in a behavior modification program under medical supervision." The Health and Public Policy Committee of the American College of Physicians has concluded that, although "drug therapy has not been found useful in smoking cessation efforts, . . . some promise has been shown for nicotine gum as a substitute for smoking and, in conjunction with other therapies, as an aid to overcoming withdrawal symptoms."

Warning: This gum should not be used during pregnancy or nursing, after a heart attack, or by anyone with peptic ulcers, cardiovascular disease, high blood pressure, angina, an overactive thyroid, or by anyone using insulin.

Table 8.1 Nicotine Replacement Therapy for Smoking

Brand	Vehicle	Doses	Dosage	Maximum Dosage
Nicorette	gum	2 mg piece	1 piece/hr	30 pieces/d
Nicorette DS	gum	4 mg piece	1 piece/hr	20 pieces/d
Nicotrol	nasal spray	0.5 mg spray	1–2 sprays/hr	40 doses/d
Habitrol and Nicoderm	patch	7, 14, and 21 mg/patch	7 mg/d (2 wks)	
			14 mg/d (2 wks)	
			21 mg/d (6 wks)	
Nicotrol	patch	5, 10, and 15 mg/patch	5 mg/d (2–4 wks)	
			10 mg/d (2–4 wks)	
			15 mg/d (4–12 wks)	
ProStep	patch	11 and 22 mg/patch	11 mg/d (2–4 wks)	
			22 mg/d (4–8 wks)*	

*For patients below 100 lbs the recommended schedule is 11 mg/d for 4–8 weeks.
mg = milligram   d = day

Behavior Modification

The variety of behavior modification programs come in various forms: self-help guides, educational courses, health-plan or government-sponsored programs, commercial ventures. The best combine techniques of self-management, contingency management, and aversive conditioning,

Self-Management Techniques   Self-management techniques focus especially on helping you eradicate the automatic, deep-seated, behavioral connections to smoking. By enhancing self-control, they give you a chance to take the driver's seat.

The very first step is simply monitoring and recording your smoking habits to become aware of your environment and what cues urge you to reach for a cigarette. Even if you can't pick out a pattern right away, writing down your observations for each cigarette (as soon as you can, if not immediately) will eventually make it clear.

Then, when you feel you understand your smoking habits and are ready to try breaking them, pick a time to start. Because people tend to smoke more during stressful times, your success will depend a great deal on what else is happening in your life when you try to stop smoking. Don't decide to give up cigarettes when you are just quitting your job or starting a new one, ending a relationship, going back to school, or moving. Choose a point when you expect things to be relatively smooth.

A helpful suggestion for a good start is writing out a contract stating all the conditions you have set out for attaining your goal. Here is an example.

Date _____

I, _____, agree to stop smoking on the morning of (_____). I have decided to stop because (list your reasons). I have enlisted the help of (wife, husband, etc.) to help me quit smoking. My helper's responsibilities are to (inquire about my progress, help me find things to do when I get the urge to smoke, etc.). To reward myself for quitting, I plan to give myself (name the treat). If I slip, I will impose (e.g., put x dollars in a pot) as punishment.

Smoker's signature _____

Helper's signature _____

We advise starting in the morning because the urge to smoke is often less frequent and less intense than later in the day as tensions build up. But no matter when you start, sooner or later during that day you will urgently long to smoke—perhaps after breakfast, or while putting your makeup on, or with your first cup of coffee or phone call at work. When this happens, breathe slowly and deeply. Try finding something to take your mind off the urge. Or pop a piece of (non-nicotine) gum in your mouth or chew on a pencil. Don't give in. This immediate urge should pass in just a couple of minutes. (But because your craving is partly due to the actual lack of nicotine in your system, you may experience some of the withdrawal effects we spoke about.)

Resisting the initial urges to smoke is—relatively speaking, of course—the easy part. Mark Twain is purported to have said, "There's nothing to giving up smoking. I've done it hundreds of times." The hardest part of stopping smoking is staying stopped. Once we have conquered "smoking as addiction," we still have to conquer "smoking as habit."

Because a habit is something we do without thinking—a deeply established automatic connection—breaking it takes time and endurance. One of the best ways to speed this process is to remove as many of your regular connections to smoking as possible. This reduces the chance of taking a cigarette "out of habit." Upset your daily routines as much as you can without turning your life into chaos.

Some suggestions: Try getting up a little earlier. Change the order in which you do things after you get out of bed—if you normally get dressed before breakfast, eat first (or vice versa). Put on your makeup in a different room. Go out for a walk on your coffee break. Two or three evenings a week, take an exercise class after work instead of going straight home. (You may also find exercise a substantial help in actually melting away the physical urge for a cigarette. And because it burns additional calories—and for many decreases their appetite for their next meal—it can help control or reverse any weight gain from stopping smoking.) Go out to a movie instead of watching television at home. Change your pre-bedtime routines, especially those involving smoking.

In addition to dissolving habit connections, the rigorous examination of one's smoking behavior that these techniques require provides an additional push. A 1978 publication on smoking control methods from the Department of Health, Education and Welfare found it clear that "when an individual begins paying unusually close attention to one aspect of his behavior, it is likely to change."

Contingency Management   Contingency management helps reinforce your desire to stop smoking. It's the carrot at the end of the stick, except that you really get the prize when you reach your destination. One common method is to collect your daily cigarette money in a piggy bank, and buy yourself something special with it at the end of specific time periods. (An example: one of the authors gave up a two-pack-a-day habit in 1969, and at the end of one year her cigarette savings paid for a ski trip to France!) The other common approach is for smokers who try to cut down their smoking before cutting it out. They put a predetermined amount of money into the piggy bank for each cigarette smoked. When they stop completely, they get it back. The smoker who cannot take that final step contributes the money to his favorite charity.

Aversive Conditioning   Aversive conditioning is designed to replace satisfying habit connections with highly unpleasant ones. The four formal approaches to aversive behavior modification are: electric shock, sensory deprivation, satiation, and rapid smoking. These require working with a trained behavioral therapist.

Use of electric shock requires that the smoker receive a somewhat unpleasant (but not dangerous) electric shock with each puff. Sensory deprivation techniques, designed to achieve a rapid attitude change, keep the smoker in bed in a dark room for 24 hours. The room remains silent except for periodic messages on the dangers of cigarette smoking. Neither of these methods has been widely used or studied.

Satiation is based on the assumption that although smoking is self-perpetuating, it becomes aversive once it goes beyond a certain frequency. The smoker doubles or triples the number of cigarettes he would normally smoke during each session with his behavioral therapist. While he smokes, warm smoky air is blown into his face. Rapid smoking, which is based on the same assumption, requires the smoker to inhale much more frequently than he usually does (let's say every six seconds) until the cigarette is finished or until he is nauseous—whichever comes first.

Although these aversive methods have some inherent danger—particularly for patients with coronary heart disease, hypoxemia, and/or hypertension—they are very effective in producing higher quitting rates at the start. But they need to be supplemented by other techniques (ideally, self-management and contingency) to achieve long-term abstinence from smoking.

An aversive technique that is both risk-free and easy to do at home involves nothing more than filling a large covered jar with your discarded cigarette butts for the week before you quit. The day before your new life begins, add a teaspoon or so of water to the jar. Then, whenever the urge for a cigarette becomes seductive, open your jar and take a sniff.

Self-Help Guides   A number of good self-help guides provide detailed programs on beating your smoking habit.

The organizations listed in the "Note" on page 90—the government Office on Smoking and Health, the American Cancer Society, the American Heart Association, and the American Lung Association—all have good self-help guides as well as educational materials.

Can a self-help program by itself do the job, or is the human element—a "stop-smoking therapist" of some sort, and the presence of others in your shoes—an essential ingredient? The importance of a "leader" seems to depend on the individual hopeful ex-smoker, according to a study comparing several different self-help programs (one of which was based on the *I Quit Kit*) used both with and without the help of a therapist. The study's authors recommend a potential two-stage process for giving up cigarettes: start on your own with a self-help program. If you continue feeling very shaky or fall off the wagon, follow up with a smoking cessation group or a behavioral therapist. Trying to kick the habit with others in the same boat provides a support system that, for some, is very helpful. Some programs actually have a buddy system, giving you someone to call when you feel about to be overwhelmed by the urge for a cigarette.

To summarize: behavior modification can be an effective way to stop smoking. The key seems to be an honest appraisal of the smoker's reasons for smoking and motivations for stopping. This allows a coherent plan to develop that combines the three necessary elements of self-management, contingency management, and aversive conditioning.

An Organized Smoke-Cessation Program   There are many stop-smoking programs, some organized by the American Lung Association, American Heart Association, or American Cancer Association, and many offered by commercial organizations. At New York University Medical Centers, for example, *Smokeless* is the program offered to employees.

Most of these programs combine behavior modification and education with a highly supportive environment. Cost and the number of sessions vary with the program. The *Smokeless* program at N.Y.U. involves six sessions for groups of 10 to 20 people. Its $200 cost is a one-time fee, which allows a registrant to retake the course if needed, and to take it anywhere the program is given.

The program is divided into seven phases, one preparatory and one for each session. The preparatory phase involves eliminating some of the most automatic aspects of reaching for a cigarette (for example, record each cigarette you smoke; wait five minutes before lighting up; buy by the individual pack, not the carton; stop using lighters, cigarette cases, etc.), and setting up a priority-ordered list of your stop-smoking goals (for example, better health, good breathing, freedom from an enslaving habit). This brings you to your first session in an optimal frame of mind. The six sessions are spread over three weeks (three the first week, two the second, one the third). Each incorporates new material with a review of important points from earlier meetings to modify behavior and attitudes.

Negative smoking—their term for aversive satiation—is part of the very first session. In general, the first sessions are geared more toward understanding why you smoke, and overcoming initial smoking temptations. There are a great variety of "urge tamer" aids to cope with cigarette urges and the situations that intensify them. Altering the many routines that involve smoking is emphasized, as are activities to keep your hands busy. Preventing overeating is dealt with in the short and long term. Success is rewarded. Support systems are encouraged. As the course progresses, the emphasis is increasingly on anticipating and coping with the potential stumbling blocks to remaining off cigarettes long enough to become a confirmed ex-smoker.

Multiple Risk Factor Reeducation Program A fascinating and unplanned discovery about smoking cessation programs popped up in the course of research studies on a very specific group of smokers—people with high cholesterol and hypertension. These major risk factors for atherosclerotic heart disease become far more potent when combined with smoking. The research was designed to see if modifying all three risk factors significantly affects the chance for a healthier future. In other words—could any of the damage be undone? These studies evaluated people both before and after the changes needed to normalize cholesterol and blood pressure, and eliminate smoking.

For giving up cigarettes, researchers typically combined behavior modification and education. The unexpected finding? Each program's success rate shot up—sometimes with more than 50% staying off cigarettes after several years! Why is the same stop-smoking program so much more effective in this context? It is believed that the overall framework of the research was responsible. The consistent and long-term follow-up, regular medical checkups, and focused emphasis on improving their health helped them personalize smoking's risk to a degree that most smokers are able to avoid. This meant they were more able to appreciate the general concept of disease prevention, and were more aware of the specific benefits available to them from giving up cigarettes.

Hypnosis

Hypnosis is a trance state that combines heightened inner awareness with a diminished awareness of one's surroundings. It can be induced artificially (by *hypnotism*), but it also occurs naturally under appropriate circumstances. Hypnosis is the state reached during daydreaming. It also describes the experience of being so completely engrossed—such as by music or a theatrical performance—that awareness of one's surroundings temporarily disappears.

Hypnosis becomes a therapeutic tool because a person in this state is especially susceptible to positive, reasonable suggestions. An unfortunate myth is that hypnotized people can be ordered to do things they would otherwise refuse. For any suggestion to be accepted, it must make sense to the individual and it must not violate his moral code.

The earliest recorded use of hypnosis in medicine is contained in a 3,000-year-old Egyptian papyrus. It had become of major medical importance in ancient Greece. Priests at Aesculepius's temple (he was the Greek god of medicine) on the Aegean island of Epidaurus used the hypnotic trance to cure pilgrims seeking help for their medical problems.

The modern use of hypnosis is said to have begun with the Viennese physician Franz Anton Mesmer (from whose name we get the word *mesmerize*) in the late seventeenth and early eighteenth centuries. He introduced the use of hypnosis into Viennese, then Parisian, medical circles. Mesmer thought that magnetism explained the effects of hypnotism, and coined the term "animal magnetism" to differentiate it from magnetism in the physical world. Reports of miraculous cures in Vienna and Paris soon won Mesmer a large popular following and the enmity of both medical establishments. They barred him from practicing medicine. After a stay in England, Mesmer returned to a life of obscurity in Austria and died in 1815.

Hypnotism's popularity was cyclical after Mesmer's death. The lack of interest following its first epidemic use was punctuated with periodic curiosity. The high point in its resurgence was between 1885 and 1910, with smaller revivals after World War I in treating war-related neuroses. Hypnosis' final decline was due to a combination of rejections. The medical profession had never accepted hypnotism as a legitimate tool, and Freud eventually rejected it as a tool in the practice of psychoanalysis (which itself was rapidly gaining popularity). Recent evidence, however, indicates that hypnosis may be valuable in helping people stop smoking.

Many people are highly skeptical about their own capacity to be hypnotized. Except for those with severe mental disturbance, it turns out that most people can be hypnotized to some degree. (Degree of hypnotizability reflects how long and how hard the hypnotist must work to achieve hypnosis.) This degree is assessed by the amount of white that shows after a person is told to roll his eyes up and keep them there while he lowers his eyelids. The higher up that the eye remains, the more hypnotizable the person is. This basic potential for hypnosis can be modified by motivation. Actual hypnotizability can be tested by hypnotizing the person to raise his arm, and recording the number of instructions and amount of time it takes. Obviously, less instructions and time go along with greater hypnotizability.

One hypnotizability and motivation are established, the person is hypnotized, given the appropriate suggestion(s) for giving up cigarettes and not replacing them with food or alcohol, and taught to hypnotize himself (called *autohypnosis*). Part of this trance ritual involves silently repeating certain antismoking points. Because autohypnosis induces relaxation, and also reinforces the suggestions implanted during the hypnosis sessions, initially it is done very frequently. One recommended schedule is every half hour plus every time the urge for a cigarette hits. It is needed less often once the urge to smoke substantially weakens. (Smoking cessation may require one or more sessions with a hypnotist.)

Effectiveness studies evaluate success for the first six-month period. Results vary tremendously, from a low of 4% (only four successful ex-smokers out of every 100 smokers trying to quit via hypnosis) to a high of 88% (hypnosis helps 88 out of every 100 smokers quit). But not all of these studies were well designed or carried out. Those that were properly done all report a 20 to 25% success rate at six months. Certain basic requirements for success include a supportive therapist, a motivated client and, most importantly, individualized hypnotic suggestions.

(Interestingly, one well-known Manhattan psychiatrist who specializes in using hypnosis for behavior modification finds that easily hypnotized people are much more likely to give up cigarettes, but least likely to stay off them. People who are more difficult to hypnotize aren't as successful in quitting, but those who do are much less likely to relapse.)

Acupuncture

Webster's dictionary tells us that the word *acupuncture*—which comes from the Latin words *acus* ("needle") and *punctura* ("pricking")—means "puncturing a bodily tissue for the relief of pain." Hair-thin needles of various lengths are inserted into one or more among several hundred points over the body.

We know that acupuncture originated in China several thousand years ago. Ancient acupuncture needles found there have been dated to prehistoric times. The third- or fourth-century Chinese medical text *The Yellow Emperor's Classic of Internal Medicine* includes acupuncture as a well-known and valuable technique, but doesn't note how it developed. Despite the test of time attesting to acupuncture's value, the American medical community relegated it to folklore, fantasy, and mysticism. It took President Richard Nixon's trip to the People's Republic of China in

1972, during which *New York Times* reporter James Reston had appendix surgery under acupuncture anesthesia, to awaken interest in acupuncture in the United States.

We know acupuncture works, although in large part we don't really understand how. We have learned that acupuncture is effective in controlling or banishing pain because of its effectiveness in stimulating the release of endorphins, the body's natural analgesics. A specialized approach to treating addictions with acupuncture uses only five points in the ear. It was adapted in the United States after dramatic success in China for coping with drug addictions, and is established in a number of centers here.

Acupuncture has been tried specifically as a stop-smoking tool. A French study used needles at points on the nose to "decongest" the respiratory tract and stimulate a feeling of disgust toward tobacco. Sixty-four percent of their smokers quit after one session. After several sessions, 78% had quit overall. The American technique twirls a needle in the earlobe, which is said to regulate the "neurovegetative" system. The smoker, who goes home with the needle still inserted, is instructed to twirl it himself whenever he craves a cigarette. Success rates in an Australian study using this technique parallel those found with other approaches. Although 95% stopped smoking after three acupuncture sessions, the rate fell to 34% at the end of one and 30% at the close of two years.

For those of you who are interested in trying this ancient treatment and do not know of a skilled, experienced practitioner in your area, there are several national organizations that will provide a list. Two reliable training organizations that can recommend acupuncturists maintain a toll-free phone number, and also have a referral section—organized by state—on the Internet. The American Academy of Medical Acupuncture in Los Angeles is at 800-521-2262 or *www.medicalacupuncture.org.* The American Association of Oriental Medicine in Catasaugua, Pennsylvania, is at 888-500-7959 or *www.aaom.org.* Unfortunately, there is no consistent insurance coverage policy for acupuncture.

Conclusion

Nothing will help you become an ex-smoker if you don't really want to do it. Your motivation is critical. The most effective program in the world cannot help you if you do not sincerely—and deeply—want to stop smoking. If the motivation is there, you will sooner or later hit upon what works for you. After this advice from the conclusion of the smoking cessation position paper issued in 1986 by the American College of Physicians' Public Policy Committee, we'll present two very different ex-smokers' stories.

A variety of methods and programs exist for the potential former smoker, and it is often best to combine a number of methods for an individualized program. Some of the most successful "programs" are those conducted largely by the individual, motivated to quit because of increasing awareness of the risks of smoking and the benefits of stopping . . . The fact remains that despite the vast array of smoking-cessation programs and methods, most people who have quit have done so largely on their own. [But] all persons who wish to quit, whether involved in a formal program or on their own, can benefit from some assistance, such as education presented in lay literature or as part of professional counseling, self-help guides, and more structured educational programs.

One Ex-smoker's Story

In February 1969, one of the authors (SSH) successfully stopped smoking with hypnosis, giving up a two- to three-pack-a-day (depending on how smoothly life was, or wasn't, going) habit of ten years' duration. I wanted to stop because I finally realized that smoking was destroying my lungs, and whatever cure "they" might find would come too late for me.

The previous September I had learned that the endless, heavily productive cough that now regularly followed my colds was repeated bronchitis. And I already had a harsh smoker's cough, pain deep in my lungs when I took a deep breath or exercised, and the audible hiss of air passing through accumulated mucus whenever I took a slow, very deep breath. In December I had learned of a woman, a heavy smoker only four years my senior, who had just died of lung cancer at age 30.

I tried quitting cold turkey, and failed—just as I had at two earlier, less motivated times in my life. Then I was told of a psychiatrist who used hypnosis with smokers, and learned coincidentally that someone I knew had just successfully worked with him. The first opening he had was in five weeks, so for the interim I smoked *without inhaling*. My one session with Dr. Herbert Spiegel lasted an hour. The hypnotic suggestions—in addition to the points I would later repeat to myself during autohypnosis—included no longer wanting to gain satisfaction from cigarettes.

I kept my half-smoked pack in my pocketbook (testing Dr. Spiegel's suggestion), yet I wasn't tempted to use it. Although in all my previous "give-it-up" attempts I used to run wildly through my apartment searching for a stale, forgotten pack or an overlooked cigarette butt, now I no longer wanted cigarettes for satisfying the needs smoking had filled for so long. And this time around, cigarette smoke from others irritated rather than tantalized me. I felt sorry for people rushing up the subway stairs, desperate to reach the street and light up.

A major discovery was exercise's effect in making my desire to smoke absolutely disappear. I had begun an adult dance class five months earlier, and happened to have a class the very evening I had just given up smoking. I began that class feeling tense and very much aware of not being able to smoke. I left feeling completely emptied of any desire to smoke. That effect was sustained for hours.

My first four days were the really rough ones, but "handle-ably" rough instead of totally crazy. Getting ready to go out in the morning and getting ready for bed at night were hardest of all, because for years I had chain-smoked through those rituals. My first morning, I think it took me three hours to get ready. I was very late for work! And exceptionally late getting to bed that night! When I woke up and opened my eyes on my fifth morning as an ex-smoker—this will sound dramatic, but it's true—I felt that an angel had passed over me during the night and cleansed me. I was at peace. That doesn't mean there weren't some very difficult situations that would take up to several years to handle well without cigarettes. I used to chain-smoke while housecleaning, and while letter writing, for example. So for a good while I wasn't very diligent at either job.

As for weight, I was an ex-fatty—terrified of gaining weight—who had relied on cigarettes to remain slim. So I ate a lot of carrot sticks and apples, put on only three pounds, then gradually took them off. Slow restaurant dinners were very hard for a while—no cigarettes to keep my hands and mouth busy before dinner was served. So I learned to eat bread s-l-o-w-l-y. Tear a roll into tiny pieces. Slowly butter each piece. Slowly eat each piece. Changing my eating and dieting habits took time and persistence. But it worked. The exercise from my dance classes certainly helped. Each class curbed the desires cigarettes had once filled, and lowered my appetite for the rest of the evening. And my thrill over how much better my body was looking and feeling became a powerful aid in preventing the abuse of food.

One more point: I used to have smoking dreams, which I later learned are quite common. My first two years as an ex-smoker, I dreamed every so often that someone offered me a cigarette—usually at a party—and without thinking I lit up, then realized in horror that I had undone all my good work. These dreams made me anxious. Could that happen in real life? Then finally I dreamed that someone offered me a cigarette, and I turned it down. "I no longer smoke," I said. That was the last smoking dream I ever had.

Another Ex-smoker's Story

Howard Otway had severe COPD, and was enrolled in the N.Y.U. Medical Centers' Pulmonary Rehabilitation program. He was kind enough to write for us his experience in trying to give up smoking.

When I was twelve years old, I promised myself I would quit smoking for my thirteenth birthday. Some forty odd years later, I managed to do it. By that time, of course, I had practically given up breathing. I had also given up climbing stairs without thinking about it, running, and getting mad enough to yell at somebody. If it took any more than survival breathing, I had given it up by the time I was fifty.

I don't remember the exact age, but I started on Catalpa tree seed pods, not a bad smoke for a six- or seven-year-old except for two rather limiting factors: they had to be relit before every puff and were available only in the autumn. But they made you nice and dizzy and I would smoke them until I was ready to fall, not unlike the lettuce cigarettes of later years that made the knowledgeable think I was a pothead.

Probably the dumbest substitution for smoking was when I decided I would take a sip of vodka every time I had the urge to smoke. That resulted in my becoming a smoking drunk who had to have a cigarette every time I had the urge for a sip of vodka.

I tried acupuncture. It cured my desire to quit smoking. But it was only temporary. I was ready to quit again a few hours later.

Hypnotism didn't work. Oh, my arms got light enough and started to float when the hypnotist suggested they were weightless, but every time he suggested I didn't want to smoke anymore it only reminded me how badly I wanted a cigarette. As I had paid him a rather handsome sum and he had virtually guaranteed a cure, he offered me additional sessions until finally one day I "woke up" in the middle of my arm flotations to ask to go to the men's room where I promptly lit a cigarette, bringing me to the realization that I was no longer only wasting his time, I was now wasting mine.

At the beginning, I was quitting once or twice a year, then I was quitting every few months, every couple of weeks, next Thursday. Tomorrow. Last Thursday, meaning the cigarette I had in my hand didn't really count because I was just having a few drags.

Finally I thought of the solution, the perfect solution. I would stop buying cigarettes and only smoke yours. After all, how long could I keep that up? Everybody would get to hating me and eventually stop giving me cigarettes. Of course in my heart I knew I was not above bumming an occasional drag. Hell, I had done that already, but there would surely be some fastidious smokers who would refuse me.

Unfortunately, I became hated sooner than I had counted on. Also, by now I was an employer and my staff could hardly refuse. And smokers as a breed are just not a particularly fastidious group. Anyway, it didn't work. I started buying everybody around me cartons of cigarettes so I could bum freely and in relatively good conscience. I now realize I carried it a bit far when I would find myself alone in a restaurant and ask the waiter what somebody at the next table was smoking so I could buy them a pack and bum one. I was always surprised that they would invariably insist I take two. But I have very strong will power. I never took more than the one I couldn't survive without.

I was now at the place where I would get short of breath from turning over in bed.

I smoked cigarettes low in tar, low in nicotine, low in taste, extra-long, extra-thin, cigarettes with holes in them. I smoked cigarettes I hated that came from badly designed, ugly packs. I smoked butts. I smoked through cotton. I smoked through plastic. I smoked through water and wool. I went to Smoke Enders.

That worked. Of course by now I was an invalid. I sat there smoking and wheezing, out of breath from the effort of getting there, learning—not to quit smoking, I knew how to quit smoking, I knew all kinds of ways to quit smoking—learning to become a nonsmoker.

I did everything I was told to do. I counted cigarettes. I wrote down the time, the place, the reason, if any, for having lit up. I saved butts. I smelled butts. I counted the days. I could hardly wait for the time I would no longer have to smoke. Finally, the night before the days of the miracle, I had my last cigarette. I didn't even finish it. I put it out more in anger than in sadness. I broke the remaining cigarettes in the pack and flushed them down the john. I washed the ashtray and went to bed. I woke up the next day a nonsmoker.

It was, indeed, a miracle . . . and so easy. I couldn't believe how easy it was. A few days later I began to wonder if a cigarette would taste the way it did when I first started to smoke, if I would get the old light-headed feeling, and, of course, I had to try it. Not that I wanted a cigarette—just to see what it was like. After all, I was now a nonsmoker. I could quit anytime. It was easy. Nothing to it. I had another.

A year later I decided I really had to stop smoking.

A cruise would do the trick. An ocean voyage. Sea breezes, and all that. I would continue to smoke until I boarded the ship.

It had been a long time since I had enjoyed a cigarette. I smoked because I had to. Now it had become painful. I had to force myself to smoke up to the day of the sailing.

I didn't get my first real urge to smoke again until I got home and then the minute my hand touched the doorknob, I wanted a cigarette. I kind of want one now. But a kindly old doctor who happens to be my brother-in-law gave me a very useful thought to remember. One drag and you're back to day one. Even I am not dumb enough to risk going back to being thirteen again.

9

Bronchodilators

The basic treatment for COPD is improving the patient's quality of life. This means reducing as much as possible his discomfort, the degree to which his disease handicaps him, and the anger this handicap has caused. Accomplishing this requires one or more of five therapeutic elements: (1) medication to relieve symptoms; (2) education of patient and family concerning this disease and its therapy; (3) environmental controls; (4) respiratory and/or physical therapy to improve physical fitness; (5) stress and anxiety management and sexual counseling.

The mainstay of COPD therapy is medication to maintain open airways and reduce bronchial reactivity. The use of drugs that loosen mucus (on a regular basis or as needed, depending on the circumstances) makes these primary medications more effective. Complications—including cough, bacterial infection, hypoxia, and *cor pulmonale*—are also aided with specific medication.

This chapter first presents the historical evolution of respiratory medication (when and how did it all really start, and where in the world), and then discusses the major bronchodilators in current use. The other types of COPD medication are described in the next chapter. The remaining four elements of COPD therapy are included in later chapters.

Note 1: All discussions of medication purposefully avoid any mention of appropriate dosage. This book is designed to help educate you, not treat you. Any questions that your reading of this book may raise concerning your medication must be taken up with your doctor.

Note 2: Whenever your doctor prescribes a new medication, it's very helpful to ask your doctor or pharmacist if there are any foods that interact with it. Scientists are continuously learning more and more about drug interactions with foods, herbs, and other supplements. (As an example: grapefruit alters the amount in your blood of certain drugs—increasing some, decreasing others.)

History of Medication for Respiratory Diseases

Greek and Roman physicians explained mucus overproduction within the prevailing concept of disease as an imbalance of some sort in the body's "humors." In this context, the famous Roman physician Galen made the following diagnostic observation: ". . . If the breath makes a raucous sound, this indicates obstruction due to an abundance of viscous or thick humors which are stuck to the bronchi of the lung and cannot be easily loosed. . . ."

Western medicine's earliest pharmaceutical attempts at treating mucus hypersecretion were directed at ridding the patient of his mucus. Paulus Aegineta wrote in the seventh century about ". . . consum[ing] the viscid and thick humor by attenuant and detergent medicines." This approach—which lasted well into our century—called for "expectorants" (which increase and liquefy mucus so it is easily coughed up) and "detergents" (which break up mucus plugs). The nineteenth century saw introduction of such useful expectorants as potassium iodide and the extract from the root of the Brazilian Ipecacuanha plant (also the active ingredient in Ipecac, used to induce vomiting to treat poisoning).

Drugs that relax the airways have been used—sometimes with vast gaps—for millennia. The Chinese were already using *ephedrine* as a bronchodilator 4,000 to 5,000 years ago. They called it "Ma Huang," an herbal remedy for coughs and colds made from the *Ephedra* plant family (Figure 9.1, right). These shrubs still grow in much of Asia and southern Europe. A record of ephedrine's use before it disappeared as a tool in Western medicine comes from the Roman historian Pliny the Elder. He noted that asthmatics took it in sweet wine for treatment of their disease.

Then ephedrine's bronchodilator properties were forgotten until Japanese investigators rediscovered them at the beginning of this century. From this they created Asthmatol, the first "modern" bronchodilator. Ephedrine also became the very first in a new class of drugs called *sympathomimetics*, which actually mimic the effects produced by the sympathetic nervous system.

Plants containing atropine were first used in India to relieve asthma, and were certainly used in Europe by the seventeenth century. The leaves

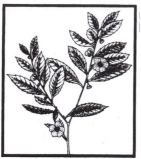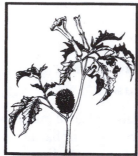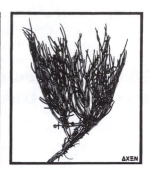

Figure 9.1   Medicinal plants (from left): tea, a theophylline source; *Datura stramonium*, atropine source; *Ephedra*, ephedrine (an early sympathomimetic) source.

were smoked until "the chest, throat, and head became light, and the cough reduced." By the nineteenth century, atropine was an important bronchodilator. The most popular atropine-containing plant used for the relief of airway obstruction was *Datura stramonium* (Figure 9.1, center). Its common names are Jamestown weed, jimsonweed, stinkweed, and thorn apple. Then atropine was in and out of favor until well into our century.

In toxic doses, atropine—a muscle paralytic—becomes a deadly poison that causes death from respiratory muscle paralysis. (The name *atropine* comes from Atropos, one of the three mythological Greek fates. Her job was severing the web of life woven and measured by her sisters, Clotho and Lachesis.) In lower doses, the drug blocks the vagus nerve (which is the path by which the parasympathetic nervous system activates the airways).

As an antiasthma medicine, atropine-like drugs have recently come into favor again after a checkered history. They have been turned to again partly because certain cases have remained unresponsive to other bronchodilators. And atropine-like bronchodilators have also been found effective in treating COPD.

In the nineteenth century, coffee came into use as a bronchodilator. The drug caffeine, coffee's effective ingredient, is closely related to theophylline, which—until recently—had been basic to asthma management for the last 60 years. Tea (Figure 9.1, left), also effective in asthma, contains both caffeine and theophylline.

At the beginning of this century, *epinephrine*—or *adrenaline*, as it is more usually called—was first discovered. At that time it was learned that the adrenal glands on the kidneys released large amounts of adrenaline into the bloodstream during periods of acute stress, and that one of adrenaline's many effects was to open up the bronchi. In the 1920s, adrenaline was developed as a bronchodilator for asthmatics. It is still often used as a drug for the emergency treatment of acute asthma attacks.

The commercial production of ephedrine and adrenaline was followed by attempts to synthesize compounds with properties similar to the natural substances. The most successful result—known both as *isoprenaline* and as *isoproterenol*—was synthesized in 1940 and is still in use.

In 1949, use of *cortisone* (one of the steroid group of drugs) became the next breakthrough in treating respiratory diseases. It was first tried on a patient with acute rheumatoid arthritis, and the results were dramatic. Then it achieved striking success in treating life-threatening asthma attacks. But the high rate of relapse once the cortisone treatment was completed led to cortisone's long-term use. Then it was discovered that maintaining patients on this drug led to serious, progressive side effects. By the 1960s, this unwitting indiscriminate use of cortisone had created a backlash against steroid drugs. Now, with greater understanding of how steroids work plus the development of steroids in aerosol form (aerosols are inhaled, and so use much smaller doses), the pendulum has returned to a sensible middle position that acknowledges both the benefits of steroids in treating asthma and the cautions needed to avoid serious side effects.

Current pharmaceutical research progresses along two directions. One is synthesizing more effective versions of existing drugs. The other is discovering new types of drugs that act on points in the COPD chain of events as yet unaffected by existing medications.

Modern Medication

The modern drugs used to treat COPD are designed to combat air flow obstruction by dilating the airways. This strategy breaks down into three avenues of approach (don't panic at forgotten or unfamiliar words, as we will carefully explain them all):

1. Induce bronchodilation by stimulating beta-receptors (which bronchodilate) and/or preventing the destruction of cAMP (which in turn reduces intracellular calcium).

2. Stop acetylcholine from stimulating cholinergic receptors (which would otherwise bronchoconstrict).

3. Prevent or reverse inflammatory events in the airways.

Although the benefits of bronchodilator therapy may not be obvious to the patient or measurable in the laboratory unless some asthma (airways that hyperreact—constrict—to certain stimuli) has also developed within the COPD mix, it is still considered the key medical treatment for COPD. Most clinicians believe bronchodilators provide subtle, yet important, benefits (perhaps by helping mucus removal) even when there is no obvious evidence of airway dilation.

The three basic types of bronchodilators (that is, the first two categories) influence the muscle encircling the airways, either by relaxing it or preventing its contraction. These muscle-directed bronchodilators make up the rest of this chapter. The remaining bronchodilator—which opens the airways by reducing inflammation of the airway lining—will be treated in Chapter 10, along with the other COPD medications.

Drugs That Stimulate Beta-Receptors

The Biochemistry of Beta-Receptor Stimulation

In Chapter 2, we described the two kinds of airway muscle-cell receptors recognized by the chemical mediators designed specifically to stimulate them: cholinergic receptors and adrenergic receptors. Adrenergic receptors subdivide into alpha-receptors and beta-receptors. Cholinergic and alpha-receptors constrict; beta-receptors relax. The degree to which airway muscle relaxes or contracts (which is what we mean by "muscle tone") depends on the balance between these two actions.

When a mediator is released, it recognizes and binds to its designated type of receptor. This binding sets off a chain of chemical events inside the muscle cell. When the cholinergic or alpha-receptor on an airway muscle cell is bound by its appropriate mediator (acetylcholine and adrenaline, respectively), *cyclic guanosine monophosphate* (*cGMP*) is eventually formed. Because cGMP raises the amount of calcium (a necessary element in muscle contraction) available to the cell's contractile proteins, muscle contraction increases.

Remember that adrenaline binds to beta-receptors when they are present in equal or greater numbers than the alpha-receptors. And when adrenaline binds to beta-receptors, *cyclic adenosine monophosphate* (*cAMP*) is eventually produced. Because cAMP lowers the amount of calcium available to the contractile proteins, muscle relaxation occurs.

The cGMP and cAMP that are produced to regulate airway muscle tone are eventually broken down by enzymes in the muscle cells. (The production and breakdown of these compounds form a regulatory cycle.) When acetylcholine comes unbound, it is inactivated by the enzyme cholinesterase. Unbound adrenaline is rapidly inactivated by the enzyme *monoamine oxidase* (*MAO*). How this is achieved, though, is not understood.

Stimulating beta-receptors also relieves cough, but the underlying mechanism is not clear. Coughing is one way in which the pulmonary system tries to rid the lungs and bronchi of excessive mucus produced during an attack. When the mucociliary system—which seems to be controlled by the parasympathetic nervous system—is stimulated, mucus production increases.

When activating beta-receptors relieves an asthmatic's cough, we don't yet know whether: the mucociliary system is being affected directly (by decreasing mucus production and increasing ciliary activity); or the effect is on the sensory neural pathways carrying information about airway irritation; or perhaps the airway smooth muscle is being directly acted upon.

Although how beta-receptors function is not completely understood, it is clear that maintaining adequate beta-receptor activity is central to managing most COPD patients. Drugs that stimulate the beta-receptors—technically called *beta-agonists*—imitate the action of adrenaline. (Table 9.1 summarizes the beta-stimulating, or adrenergic, bronchodilators currently available.)

General Beta-Receptor Stimulating Drugs

"*Imitate* the action of adrenaline" is a key phrase defining the value of today's beta-receptor stimulator drugs. If adrenaline has the effect we want, why do we need to use an imitator? Drawbacks limit adrenaline's use to asthma emergencies. The drawbacks: it cannot be taken orally because the digestive tract inactivates it; its injected and inhaled effects are relatively short-lived because enzymes in the blood destroy it very quickly; it also stimulates beta-receptors in the heart, sometimes disturbing the heart's normal rhythm; it also stimulates alpha-receptors, sometimes constricting artery and vein smooth muscles (increasing blood pressure), constricting the bladder opening (causing urine retention), and causing headaches and brain overstimulation.

The search for a beta-stimulating drug that ignores alpha-receptors led to *isoproterenol*. It replaced adrenaline in popularity because of its potent beta-stimulant properties plus the virtual absence of alpha effects. But this adrenaline derivative retains other disadvantages of its parent compound, that is: ineffectiveness when taken orally, relatively short duration of action, and undesirable cardiac effects. This last limitation is the most troublesome.

Table 9.1 Commonly Used Prescription Bronchodilators

The evaluations range from "+" (least effective) to "++++" (most effective)

Generic Name	Brand Names	Preparation	Relative Bronchodilation Effectiveness	Time to Response	Duration of Effect	Remarks
Beta-adrenergic						
Isoetherine	Bronkometer	MDI*	++	5–15 min	1.5–2.5 hr	Less effective than new drugs
	Bronkosol	Nebulizer	++	5–15	1.5–2.5	
Metaproterenol	Alupent	MDI	+++	30–45	3–5	Can cause tremor, tachycardia, nervousness
	Metaprel	Nebulizer	+++	30–45	3–5	
Terbutaline	Bricanyl	MDI	++++	10–30	4–6	Can cause tremor
	Brethine	Tablets	++++	120–150	5–6.5	
		Injection	++++	30–45	2–4	Can cause tachycardia
	Breathaire	Nebulizer	++++	10–30	4–6.5	
Albuterol	Ventolin	MDI	++++	30–60	4–6	Fewer side effects
(Salbutamol)	Proventil	Nebulizer	++++	30–60	4–6	
		Rotocaps	++++	30–60	4–6	Inhaled powder
		Tablets	++++	120–180	6–8	
Bitolterol	Tornalate	MDI	++++	60–90	6–8	Long-lasting
Pirbuterol	Maxair	MDI	++++	30–60	5–6	

Long lasting beta-adrenergic						
Salmeterol	Serevent	MDI	+++++	120–180	12	Longest-lasting; use as maintenance drug
Anticholinergic						
Ipratropium bromide	Atrovent	MDI	++++	60–90	2–4	More effective than beta-agonists in some patients.
Combination bronchodilator						
Ipratropium bromide + albuterol	Combivent	MDI	++++	30–90	3–5	More effective than ipratropium or albuterol alone

MDI = metered dose inhaler

Beta-2 Specific Stimulating Drugs

Happily, though, it turns out that there is more than one type of beta-receptor. Beta-1 receptors are abundant in the heart, and activating them causes the heart to beat more quickly and forcefully. Beta-2 receptors are the primary ones in the airways, and their activation causes bronchodilation. Pharmaceutical research is now looking for cardiac medication that blocks beta-1 receptors—to prevent the heart from beating too fast—and has no effect on beta-2 receptors. The goal for bronchodilator drugs is potent beta-2 stimulation with minimal beta-1 action.

Currently, there are six major "beta-2 selective" bronchodilators available. Although they vary in potency and duration of action, they all last longer than isoproterenol and their cardiac effects are less pronounced. Five have been available for a while. They are *isoetharine, metaproterenol, terbutaline, albuterol* (known as *salbutamol* everywhere except in the United States), and *bitolterol.* The sixth—*salmeterol*—has recently become available in the United States. Studies comparing it to the earlier five indicate that it is even more beta-2 selective, more potent, and longer-acting. Although it takes longer to reach its maximum bronchodilation effect, it lasts for 12 hours—twice as long as the others. It's not a substitute for them, however. The current recommendation is to use salmeterol on a regular twice-a-day maintenance schedule, and use albuterol as a "rescue" drug to relieve an acute bronchospasm.

It has been observed that beta-2 receptors in airway muscle lose sensitivity after a patient begins using a beta-stimulator drug. This explains the noticeably decreased effectiveness of these drugs over the first several weeks of use. After this initial change, though, response to the drug becomes relatively stable. This sensitivity loss is the body's attempt to reduce what it perceives as overstimulation of the beta-receptors. It reacts by actually decreasing their number. We are not aware, though, of any studies that suggest increasing the dosage of beta-2 stimulating drugs to counter this loss of sensitivity. (The long-term implications of this phenomenon for the patient are not yet clear.)

Administration   The effectiveness of these drugs is partly determined by how they are taken: orally, by injection, or by inhalation. Inhalation—which is the most common—has two big advantages: (1) because the drug is deposited directly in the airways, less of the drug is needed for a given result than when it has to be distributed throughout the body to reach the airways; and (2) because less of the drug travels throughout the body, the side effects are lessened. But inhalation also has two disadvantages: (1) because the drug lands primarily in the large airways, the dilation benefit is concentrated in the central airways; and (2) a severe respiratory obstruction prevents inhaled drugs from reaching obstructed airways (but oral and injected medication will, because they travel in the blood).

Side Effects The degree of side effects is determined by the amount of a drug that reaches organs other than the lungs. With the typical inhaled doses, side effects—aside from a rare case of local irritation from the propellant in the spray—are minimal. But with oral and injected medication, and with higher doses of inhaled drugs, side effects become more common.

Because selective beta-2 stimulators are only *relatively* selective, heart-rate increases from activated beta-1 receptors in the heart. Because of the relaxing effect on smooth muscle encircling the blood vessels, blood pressure may fall slightly and nasal congestion is sometimes aggravated (from relaxed blood vessels in the nose). Since these drugs do not reach the brain, effects on the central nervous system are slight. These effects—if they occur—include occasional restlessness, sense of apprehension, headache, and neurally induced muscle tremor.

Skeletal muscle tremors are a much more common side effect. Activation of the beta-2 receptors in these muscles causes tremors. This occurs with lower drug doses than the other side effects do, but it does not warrant concern from patient or physician. In fact, this tremor can be useful. Its occurrence is often a concrete indicator that an effective dose has been achieved. And the degree of tremor usually diminishes within a few weeks because the beta-2 receptors in these muscles lose sensitivity.

Interaction of Beta-2 Stimulators with Other Drugs

Theophylline Beta-2 stimulators and theophylline (a bronchodilating drug discussed in a section to follow) are often used together. In combination they act synergistically, meaning that the presence of each one makes the other more effective. Because of this synergistic action, the dose of each can be reduced when they are combined. And the combination often achieves greater bronchodilation than the higher dose of either drug alone, plus the lower doses make side effects less severe.

Cortico'steroids These anti-inflammatory drugs intensify beta-2 effects by raising beta-2 receptor sensitivity, possibly by increasing their numbers.

Monoamine Oxidase (MAO) Inhibitors These drugs are used in the medical treatment of severe emotional depression. Since they inhibit the enzyme that would otherwise destroy excess adrenaline, the concentration in the body of this natural beta-receptor stimulator becomes much greater than usual. Caution is advised in considering the use of oral beta-stimulators for COPD patients already taking MAO inhibitors because of possible intensification of cardiovascular effects from adding a synthetic beta-stimulator to an already high concentration of adrenaline.

Beta-Blocking Drugs   Beta-blockers (designed to inactivate beta-1 receptors) are increasingly popular for treating cardiovascular disorders. In sufficient doses, though, they block the effects of beta-2 stimulators. For the COPD patient who has developed a significant asthma component, the result can be dangerous. This strongly applies to the nonspecific beta-1 blockers (for example, *propranolol, nadolol, pindolol, timolol*), and somewhat less to the specific beta-1 blockers (for example, *metroprolol, atenolol*). Even when used as a topical eye medication (Timoptic) for the treatment of glaucoma (a potentially blinding eye disease), enough of the beta-blocking agent can be absorbed into the blood to cause clinically significant bronchospasm. When at all possible, every attempt should be made to exclude use of beta-blocking medication with COPD patients who have a significant asthma component.

   Note: Make it a rule to clear *any* medication—including over-the-counter drugs—with the doctor treating your COPD before you use them. This becomes especially important to remember if you are seeing more than one doctor, because then the chance increases of being on conflicting medications. Such common problems as anxiety, insomnia, indigestion, and hypertension require especially careful management to avoid discomfort or hazard from drug interactions.

Anticholinergic Drugs

The vagus nerve is the parasympathetic nervous system's pathway to the lungs. It affects airway muscle tone and mucus secretion. When the vagus nerve is stimulated, it releases *acetylcholine*, the cholinergic mediator. This mediator contracts the airway muscle and increases mucus production. Because this whole mechanism involves nerves, its effects are termed *neurally mediated.*

   These cholinergic mediator effects can be stopped by a drug that blocks the action of acetylcholine. *Atropine*, which we described in our historical survey of treatments, does just that. In fact, atropine inhalation was a standard asthma treatment until the 1930s, when the first crop of beta-stimulators (the general adrenaline imitators) rendered the side effects of atropine unacceptable. But though atropine was pushed off center stage, it never quite disappeared.

There is now new interest in anticholinergic bronchodilators spurred by two developments over the past 35 years. One is better understanding of the ways in which acetylcholine influences the diameter of healthy and diseased airways. Second has been development of effective atropine-like drugs that—unlike their parent—are not absorbed into the general circulation. Local administration (by inhalation) of these atropine-derived drugs means much smaller doses are needed, and therefore side effects are much gentler.

The most extensively studied atropine derivative, *ipratropium bromide*, has been available in the United States since the early 1980s as an MDI under the brand name Atrovent. COPD patients were among the first test subjects for this drug. Its action and side effects were compared to the two commonly used bronchodilators. Most studies found COPD patients more responsive to ipratropium bromide than to beta-adrenergic and theophylline bronchodilators, either alone or in combination.

The time span is different, though. One dose of a beta-stimulator takes less than 30 minutes to achieve the maximum amount of bronchodilation, but it lasts for only 3 to 4 hours. One dose of the anticholinergic drug takes from 30 minutes to 3 hours to achieve maximum bronchodilation, but the effects last for 4 to 8 hours.

A growing number of doctors now prescribe these two different bronchodilators together to provide the best of both worlds. Combining the beta-stimulator's rapid onset with the anticholinergic's long-lasting activity is more effective than using either one alone (and permits beta-stimulator dosage to be lowered). (Theophylline and steroids also increase the potency of anticholinergic drugs.)

At present, though, there is little evidence to tell us whether ipratropium bromide and the beta-stimulator should be taken one right after the other or separated by a brief interval, or in which order they should be used. Most doctors we spoke with in the metropolitan New York area have their patients inhale Atrovent 15 to 30 minutes before using their prescribed beta-adrenergic bronchodilator. European pharmaceutical companies' solution is the production of "combination inhalers," now available in the United States.

For COPD patients with an obvious asthma component, anticholinergic therapy is most effective with bronchospasm triggered by inhaled irritants (such as cold air and cigarette smoke), and in patients whose symptoms become worse during stress. It is also particularly effective for COPD patients whose major symptom is coughing. Ipratropium bromide works well with any age patient but is at its best with adults over 40.

The initial introduction of ipratropium bromide met with concern that it would produce side effects similar to those of atropine. Atropine's undesirable consequences appear at doses equal to, or just slightly above, those needed to produce bronchodilation. Of particular concern for COPD patients are the severe inhibition of airway mucus secretion and mucociliary transport. Also, atropine is contraindicated—warned against—in two conditions common in elderly patients: narrow-angle glaucoma and obstruction of the bladder's neck.

But this early concern was unfounded. Because so little inhaled ipratropium bromide crosses into the blood, side effects are almost nonexistent. Studies in asthmatic and chronic bronchitis patients taught us that ipratropium bromide does not substantially affect mucus production or consistency even with larger than normal doses. And inhaling four times the recommended dose does not increase intraocular pressure (a major worry with glaucoma's already dangerously increased pressure within the eye) or weaken the bladder muscle that maintains urinary continence.

In summary: ipratropium bromide is a safe, well-tolerated bronchodilator. Although with asthma it is less potent than beta-stimulators, in chronic bronchitis and emphysema it is usually equal or greater in potency.

Use and Care of Metered-Dose Inhalers

Beta-stimulators (as well as anticholinergic and steroid drugs) can be inhaled as an aerosol using a *metered-dose inhaler* (*MDI*). This is a hand-held, pressurized cartridge type of device in which the drug is either carried in a propellant gas (such as freon), or turned into a spray by passing a stream of air over a solution containing the drug. The MDI's advantages are its easy portability and its ability to deliver a fixed dose of medicine. Its disadvantage is the degree of coordination needed to get the most effective amount of medicine into the lungs. This means that anyone who has difficulty coordinating complex maneuvers cannot use this technique effectively. (Then a home nebulizer should be used. This larger unit does not require any dexterity. Patients simply breathe their medicine from it for several minutes.)

Another frequent handicap to using an MDI effectively is not knowing the proper technique. *This is the proper way to use a hand-held MDI* (also look at Figure 9.2): hold the device right in front of your *open* mouth. Do not close your lips tightly around the mouthpiece no matter what the written instructions say! Then blow out all the air that you can, and depress the MDI—which automatically releases the right amount of medicine—as you start breathing in. Slowly keep the inhalation going (think of slowly sipping hot soup from a big spoon). Then hold your breath for 10 seconds. Then slowly breathe out.

No matter how good you are at using an MDI, though, most of the medicine ends up on the back of your throat—perhaps as much as 90%. It is absorbed through the surface of the mouth and throat instead of reaching the lungs directly. One reason for this is that the medicine jets out too fast. An *ineffective* solution to this problem is holding the MDI one or two inches away from your mouth. This just makes coordination harder.

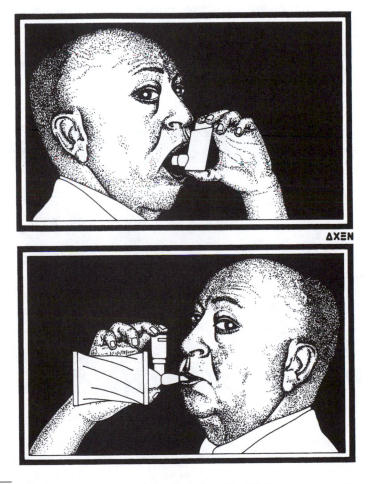

Figure 9.2 How to use a metered-dose inhaler. *Top:* Without a spacer. *Bottom:* With a spacer.

What we find really helps is to use a *spacer* between the MDI and your mouth. A spacer is simply a tube about three inches long and about two inches wide. Because it slows the speed at which the medicine travels before it enters your mouth, evaporation makes the aerosol droplets smaller and so able to penetrate deeper into the lungs. This kind of aid has been shown to deposit more of the medicine in the lungs more effectively.

Several companies build a spacer into their steroid MDI. Rorer Pharmaceuticals, Inc. (in Miami, Florida), distributes Inspirease (Figure 9.2), an add-on device that can be used with any MDI. The Inspirease is an inflatable plastic bag with a reed-containing mouthpiece that whistles if you inhale too quickly. The medicine is released into the inflated bag, and you inhale from the bag slowly enough to keep the whistle from blowing. After holding your breath for ten seconds, you exhale back into the bag. (Repeat the procedure if more than one puff is needed.)

Unfortunately, the patients we have spoken to complain that these commercial aids break too easily. They may be most appropriate, then, for those who need an easily portable inhaler but have difficulty mastering the use of an MDI without such an aid.

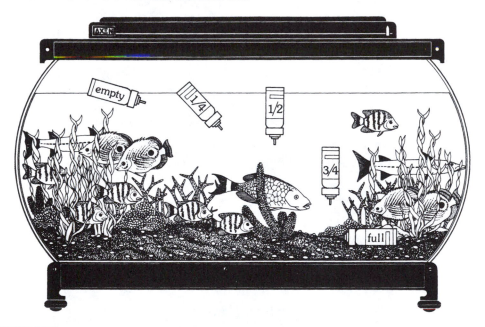

Figure 9.3   Checking how much medicine remains in a metered-dose inhaler. Drop the *canister only* in a *glass of clean water. Empty:* it floats on top. *Partially full:* it floats submerged. *Full:* it sinks to the bottom. (Note: Use a glass, not a fish tank. The fish tank was used in this illustration strictly to add a touch of humor.)

A practical problem in using an MDI is not knowing when it is almost empty and your prescription needs renewing. There is a way! Place your MDI cartridge—the part containing the medicine—in a glass of water (Figure 9.3). If the MDI sinks, it is full; if it floats fully submerged, it is three-quarters full; if the bottom breaks the top of the water, it is one-half full; if more shows, it is one-quarter full; and if it floats horizontally, it is empty.

The dispenser in which the MDI cartridge fits should be cleaned periodically. One technique involves an initial cleaning with liquid detergent and hot water, then soaking the dispenser for 30 minutes in a solution that is one-half water and one-half white vinegar. Dry with a towel afterwards. The tip of the MDI cartridge should simply be rinsed in hot running water after each day of use.

Theophylline

Theophylline has fallen out of favor since the earlier edition of this book. Scientific opinion now sees only marginal bronchodilating effects in COPD, in addition to the difficulty of maintaining effective levels in the blood without encountering potentially toxic side effects. Many physicians, however, still prescribe the various forms of this drug. Some focus on research suggesting possible benefit to the respiratory muscles, some physicians like the experience their patients tend to have on this drug, and for others, it's simply become a habit. Consequently, we decided to retain the section on theophylline just in case your physician advocates it. This will help you discuss it, and make your own informed decision about taking it.

Theophylline is a drug chemically similar to caffeine. Caffeine, as we know, is found in coffee and tea, and is added to most cola beverages. Both theophylline and caffeine belong to the class of chemicals called *methylated xanthines.* They stimulate skeletal muscles, the central nervous system, and the heart. They relax smooth muscles, especially the airway muscles. Both theophylline and caffeine are an effective diuretic. But the relative emphasis of their effects in different.

Caffeine is primarily a stimulant for skeletal muscles and the central nervous system. Theophylline is most potent as both a heart stimulant and a relaxer of smooth muscle. More recently, theophylline's ability to strengthen the diaphragm and reduce its fatigue has come to be appreciated. It has also been recently learned that theophylline stimulates mucociliary clearance of the airways, inhibits the release of mediators causing anaphylaxis (a life-threatening allergic reaction involving all bodily systems), and suppresses the edema that often accompanies asthma.

So theophylline holds two benefits for COPD patients even when there is no asthma component. For one, it helps get rid of mucus. This is a daily need for some COPD patients, while others need it only during respiratory infections. Theophylline also strengthens the diaphragm; our main inspiratory muscle. The COPD patient's normally hard-pushed respiratory muscles must labor far more intensively during an acute exacerbation. This can exhaust them, precipitating respiratory failure. But a strengthened diaphragm can resist this extreme, possibly life-threatening, fatigue.

How Theophylline Works

For a long time, researchers thought they understood how theophylline works. They were confident that it simply maintained a high level of cAMP in the body by blocking the enzyme that would otherwise destroy it. This, in turn, would lower the amount of calcium available for smooth muscle cell contraction.

But more recent investigations have thrown serious doubt on this enzyme-blocking explanation, and also raised other possibilities. Some researchers believe theophylline may change the way in which calcium actually enters and leaves smooth muscle cells. Some think it may inhibit certain compounds—called prostaglandins—which are now tentatively implicated in some forms of asthma. Others suggestions have been raised as well. Now nothing is certain beyond acknowledging the complexity of the way in which theophylline produces bronchodilation.

Effective Dose Range

The beta-2 bronchodilators that we just finished discussing are effective over a relatively broad range of concentrations in the blood. But for theophylline, the range between effective and toxic doses is extremely narrow. With a concentration of less than ten milligrams of the drug for each liter of blood plasma, most patients receive little or no therapeutic value even though some side effects may occur. (An occasional patient, though, may benefit from these low doses.) Above 20 milligrams per liter of plasma, the drug is toxic. It can become life-threatening if the blood concentration is allowed to rise high enough beyond this.

A drug's concentration in your blood depends on how much of it is taken, how fast it is absorbed, which organs it enters, and how fast it is then removed (metabolized) from your blood. Several factors can dramatically alter this removal rate. Smokers—both tobacco and marijuana—remove theophylline twice as fast, on the average, as nonsmokers do. So smokers need a higher standard dosage to compensate for this rapid elimination. What you eat is also important. A high-protein, low-carbohydrate diet means that theophylline will be eliminated 25% faster than otherwise. And a low-protein, high-carbohydrate diet slows its removal by 25%. Although we don't yet know why, eating a charcoal-broiled steak also speeds up theophylline's removal!

Viral illness and certain medications also affect the rate at which theophylline is removed. These circumstances all require an appropriate dosage change. Theophylline's removal rate is slowed by: fever from viral infections, drugs used for heart disease (such as Inderal), some antibiotics (for example, *erythromycin*) and drugs used for some digestive tract problems (for example, *cimetidine* [Tagamet]). This rate is slightly increased by: intravenous use of isoproterenol (during severe asthma attacks), and *phenytoin* (Dilantin) or high doses of *phenobarbital* (a barbiturate) for convulsions. A slight increase in removal rate only becomes important if the blood concentration is already at the low end of the effective range.

A precise technique for accurately determining theophylline's concentration in a patient's blood (called *serum theophylline*) minimizes the chances of ineffective or toxic doses. But this means that—if you are using a theophylline preparation—the level of the drug in your blood must be monitored periodically, and additionally whenever your symptoms of airway obstruction become unexplainedly worse or symptoms of toxicity appear. *The only reliable information for warning your doctor of impending toxicity is the level of theophylline actually in your blood.*

Side Effects

Theophylline can produce a wide range of negative effects on a variety of organ systems. When a patient first starts using this drug, central nervous system stimulation and slight nausea or queasiness are a common experience. These effects usually disappear, though, as tolerance for the drug develops. At the higher therapeutic doses (and beyond), a racing heartbeat—called *tachycardia*—and heart palpitations are frequent.

Theophylline Overdose

When the dose level goes beyond 40 milligrams of theophylline per liter of blood plasma, the heart can lose its normal rhythm or stop altogether. The initial central nervous system effects are restlessness, irritability, and increased nausea. They can progress to severe insomnia, agitation, and vomiting, and culminate in convulsions and coma. Intestinal pain and diarrhea occur, and the kidneys increase urine production.

Prompt emergency treatment is essential after overdosing with theophylline. First, syrup of ipecac is given to induce profuse vomiting. Then the patient is given at least 30 grams of charcoal (an absorptive poison antidote) and 10 grams of sodium sulfate (a laxative).

Even low effective doses of theophylline can have grave consequences if a COPD patient also suffers from heart failure or liver dysfunction. These conditions slow the rate of theophylline removal to such a degree that low doses automatically become high ones. Then the intense side effects also seriously exacerbate the other medical condition.

Using Theophylline Effectively

Theophylline products exist in numerous forms (Table 9.2). A recent listing of all FDA-approved prescription drugs lists 126 different preparations that contain theophylline. This gives your doctor great flexibility if he needs to prescribe theophylline for you.

Selecting a theophylline product, and determining the best dose and time between doses, must integrate the patient's clinical needs, the absorption characteristics of different formulations, and the drug's removal rate in the particular patient. The dose and dose interval decided on, plus the rates of theophylline's absorption and removal, each affect the fluctuation of its concentration in the blood. For maximum benefit from the drug, the blood concentration must be maintained within the narrow therapeutic range around the clock. This means that the above four factors must be coordinated to keep fluctuations at a minimum.

Confusion has been created, though, by the rapid proliferation of sustained-release formulations and by manufacturers providing inconsistent dosage guidelines and inappropriate dose interval recommendations. The rate and extent of absorption differ between different slow-release formulations, and sometimes even between different doses of the same brand. (The absence of meaningful FDA regulation plus the promotion of generic drug substitution have only increased the difficulty.) The optimal theophylline formulation, dose, and dosage interval can only be determined via the patient's blood concentration measurements.

Once a patient has invested the time and money that this requires, he should continue using the brand that was finally decided upon. The generic equivalent is not equivalent when it comes to theophylline. Your doctor's prescriptions should always include the instruction: *Do not substitute.*

Understanding the relative strengths of different types of theophylline preparations is very important for the patient. A preparation's strength is determined by the actual amount of theophylline in it (called *anhydrous theophylline*). The amount of medicine that you take each time refers to the amount of your preparation, not the amount of anhydrous theophylline. So the identical dose of different preparation will not each give you the same amount of anhydrous theophylline. If your doctor changes your theophylline medication, don't be alarmed if your dose and/or dose interval are also changed.

For example, if you have been taking 400-milligram doses of a pure theophylline preparation and then switch to 400-milligram doses of a theophylline salt (for example, Choledyl), you would suddenly get only 256 milligrams of anhydrous theophylline per dose—one-half the previous amount. To get the same therapeutic benefits as you did with the pure theophylline preparation, you would have to take about 626 milligrams on the same schedule, or 315 milligrams twice as often.

Administration

Theophylline preparations basically fall into two groups: rapidly absorbed and slowly absorbed. The rapid absorption products—normally given intravenously—are usually used during an acute asthma attack. The sustained-release (or slow release) theophylline preparations are used for COPD maintenance therapy because they can be scheduled for longer intervals. They also reduce fluctuation in blood concentration, which in turn improves symptom control. And the longer dosage intervals result in better patient compliance.

The patient's drug removal rate must be accounted for in determining this interval. Patients with particularly rapid removal rates and a strong asthma component may have to take a sustained-release preparation every 8 hours instead of every 12 to prevent symptoms from breaking through before the next dose. COPD/asthma patients with particularly slow rates can control their symptoms adequately with one dose every 24 hours.

Slow-release theophylline products are given by mouth, usually in a tablet or a bead-filled capsule. The beads can be sprinkled on soft food (for example, applesauce or yogurt) for people who find tablets difficult to swallow. If you prefer a liquid syrup (which is generally for children, despite the extremely bitter taste), your prescription should state the dose in milligrams. And ask your pharmacist to give you a measuring device to use that will ensure accurate dosage.

Table 9.2 Commonly Used Sustained-Release Theophylline Preparations

Brand Name	Distributor	Manufacturer	Remarks
Bronkodyl	Breon	Cord Labs	300 mg capsules
Choledyl SA	Park Davis	Warner-Lambert	400 and 600 mg tablets equivalent to 256 and 364 mg theophylline, respectively
Constant-T	Ciba-Geigy	Cord Labs	200 and 300 mg tablets scored for fractional doses
Elixophylline SR	Berlex	Cord Labs & K-V Labs	125, 250, and 500 mg capsules
Quibron T/SR (Dividose)	Mead Johnson	Central Pharmaceuticals	130, 260 mg capsules
Quibron bid	Mead Johnson	Central Pharmaceuticals	130, 260 mg capsules
Respid	Boehringer-Ingelheim	Riker Labs	250, 500 mg scored tablets
SloBid Gyrocaps	Rorer	Rorer	100, 200, 300 mg capsules, long-acting dye-free beads
Slophylline	Rorer	Cord Labs	60, 125, 250 mg capsules, long-acting dye-free beads
Somophyllin CRT	Fisons	Graham	50, 100, 250 mg capsules
Sustaire	Roerig	Key Pharmaceuticals	100, 300 mg scored tablets

Theobid	Glaxo	K-V Labs	130, 260 mg capsules
Theodur LA	Central	Central Pharmaceuticals	130, 260 mg capsules
TheoDur	Key	Key Pharmaceuticals	100 mg tablets and 200, 300 mg scored tablets
TheoDur Sprinkles	Key	Key Pharmaceuticals	50, 75, 125, 200 mg capsules; capsules are opened and medication is sprinkled on food
Theolair-SR	Riker	Riker	250, 500 mg scored tablets
Theon 300	Bock Pharm	Central Pharmaceuticals	130, 260 mg capsules
Theophyl-SR	Johnson and Johnson	Cord Labs	125, 250 mg capsules
Theophylline anhydrous TD	Stayner	Central Pharmaceuticals	130, 260 mg capsules
Theospan SR Laser	Laser	Central Pharmaceuticals	130, 260 mg capsules
Theo-24	Searle	GD Searle	100, 200, 300 mg capsules; one dose/day for some patients
Theovent	Schering	K-V Labs	125, 250 mg capsules
Uniphyl	Purdue-Frederick	Perdue-Frederick Labs	200, 400 mg scored tablets designed for one-a-day dosing

Interactions with Other Drugs

Beta-2 Stimulator   The first type of interaction to consider is the synergistic reaction when theophylline is teamed with a beta-2 stimulator. Theophylline is certainly an important drug for patients with advanced COPD because of its help in clearing mucus and strengthening the diaphragm. At the same time, its bronchodilating effects counter any tendency toward the asthmatic's hyperreactive airways. But some COPD patients with a substantial asthma component may find that theophylline alone cannot satisfactorily control their asthma symptoms. Then a beta-2 stimulator is added to their "menu." We have already mentioned that giving these two asthma drugs together means the effective dose of each can be lowered, which then reduces the risk of side effects. This is particularly helpful when the optimum theophylline dose otherwise needed for maximum bronchodilation is above the nontoxic range.

Drugs Affecting Theophylline's Removal   A different type of drug interaction involving theophylline occurs when another medication that the patient is taking changes theophylline's removal rate. See the earlier section on "Effective Dose Range" for a listing of the kinds of drugs that slow this rate down or speed it up.

Theophylline's Effects on Other Drugs   In two cases, theophylline alters the effect of another drug. *Phenytoin*—an anticonvulsant—seems weakened when it is taken together with theophylline. *Lithium*—taken to control manic-depressive psychosis—is eliminated from the patient's system much more quickly. Because researchers are not yet sure whether it is only the initial simultaneous dose(s) or each individual dose that acts so dramatically, lithium blood levels should be monitored regularly whenever a patient is also using a theophylline preparation.

10

The Rest of the COPD Drugs

The previous chapter discussed the various bronchodilators used in treating COPD. This chapter presents the other appropriate COPD medications: corticosteroids to reduce airway inflammation; antibiotics and vaccination to control respiratory infections; cough suppressant medications; and mucolytics and expectorants for mucus. Before ending, we highlight promising experimental drugs.

Caution: Whenever your doctor prescribes a new medication, it's very helpful to ask your doctor—or pharmacist—if there are any foods that interact with it. Scientists are continuously learning more and more about food-drug interactions. (As an example: grapefruit alters the amount in your blood of certain drugs—increasing some, decreasing others.)

Corticosteroids

Steroids and Respiratory Disease

Natural corticosteroids—usually simply called *steroids*—are hormones produced in the body by the outer layers (the cortex) of the adrenal glands, which are located on the kidneys. These hormones are essential to life. They play a critical role in such diverse bodily processes as energy metabolism, kidney function, and the immune system.

The corticosteroids fall into two groups. One of them—called the *glucocorticoids* for their effect on glucose (a kind of sugar) metabolism—has strong anti-inflammatory properties. When we talk about *steroids* in relation to COPD, we are really referring to this particular group of steroids.

Soon after the glucocorticoid hormones were synthesized in the laboratory and their dramatic anti-inflammatory characteristics identified, they were brought into the treatment of asthma, a chronic respiratory disease. In the early 1950s, steroids revolutionized life for many asthmatics whose symptoms responded poorly to the other drugs then available. Instead of being incapacitated by their disease, their symptoms suddenly disappeared and their dependence on other forms of treatment lessened.

But the unexpectedly high price paid for this miracle soon became obvious. The catalogue of far-ranging side effects included many that were extremely serious: for example: poor wound healing, loss of calcium from the bones, severe stomach bleeding, psychosis, and stunted growth in children. The use of steroids in asthma was rejected about ten years after they were first introduced.

Now the situation in regard to asthma has changed again. A deeper and more objective understanding of steroids' therapeutic effects has clearly established them as a first-line drug in controlling this respiratory disease. The new inhaled steroids greatly lessen side effects. And advances in our understanding of the body's response to steroids have led to auxiliary techniques that also help in minimizing side effects.

The use of steroids in COPD, however, is unresolved. Those supporting it feel that the same anti-inflammatory properties so important in managing severe asthma can also help chronic bronchitis patients. There are two potential situations for adding steroids to the drug regimen of a COPD patient with a substantial chronic bronchitis component. One involves intravenous steroids during hospitalization for a temporary worsening. The other would add oral or inhaled steroids to the regular medication menu of a stable patient.

The first scenario—intravenous steroid use to bring the patient more quickly through acute episodes and minimize the increase in blood gas imbalance—has not yet been adequately examined. But there is a reliable study demonstrating steroids' benefits in bringing patients through the acute respiratory failure that exacerbations can provoke. Although this does not warrant adopting intravenous steroids as a regular therapy for acute episodes, it certainly underscores their value for patients who are not responding to standard therapy.

The use of steroids by stable COPD patients has, by contrast, been thoroughly evaluated. Most reliable studies find steroids effective for only a minority of patients. But the lack of any means for predicting which patients will benefit prevents specific recommendations. The general sense, however, is that steroids should be tried for all patients with very severe airflow obstruction (that is, their FEV_1 is only 1 to 1.5 liters).

The following example indicates how a two-week steroid trial should be conducted. For two to three months before starting medication, FEV_1 is measured several times. After two weeks of medication, the patient's

FEV_1 is measured again. If it is not at least 25% larger than the best pre-steroid value, discontinue steroids. But if the patient's airflow is significantly improved, then continue treatment. Taper the dosage to the lowest one that works. Discontinue using steroids periodically to see if the patient still needs them to do his best.

How Steroids Work

Steroid production is controlled by the body's master gland, the pituitary, via its secretion of *adrenocorticotrophic hormone* (*ACTH*). The pituitary releases ACTH into the bloodstream, which brings it to the adrenal glands. The arrival of ACTH at the adrenal cortex is its signal to immediately manufacture and release steroids. (Their release then temporarily stops any further release of ACTH.)

Steroids are produced in their greatest amounts shortly after waking up. They are lowest during sleep, with the lowest production of all usually between 2 A.M. and 4 A.M. (As we will see, this diurnal variation must be kept in mind when steroid drugs are prescribed.) The amount of steroids normally produced at any given time of the day or night can be increased by stress.

Steroids work along two different avenues simultaneously. Their action is rapid by one route, and slower by the other. The net effect is that steroids inhibit the release and further formation of the body's inflammatory chemicals.

Steroids also prevent the initial decrease in beta-receptor sensitivity that otherwise happens when beta-stimulating bronchodilators are used. In addition, some investigators feel that steroids directly relax airway muscle, inhibit bronchoconstricting cholinergic mechanisms, increase mucociliary activity, and decrease mucus production.

Using Steroids

Because of the side effects that must be dealt with, though, steroids should only be added to your drug regimen if the highest tolerable doses of all other available medications cannot control your symptoms adequately. And they should be discontinued—or at least reduced—as soon as it is appropriate to do so.

When during the day you take your steroid preparation, and how much you take, are extremely important in minimizing an otherwise critical side effect. Remember that the natural production of steroids temporarily cuts off the pituitary gland's production of ACTH. And until ACTH starts up again, no further steroids are produced.

Steroid drugs participate in this negative feedback cycle because the pituitary gland does not distinguish between natural and synthetic steroids. So when you start taking a steroid drug, the pituitary gland immediately decreases or stops its production of ACTH. This means that the adrenal glands decrease or stop producing steroids. Your body's own source of steroids temporarily dries up, so to speak. But this effect will be minimized if your dose schedule is properly dovetailed with your body's natural steroid-production rhythm. Taking steroids in the morning—which is the high point of ACTH production—interferes the least with the adrenal glands' natural activity.

Only minor interference occurs when steroid therapy lasts for just a few days—and this disappears rapidly as soon as the drug is stopped. Natural steroid suppression is greater, and lasts longer, as both dose level and length of therapy increase. (No one is sure, though, at exactly what drug dosage such suppression begins.) After a relatively short course of steroid medication, it takes about three days for the adrenal glands to resume their normal steroid activity. But if steroid treatment lasts for months or years, it may take six months or more before the adrenal glands are functioning normally again.

Because there is always a time gap between ending steroid treatment and the body's resumption of its own steroid production, the drug should never be ended abruptly. It should be tapered off little by little as the adrenal glands gradually regain their capacity to produce the amount of steroids normally needed.

Only several days are needed to taper off after a relatively short, low-dose treatment. But as dose and/or length increase, the tapering-off time becomes proportionately longer.

Short-term steroid therapy consists of one dose each morning for four to ten days. If longer treatment is needed, one dose is taken only every other morning. But if symptoms start to break through, then a daily morning dose must be tried. If symptoms still reappear between doses, the only alternative left is taking several doses spread over the day. This should be changed to one of the less frequent schedules as soon as symptom control improves.

Administration

Steroids can be taken orally or by injection, or by using an MDI to deliver them directly to the airways. Since an inhaled steroid penetrates into the lungs most effectively when the airways are dilated, it should be used 5 to 15 minutes after an inhaled bronchodilator.

Oral preparations are used far more often than injected steroids (see Table 10.1). The most common oral steroids are *prednisone, prednisolone,* and *methylprednisolone*. Because prednisone is changed to prednisolone once the body metabolizes it, some experts feel that using prednisolone or methylprednisolone to start with makes it easier to predict the blood concentration of this drug that a particular dose will achieve. Methylprednisolone may also have better inflammatory properties than the other two, and it definitely causes less salt retention. (Salt increase in the body can raise blood pressure.)

Using inhaled steroids dramatically reduces the frequency and severity of side effects. This is in part the nature of an inhaled drug, and partly because—for patients with asthma—inhaled steroids clearly help reduce the need for oral forms of the drug. *For COPD patients in general, though, the few studies evaluating inhaled steroids show even fewer predictable benefits than oral steroids produce.* In a recent study that followed stable COPD patients for 4 weeks of inhaled steroid treatment, only 25% of the overall group showed some degree of improvement, but 75% of those patients who also had a strong asthma component improved. *Although some doctors now prescribe inhaled steroids to all their advanced COPD patients, this should really be done only for the patient who also has a strong asthma component.*

The available inhaled steroid preparations (see Table 10.2) are *beclomethasone dipropionate* (Vanceril and Beclovent), *triamcinolone acetonide* (Azmacort), and *flunisolide* (Aerobid).

Interactions with Other Drugs

Drugs That Affect Steroids Certain drugs change the rate at which steroid drugs are removed from the body. Steroids are metabolized more quickly when they are taken together with *barbiturates, ephedrine,* and *rifampin* (a type of antibiotic). Steroids are metabolized more slowly when they are used at the same time as *estrogen,* certain other *antibiotics,* and the anti-allergy medication *cromolyn sodium* (although this effect is slight). In another type of effect, *indocin* (used in treating arthritis) increases steroids' potential for causing stomach ulcers.

Drugs Affected by Steroids Steroids also affect other drugs. As we pointed out earlier, they enhance the action of *beta-stimulating bronchodilators* by preventing the beta-receptors from becoming less sensitive. Caution should be used when diabetic asthmatics use steroids, because they can dangerously reduce the action of the *oral hypoglycemic* medication many diabetics depend on. Taking steroids along with *potassium-depleting diuretics* increases the risk of dangerously lowering the body's potassium level. This in turn also increases the likelihood of toxicity for

Table 10.1 ORAL GLUCOCORTICOIDS IN COMMON USE

Drug	Brand Name	Remarks
Hydrocortisone (cortisol)	Generic Cortef TM Hydrocort	All are short acting (8–12 hrs), with limited anti-inflammatory potency and significant salt-retaining potency.
Cortisone	Generic	Same as hydrocortisone, except slightly less anti-inflammatory potency than hydrocortisone.
Prednisone	Generic	Intermediate-acting drugs (12–30 hrs). Compared to hydrocortisone, they have 3.5 to 4 times the anti-inflammatory potency and a much reduced salt-retaining potency.
Methylprednisolone	Medrol	Five times the anti-inflammatory potency of hydrocortisone with negligible salt-retaining potency.
Triamcinolone	Aristocort Tab	Similar to methylprednisolone in effect, and somewhat longer lasting (12–48 hrs).
Betamethasone	Celestone Tab	This long-acting corticosteroid (48–54 hrs) has 25 times the anti-inflammatory potency of hydrocortisone and no salt-retaining potency.
Dexamethasone	Decadron	Similar to betamethasone, but with slightly higher anti-inflammatory potency.

Table 10.2   INHALED GLUCOCORTICOSTEROIDS

Preparation	Brand Name	Remarks
Budenoside	Pulmicort Turbuhaler	The most potent of the inhaled glucocorticosteroids.
Beclomethasone dipropionate (BDP)	Beclovent Vanceril Vanceril DS	60% of the relative potency of budenoside.
Triamcinolone	Azmacort	35% of the relative potency of budenoside. Comes with its own spacer.
Flunisolide	Aero Bid	Similar potency as Azmacort.

heart patients taking any of the *cardiac glycosides* (a group of heart medications that includes *digitalis*).

Side Effects with Long-Term Use

The exact nature and degree of these problems are determined by a variety of factors. These include each patient's individual biological reaction to steroids, the particular steroid preparation used, dosage size and schedule, and the use—or lack—of measures to counter specific effects.

The single most important side effect of inhaled steroids is thrush, which is a yeast infection in the mouth. It has occurred in up to 77% of oral steroid users. Large doses, diabetes, poor dental hygiene, and the simultaneous use of antibiotics all increase this risk. It is extremely important to gargle and rinse your mouth carefully with water after each inhaled dose.

The milder negative effects from all systemic steroids (referring to oral or injected preparations, because they travel throughout the body system) include increased appetite, some facial bloating, and acne. Moderate effects include leg cramps, insomnia, headaches, and unexplained mood changes.

The group of serious side effects includes such hazards as: skeletal muscle weakness (which responds to exercise); poor wound healing (countered by meticulous wound care plus vitamin A supplements); poor control of diabetes (countered by increasing the insulin or oral hypoglycemic agent); suppressed adrenal glands (countered by increasing steroid doses during stress); weakened immune response (countered by meticulous surveillance for infection); potassium loss (countered with potassium supplements); calcium loss from bones (minimized with calcium + vitamin D supplements and exercise). People who are susceptible to diabetes risk increasing the likelihood that they will develop it.

Stomach ulcers, gastric hemorrhage, intestinal tears, pancreatitis, cataracts, high blood pressure, and psychosis all require more sophisticated medical attention. And for COPD patients who already suffer from any one of these conditions, steroid drugs should be completely avoided if at all possible.

Antibiotics and Airway Infections

COPD patients are more susceptible to respiratory infections, and vulnerable to severe consequences from them. Frequent unchecked lung infections can accelerate pulmonary destruction in all these patients, and precipitate a life-threatening crisis in advanced cases. So it is critical for

COPD patients to protect themselves against airway infections. *Avoidance* measures (which are outlined in Chapter 15) minimize their number. *Control* measures—meaning the most effective use of antibiotics—minimize the impact of those airway infections that can't be prevented.

Arrival of a chest infection is always heralded by warning signs: malaise, easier fatigability, worsening dyspnea, fever, nasal congestion, increased coughing combined with more difficult expectoration (clearing the mucus out) as the mucus becomes yellow or green and much more viscous. These infections are typically caused by certain bacteria (*Haemophilus influenza, Streptococcus pyogenes, Diplococcus pneumonia, Klebsiella pneumonia*) and/or viruses (*influenza, adenovirus, respiratory syncytial virus*).

Because these airway infections are a major cause of exacerbated symptoms for a COPD patient—especially one with substantial chronic bronchitis—it is critical to control them. This is done with appropriate medication. *Antibiotics*—also called *antimicrobials*—is the general term for agents used to treat infection. Since microbes come in two different kinds, so do antibiotics: *antibacterial* and *antiviral*. In common use, though, people interchange *antibiotic* and *antibacterial*. We will adopt this habit, applying *antibiotic* only to antibacterial drugs.

The History of Antibiotics and Respiratory Infection

The very first drug used to treat pulmonary infections were the *sulfonamides*. The German dye industry actually developed them, at the turn of the century, in its search for better colorfastness. The sulfonamides were highly successful dyes because they bonded to wool and silk proteins. Some observant medical researchers of the day wondered if these new dyes might also react with bacterial proteins. The first medical report on the sulfonamides, in 1913, found them effective against pneumococcal and staphylococcal bacteria.

In 1928, London scientist Alexander Fleming accidentally discovered that something in the common greenish-colored *Penicillium notatum* mold kills bacteria. Eleven years later at Oxford, H. W. Florey finally isolated the actual "bactericidal" substance from this mold. Although the yield from this process was tiny, he eventually accumulated enough penicillin to treat a patient desperately ill with staphylococcal and streptococcal infections. The patient lived.

The decades since Florey first used penicillin to save a life have seen proliferation in two related directions. On the one hand, bacteria have shown that they can alter the aspect of their structure that is vulnerable to a particular antibiotic. So bacterial strains now exist that are resistant to all but the newest drugs. Also, as pharmaceutical companies continue their battle to regain the forefront, they are coming up with both new types of antibiotics and improved versions of older ones.

COPD and Antibiotic Use

You should start your prescribed antibiotic *quickly*—no more than 24 hours after you first notice the early signals of a chest infection: a lot more coughing and mucus, with mucus becoming yellow to green. So call your doctor right away. (Don't delay because you fear not having an infection and wasting his time. If you have chosen your doctor well, he prefers risking a few minutes of his time over the consequences to you of failing to control a respiratory infection.) Then follow your doctor's instructions for letting him know your progress—or lack of improvement—and for taking your medication.

As long as there is no reason to switch your antibiotic, your doctor will have you take it for one week to ten days. But if your infection does not improve quickly, most likely the bacteria causing it is not highly vulnerable to this antibiotic. Your doctor will prescribe a different antibiotic, and he may also send a sample of your sputum to the pathology laboratory for "culture and sensitivity" tests. "Culturing" the bacteria in your sputum means growing them until the different bacterial groups, or colonies, become large enough to be identified under the microscope. "Sensitivity" testing determines the antibiotic(s) most lethal to these particular bacteria. These tests take time, yet you must continue taking an antibiotic. So your doctor will combine knowledge and instincts to choose an alternative, revising this choice only if necessary once the results are in.

Several types of antibiotics effectively subdue the COPD patient's typical lung infections: the main ones are the *penicillins*—also called *beta-lactams* (such as Ampicillin), the *macrolides* (such as Biaxin), the *cephalosporins* (such as Keflex), the *fluoroquinolones* (such as Cipro), and the compound antibiotic *trimethoprim-sulfamethoxazole* (called Bactrim or Septra). Each type of antibiotic attacks bacteria in a different way.

Although antibiotics can have side effects, they are usually minimal. The most common is some degree of stomach discomfort and/or diarrhea. A small amount of food (crackers are excellent) along with each pill can calm a distressed stomach for some. Diarrhea can occur because bactericidal drugs often destroy helpful as well as dangerous microbes. This includes friendly bacteria that live in our large intestine and regulate the consistency of our bowel movements. Yogurt, however, contains these same helpful bacteria if it hasn't been cooked at too high a temperature. So a daily portion of bacteria-containing yogurt for the duration of antibiotic therapy usually minimizes or stops diarrhea. In fact, many doctors now instruct their patients to add yogurt to their diet as soon as they begin an antibiotic. It is critical, though, to choose a brand of yogurt that states "live cultures" clearly on the container. Most such brands contain one or two of the bacteria your intestines need. At the writing of this book, the best brand for this purpose is *Stoneyfield*, which contains six.

Note: Your stomach contents can interfere with antibiotic absorption into your system. Try to schedule meals, milk, and/or antacid use to come at least one hour after taking an antibiotic dose, or two hours before. If you are unsure about this food-medication separation for a particular antibiotic, check with your pharmacist. If your eating pattern makes it difficult to coincide antibiotic medication with an adequately empty stomach, let your doctor know. He may be able to prescribe an equally effective antibiotic that does not require an empty stomach.

It is important for those of you who take theophylline to know that some antibiotics will slow its removal. Ask your doctor about this possibility if he prescribes an antibiotic that you have not taken before. If you ever do find yourself having to take an antibiotic that is going to increase the theophylline level in your blood, be alert for early signs of theophylline toxicity: irritability, restlessness, nausea. If they appear, *do not* take your next theophylline dose; *do* call your doctor immediately.

You may not initially recognize these theophylline toxicity symptoms. But as they intensify to severe insomnia, agitation and vomiting, it becomes difficult to mistake them for anything benign. *Do not* take your next theophylline dose. *Do* get immediate medical help. If your doctor is unavailable, go to the emergency room at the hospital where he is affiliated.

Antiviral Drugs and Airway Infections

The emergence of antiviral drugs is very recent. Their development has lagged way behind antibacterial antibiotics, but not for lack of concern. Both the structure and tiny size of viruses make them far more difficult than bacteria to destroy. But now that a start has been made, many more antiviral antibiotics are expected in the next several years as a spinoff of the tremendous effort in developing drugs to kill the AIDS virus.

Amantadine and rimantadine—the two antiviral drugs currently available—can lessen a viral infection's severity. So some doctors prescribe one or the other whenever a COPD patient catches a cold (or flu, if the annual vaccination was neglected).

Your doctor may regularly put you on an antibacterial antibiotic even when you are clearly ill with a cold or flu. This is precautionary. He is using it prophylactically, taking care to prevent a bacterial infection from settling in while your immune system is occupied fighting your viral infection.

Anticough Medication

One of the most common complaints among COPD patients is a constant, highly irritating—to themselves and others—cough that does not even provide the satisfaction of bringing up much sputum. The cough is weak, but the sound isn't. It can be intolerable to companions by day. At night such a cough can disturb sleep—for both patient and spouse. So the benefits of suppressing such a miserably disturbing cough usually outweigh potential problems from over-the-counter (OTC) medications.

The biggest problems are not so much from the cough suppressant agent itself, but from other ingredients common to many cough medicines. These may include: an antihistamine (it can thicken sputum, making it even more difficult to bring up; it can depress the central nervous system, causing sleepiness and dizziness; it can slow the respiratory center); a drying agent (which also thickens sputum); a vasoconstrictor (which further narrows the lungs' blood vessels, adding to the heart's pumping effort); an expectorant (which increases mucus production).

Some doctors find a nonnarcotic cough suppressant acceptable as long as the lowest effective dose of the simplest formulation is used. This does not mean that you should decide on your own about using a cough medicine. You need to talk it over with your doctor, as the fine print on cough-medicine wrappers instructs. The most popular OTC anticough agent, *dextromethorphan*, is found in a number of brands and formulations (see Table 10.3). Some brands (for example, Romilar, Robitussin) label their dextromethorphan-only formulation *DM*. Others (for example, St. Joseph's) require you to read the fine print to learn the ingredients. Stay away from anything warning: "This product may make you sleepy or dizzy." That warning indicates ephedrine, pseudoephedrine, or one of the other sympathomimetic (adrenaline-like) agents.

In those particularly severe cases requiring a narcotic cough suppressant, *codeine* and *hydrocodone* are relatively safe when used according to your doctor's careful instructions. But keep in mind that these compounds can be potent respiratory center and central nervous system depressants. Immediately report any intrusive side effects—especially involving breathing—to your doctor immediately. The two strongest

Table 10.3 COMMON ANTICOUGH MEDICINES

Agent	Remarks
Codeine	Effective and most commonly used narcotic cough suppressant. Because it is a narcotic, and so can be habit forming, it requires a prescription.
Hydrocodone	Narcotic, requires a prescription.
Hydromorphone	—
Morphine	Powerful narcotic. Must be used with great care.
Benzonatate	Non-narcotic cough suppressant. Sold as Tessalon Perles, which must be swallowed. By prescription.
Caramiphen	Non-narcotic cough suppressant combined with antihistamine. Sold as Tuss-Ornade. By prescription.
Dextromethorphan	Non-narcotic, over-the-counter cough suppressant. The active ingredient in Delsym, DM cough, Romilar, and others.
Noscapin	Non-narcotic over-the-counter cough suppressant. Used in Tusscapin, for example.

narcotic suppressants—*morphine* and *hydromorphone*—should be used only in a closely supervised environment (meaning a hospital).

Coping with Mucus

COPD patients with a significant asthma component to their disease have a big problem with the heavy flow of thick bronchial mucus that typically accompanies their bronchospasm episodes. Because bronchospasm's temporary narrowing on top of COPD's permanent narrowing constricts their bronchi to an exceptional degree during these episodes, additional mucus blocks them very easily. We know that severely narrowed, obstructed airways weaken expiratory airflow. Then coughing is less effective in bringing this mucus up.

During an asthma attack, then, drugs that make this outpouring of thick mucus easier to expel are a major help. Over the years, a large number of pharmacologic agents have been tried in this regard. They are called *mucokinetic drugs.* The entire process of easing the mucus-clearing difficulty is called *mucokinesis.*

Several of the antiasthma drugs we already discussed are also somewhat mucokinetic: the beta-2 stimulators, theophylline, and the glucocorticoid steroids. Seven other kinds of drugs are devoted exclusively—with greater and lesser success—to mucokinesis.

1. *Antibiotics:* Mucus becomes thicker and stickier (more viscous) during an infection. Because antibiotics fight infection, they ensure a mucus that is less viscous, and therefore more easily cleared from the airways.

2. *Diluents:* Diluents work on the theory that increasing the water content of mucus—hydrating it—makes it less viscous. Hydration is a wise precaution for the COPD patient with asthma. Some diluents, such as water or a salt solution, can be administered directly into the airways with a nebulizer.

3. *Surfactants:* Surfactants act as a detergent or wetting agent, somewhat like dishwashing soap. Soap weakens the sticky hold of fats and food adhering to dirty dishes. Surfactants weaken the sticky hold of mucus adhering to the airway walls. *Sodium bicarbonate*, a surfactant, is delivered directly to the airways via aerosol.

4. *Bronchomucotropics:* Bronchomucotropics increase two things. One is the amount of mucus, the other is the amount of respiratory tract fluid that is secreted. Familiar examples are *eucalyptus* and *menthol,* the aromatic inhalants found in Vicks VapoRub. Although these products have an amazingly large following, there is no proof of their effectiveness. But since they have not been disproved either, we should not automatically equate lack of proof with lack of value. Any COPD patient with asthma who finds bronchomucotropics useful should not let himself be dissuaded from using them.

5. *Mucolytics:* These agents make mucus less viscous by breaking down mucus molecules. The most effective mucolytics are the amino acid *L-cysteine* and its derivative, *acetylcysteine.* This derivative is marketed in the United States as Mucomyst, and elsewhere as Airbron, Mucolyticum and Nac. This agent, however, may cause problems as well as solve them. Because the solution smells like a cross between rotting eggs and burning hair, the aerosol may be so irritating that it actually causes a bronchospasm.

   In the United States, enzymes—particularly *dornase*—have also been used to break down mucus molecules. Enzymes once had many proponents, but their value in treating asthma has never been satisfactorily demonstrated.

6. *Expectorants: Expectoration* means bringing up mucus from your airways. Expectorants are taken by mouth to produce a greater amount of mucus of a consistency that can be coughed up more easily (see

Table 10.4). Although expectorants were the mainstay of the nineteenth-century version of asthma therapy, there has been little hard evidence—until recently—that these drugs actually do increase an easily cleared mucus. The most effective expectorants may actually combine the characteristics of the bronchomucotropics and the mucolytics. This list includes *iodide, terpin hydrate*, and various salts, herbs, and plant derivatives.

7. *Mucoregulators:* Mucoregulators alter the action of the mucous glands so that they produce less viscous mucus. (These drugs may also affect the airways directly to reduce bronchospasm.) Many of the herbs and plants used in folk medicine have been studied in this context.

Table 10.4 COMMON ORAL EXPECTORANTS

Agent	Brand	Remarks
Guaifenesin	Breonesin, Robitussin, etc.	Over-the-counter
Ammonium salts	Variety of brands	Over-the-counter
Hydriodic acid	Hydriodic Acid Syrup	By prescription
Potassium iodide	Pima, SSKI	By prescription
Calcium iodide	Calcidrine	By prescription (contains morphine)
Iodinated glycerol	Organidine	By prescription
Sodium citrate	Tussar-2	By prescription (contains codeine and antihistamine)

Miscellaneous Mucokinetic Agents

A long list of items has been tried over the years in the continuing search for a good mucokinetic agent. Some continue in use although there is little, if any, proof of their effectiveness. Some run more risks than benefits, and many others have long ago fallen by the wayside.

But two items from Grandma's pharmacopoeia are still successful after hundreds of years. One is *garlic*. Folk tradition considers this potent herb of great value in treating asthma and bronchitis. And many formal pharmacopoeias throughout the world list garlic among the expectorants.

The primary component of garlic is the nonodiforous compound alliin (S-allyl-L-cysteine sulfoxide). When garlic is crushed, an enzyme breaks down the alliin into allicin, the aroma of which we all know. Interestingly, the alliin molecule bears a remarkable resemblance to S-carboxy-methylcysteine. Similar molecules exist in horseradish, radishes, onions, hot peppers, and mustard—all edibles that stimulate respiratory mucus production. Garlic, and other pungent herbs and spices, may act by stimulating mucus-producing vagus nerve reflexes. The odiforous component of garlic obviously leaves the body via the lungs, where it may have a local bronchomucoregulatory effect.

The second item—*hot chicken soup*—was first prescribed in writing centuries ago by Maimonides. His twelfth-century *Treatise on Asthma* contained his humble apology for not being able to cure the disease, plus his suggestion that "the soup of fat hens is (an) effective remedy." Chicken soup (also known as "Jewish penicillin" and "Bubbemycin") is a proven potent mucociliary stimulant. So it is reasonable to regard a pungent, peppery, garlic-laden, onion-enriched chicken broth to be the ultimate in mucokinesis. This is obviously the standard against which all potential candidates for the honor must be compared.

Experimental Emphysema Treatment

An intriguing study done with laboratory animals in 1997 raised the possibility that emphysema damage may be reversible with a treatment derived from vitamin A called *all-trans-retinoic-acid* (*ATRA*). The following year, very preliminary tests began with patients at UCLA. The results stimulated additional interest and support, and now the federal government—through the National Institutes of Health—is supporting a large-scale preliminary study that will be carried out in five centers across the United States. If the results are good, then a large controlled clinical trial will be mounted.

As of the writing of this book, recruitment of volunteers for this initial preliminary phase isn't expected to begin before May 2000 at the earliest. By the time you are reading this, that date will be in the past—but remember that these studies take time to conduct, and new volunteers are enrolled over an extended period of time. So if you are interested in participating in whatever phase of this study is currently in progress, call one of the contacts listed here to find out if they are still in the preliminary stage, or if a clinical trial is already under way.

Michael D. Roth, M.D.
Department of Medicine, Division of Pulmonary and Critical Care
UCLA School of Medicine, Los Angeles, CA
Contact: Carlena Leuffroy, 310-825-0759

Frank Sciurba, M.D.
Division of Pulmonary, Allergy and Critical Care Medicine
University of Pittsburgh, Pittsburgh, PA
Contact: Betsy George, 412-648-6388, then, press "2"

Neil W. Schluger, M.D.
Chief, Clinical Pulmonary Medicine
Columbia University, New York, NY
Contact: Pactricia Jellen, R.N., 212-305-1158

George T. O'Connor, M.D.
Pulmonary Center
Boston University Medical Campus, Boston, MA
Contact: Laura Agreda, 617-638-4479

Joe W. Ramsdell, M.D.
University of California, San Diego Medical Center, San Diego, CA
Contact: Arlene Yoffe, 619-543-7736

Stress and Anxiety Requiring Medication

Some COPD patients will need psychiatric care. And some of these individuals will need to take temporary or long-term medication—called *psychotropic,* or "mood-altering," drugs—to help control their symptoms. For some patients, in fact, this is the only workable alternative.

Because overdose of narcotics, sedatives, tranquilizers, and antidepressants continues as one of the most frequent causes of acute respiratory distress among COPD patients, *these drugs must be dispensed to them with particular caution* (see Tables 10.5–10.7). Dosage and schedule must be carefully individualized according to age, stage of the disease, any coexisting disease, and any previous reaction to a given medication. As a rule: the older the patient and/or the more intrusive his COPD symptoms and/or the more coexisting diseases he has, the lower the dose should be of the recommended psychopharmacological agent. (For severe COPD patients, for example, dosage should be one-third, or even less, than that prescribed for a healthy individual.)

Table 10.5 EXAMPLES OF ANTIDEPRESSANTS

Generic Name	Brand Name	Category
Amitriptyline	Elavil	Tricyclic
	Endep	
Doxepin HCl	Adapin	
	Sinequan	
Imipramine HCl	Tofranil	
Imipramine pamoate	Tofranil PM	
Desipramine	Norpramin	
	Pertofrane	
Nortriptyline	Aventyl	
	Pamelor	
Protriptyline	Vivactil	
Maprotiline	Ludiomil	Tetracyclic
Trazodone	Desyrel	
Amoxapine	Asendin	Dibenzoxapine

Side Effects		Precautions*
Dry mouth	Nausea	Cardiovascular disorder
Potential difficulty	Heartburn	Thyroid disease
handling secretions	Hypotension	Concurrent use of
Blurred vision	Sexual dysfunction	sympathomimetic amine
Constipation		drugs

*To be used with caution when any of these conditions exists.

Table 10.6 COMMON MINOR TRANQUILIZERS (ANTIANXIETY OR SEDATIVES)

Generic Name	Brand Name	Category
Chlordiazepoxide	Librium	Benzodiazepine
Diazepam	Valium	
Oxazepam	Serax	
Chlorazepate	Tranxene	
Alprazolam	Xanax	
Triazolam	Halcion	
Tremazepam	Restoril	
Flurazepam	Dalmane	
Lorazepam	Activan	
Lalazepam	Paxipam	
Hydroxyzine chloride	Atarax	Diphenylmethane
Hydroxyzine	Vistaril	
Buspirone	Buspar	Buspirone

Side Effects		Precautions*
Drowsiness	Blurred vision	Glaucoma
Ataxia	Dry mouth	Concurrent use of
Confusion	Potential difficulty	anticoagulant drugs
Slurred speech	handling secretions	Renal impairment
Headache	Sexual dysfunction	Respiratory depression
Dizziness		

*To be used with caution when any of these conditions exists.

Table 10.7 COMMON NEUROLEPTICS OR MAJOR TRANQUILIZERS

Generic Name	Brand Name	Category
Thioridazine	Mellaril	Phenothiazine
Chlorpromazine	Thorazine	
Fluphenazine	Permitil	
	Prolixin	
Prochlorperazine	Compazine	
Trifluoperazine	Stelazine	
Molindone	Moban	Dihydrolindoles
Thiothixene	Navane	Thioxanthanthenes
Haloperidol	Haldol	Butyrophenones

Side Effects		Precautions*
Blurred vision	Potential difficulty	Depression
Constipation	handling secretions	Respiratory diseases
Postural hypotension	Changes in temperature	Cardiac diseases
Photosensitivity	control	Respiratory depression
Fatigue	Sexual dysfunction	Concurrent use of some
		vasoactive drugs

*To be used with caution when any of these conditions exists.

The list below will familiarize you with the four basic kinds of medication that can be useful in treating psychiatric disease or sustained emotional upsets (such as death of a spouse) in COPD patients. Even if this information is not relevant for you now, having a general sense of the drugs and the conditions they treat will help you ask the right questions if a future need arises for you or a family member.

1. *Neuroleptics*, also called *major tranquilizers* or *antipsychotic agents*, are used in psychiatric diseases such as schizophrenia and in acute psychotic reactions.

2. *Antidepressants* are used to treat depression both as an entity in itself and as part of manic depression.

3. *Mood modulators* are designed to control disruptive mood swings, such as those occurring in manic depression.

4. *Anxiolytic agents* are used to reduce anxiety for people who are acutely or chronically distressed. In more extreme psychiatric conditions, they are used together with drugs from one or more of the other categories.

Tables 10.5 to 10.7 list—for each kind of medication—examples of popular names, common side effects, and precautions.

11

Complementary Therapies for COPD: Old Treatments Have New Life

The COPD treatments we have been discussing—medications, the various physical therapy modalities, oxygen, and so on—are all tools prescribed by Western medicine, which is heavily dominated by a modern perspective and technology. Western medicine has benefited greatly from this century's scientific progress and from health care discoveries and innovations fueled by this century's wars. But these enormous advances unfortunately displaced still-valuable traditional treatments that had been practiced for hundreds or thousands of years. If they weren't scientifically provable, explainable, or at least reasonably modern, they ended up on the cutting room floor. The impact was greatest in the United States. We not only lacked the centuries of history that elements of traditional medicine had in Europe, we also had the American Medical Association, which took the lead in pushing these treatments out of the mainstream to do away with competition to physicians. A great many treatments—such as herbal medicine, hypnosis, massage, chiropractic, and homeopathy, to name just a few—came to be regarded with disfavor and suspicion, and existed on the fringe.

When health care was touched by the activism and anti-establishment attitude of the 1960s, a growing number of people began investigating this medical fringe, which by then included newcomers as well as traditional treatments. Some approaches gained temporary fad popularity. Others—those that help significantly to cope with health problems little responsive to Western medicine—have made a substantially increasing impact. And now the AMA itself has finally come to realize that *alternative* or *complementary* therapies—as they are called—can work extremely well in partnership with Western medicine. They acknowledge that treatments in use for several thousand years have value—whether or not we understand how they work—or they would have fallen by the wayside in the ancient past. The growing use of the term *complementary* to replace *alternative* reflects this current emphasis on the value of partnership instead of the antagonistic either/or mentality that held sway for a long time.

Although it is a slow process, with large areas of ignorance and resistance, complementary medicine is finally starting to gain legitimacy in the medical establishment. We are beginning to see the emergence of physicians who practice *integrated medicine*—meaning that they provide Western and a range of complementary therapies under one roof. More and more good research is taking place, and top medical journals are starting to publish it. The federal government has established a center for funding such research, and a core of medical schools have added courses in complementary medicine to the curriculum. Recognition of the value these ancient therapies offer has now become one of the modern revolutions in health care.

Because much of this progress has occurred since the book's first edition, this is a good time to bring you information on complementary treatments you may want to add to your health care regimen. An advantage of complementary therapies is that they are often gentle—and inexpensive—enough so that you can experiment. If complementary treatments appeal to you, see what is helpful and can comfortably become part of your routine. Those that are more costly (such as hypnosis) and not guaranteed to be covered by insurance are not usually needed on a regular basis. We have consulted with experts in the field, and bring you highlights of the treatments they use in helping COPD patients live in the best health that they can attain.

Do's: We want to emphasize two points. *Do* feel confident about trying treatments we mention here unless we include a need for caution (as with lobelia and wild indigo). Most of the treatments we discuss here are not dangerous to use without professional supervision. And when you see a dosage range, it means that you have to find what is right for you, i.e., start at the low end, and gradually work up if this doesn't seem to be enough. (And if the high end still doesn't work, then it's not a treatment that works for you.) And whatever you do decide to try—please *tell your doctor* and any other health care professionals you see. It helps them to give you the best care, and your experiences may benefit other patients. And if your doctor is one who tends to dismiss complementary treatments, perhaps any positive results you experience will help to expand his perspective. (National surveys document that the great majority of people who use complementary treatments actually hide this information from their doctor, typically because they fear disapproval. That doesn't help patient or doctor.)

Don'ts: When it comes to choosing nutritional or herbal supplements, there are certain things *not* to rely on. One is the term *natural*—which advertising companies unfortunately use in a manipulative way to imply a guarantee that a health care product is helpful and safe. Looking at the range of medicinal plants, for example, *all* are natural, but some are therapeutic, some are poisonous, and still others are good *or* bad for you depending on the dose and/or your particular circumstances. Do *not* choose a nutritional or herbal supplement—or select a dosage—by reading manufacturers' recommendations. Some may be reasonably accurate, but many are not. And *never* seek the advice of health food store employees. The employee who really knows his herbal/nutritional medicine is rare indeed. Far too many are simply parroting misinformation they have read or heard elsewhere.

Contributors: The two people we relied on most heavily for information are Donald Yance, Jr., MH, CN, AHG (*M*aster *H*erbalist, *C*ertified *N*utritionist, *A*merican *H*erbal *G*uild) and Tieraona Low Dog, M.D., AHG (former president) both highly respected holistic health care practitioners and among this country's top herbalists. Mr. Yance has practiced complementary approaches to health care for 15 years, both as an addition to standard physician-prescribed care and as primary care. He founded the *Wellsprings Center for Natural Healing East* and *West*, which are busy nonprofit health care facilities in Fairfield, Connecticut, and Ashland, Oregon. He is solidly grounded in both the traditions and science of herbal medicine and nutrition. Mr. Yance works with oncologists and lectures on his approach to cancer at hospitals in and around the Fairfield area and at national conferences, and recently published *Herbal Medicine, Healing & Cancer* (Keats Publishing).

Dr. Low Dog—who has spent most of her life learning about the medicinal properties of plants from Native American healers—established her own practice 17 years ago. Most recently she founded the Tree House Center for Integrative Medicine in Albuquerque, New Mexico, where she regularly sees patients and teaches medical students, residents, and naturopathic students who train with her. She also founded the New Mexico Herb Center (a professional training facility) and is Director of Education at Foundations in Herbal Medicine in Albuquerque. Dr. Low Dog is Albuquerque's local "alternative medicine doctor" on TV. Her detailed clinical expertise is matched by her understanding of the biochemistry of plants used in herbal systems from cultures around the world and her knowledge of the research literature, and she is chairperson of the Botanical Medicine Committee for the *United States Pharmacopeia* and part of the faculty for Columbia University's course on Botanical Medicine for

Physicians. She is in great demand for lectures and workshops, and spoke at over 52 medical conferences throughout the United States and Europe in 1999 alone.

We'll describe their recommendations for thinning and bringing up mucus, for combating respiratory infections, for controlling coughs safely, for counteracting some of the side effects of steroid drugs, for improving the overall health of your lungs, for coping with panic/anxiety, and for improved sleep.

The Plant Advantage

Jim Duke, Ph.D., author of *The Green Farmacy* (Rodale Press), is an internationally known ethnobotanist who studies medicinal plants from cultures around the world and worked with the Department of Agriculture and the National Cancer Institute for a number of years. He explains a basic difference between synthetic drugs developed by pharmaceutical companies and medicinal plants. And though he was talking specifically about herbs at the time, this includes our fruits, vegetables, and dietary herbs as well.

Because a drug results from isolating an active substance—and altering it to make it stronger and stronger—drugs are highly concentrated substances narrowly targeted to affect a specific biochemical pathway in the body. Because this high concentration at full strength tends to cause unacceptable side effects, the dosage actually prescribed for patients is significantly lower. But in doing this to diminish side effects, effectiveness is sometimes also reduced and side effects—although less—may still be a problem for many patients.

Because plants each combine an often formidable number and variety of chemical compounds, a single herb affects a variety of biochemical pathways—and so can help with several problems—simultaneously. Although the impact of these compounds is often milder than drugs, sometimes several coexisting compounds function to boost each other significantly, still without creating difficult side effects. Side effects are not troubling with a great many medicinal plants. Sometimes a plant contains the very ingredient that neutralizes a potentially unpleasant effect of one of its main compounds! And it is frequently possible to add an herb that will counterbalance any side effect.

This does *not* mean that pharmaceutical medicines are bad and herbal medicines are good. It *does* mean that each type of medicine has its place. Some drugs are miracle workers. Some are essential. Dr. Low Dog would not think of replacing your bronchodilator. She acknowledges that there are herbs with the anticholinergic properties needed to open constricted airways. "But just because we have herbs that can accomplish this does not mean that herbs are the best treatment to use," she cautions. "I think that Atrovent works best." We need pharmaceutical drugs. But they are not the whole story.

Nor does this mean that all herbs—simply because they are *natural*—are *safe* or *healthy*. We cannot stress this too often—and you will find this warning repeated. Although the majority of plants will not cause irreparable harm even if overdosed, some plants are dangerous in high doses. And some are dangerous at any dose.

Another plus for plants comes with finances, especially for patients who must pay for their medications out of pocket, including those on Medicare. Drugs tend to be costly, reflecting the pharmaceutical company's substantial earlier investment to develop the drug, then gain FDA approval, and then market it. Foods and medicinal plants, on the other hand, are significantly cheaper.

Herbal Formulations

Herbs come in several types of preparations, most commonly: dried and packaged in loose form, for making a tea; dried and packaged in capsules, to swallow with liquid; and as a liquid called a *tincture* or *fluid extract*. They are not simply duplicates in different form, because the method of preparation has some influence on which of a plant's various compounds end up in the final product. Some herbalists are very strict about which way a particular herb should be taken by an individual patient for a specific problem; others give more weight to personal preference. Capsules are obviously the simplest to take, and avoid any unpleasant taste, but they are not as bioactive as a tea, and neither is as bioactive as a tincture or fluid—which are highly concentrated and very readily absorbed. Some people love to sip their herbs in tea form, and enjoy the ritual of preparation. Others find the process time-consuming and messy, and much prefer a tincture or capsules.

To make a *tea*, use 1–2 tsps. of dried herb per cup of water. With bark, seeds, or root, bring cold water to a gentle boil, then simmer—covered—for 10 minutes. For dried flowers or leaves, pour boiling water over the herb and then let it sit—covered—for 10 minutes. Strain and drink within 24 hours.

A *tincture* has been made by steeping the herb in a water-alcohol mixture. The strength should be listed on the label, usually as a ratio—most typically, 1:5. This ratio tells us that 5 ml of the tincture equals roughly

1 gram of the herb. Sometimes the liquid preparation is in *fluid* rather than tincture form, which is a 1:1 ratio—and tells us that only 1 ml of the fluid is needed to equal 1 gram of the herb. The appropriate dose of tincture or fluid is mixed with a little bit of water, then drunk. *A word about dose:* tinctures and fluids come with an eyedropper, and label instructions usually give a recommended dose in terms of number of drops. *Ignore this.* It's far more effective to measure your dose by *milliliters* (abbreviated *ml*). Dr. Low Dog recommends two easily available—and very inexpensive—tools for doing this. One is the kind of teaspoon or eyedropper used for giving liquid medication to small children, available in supermarkets and drugstores at somewhere under $2. It doesn't matter if it is calibrated in ml's or cc's, as they are equivalent. Or you can ask your pharmacist for a 5 cc syringe without the needle attached. The syringes are marked more finely, in gradations of 1/10 cc, and can be easily washed out between uses.

Caution: The quality of herbal products varies tremendously, from excellent to nonexistent. Do *not* go into your local health food store or vitamin shop and choose by price or the most authentic-sounding label. Dr. Low Dog and Mr. Yance have both spent substantial time investigating various manufacturers. You'll find approved resources—some available by mail order—at the end of this chapter.

Coping with Mucus

Mr. Yance uses a nutritional supplement called *N-acetyl cysteine*, or *NAC*, to help thin mucus that is otherwise difficult to bring up and get out. It works by dissolving the chemical bonds that normally link mucus molecules together to form the tenacious, gluey substance that—especially in chronic bronchitis—can resist all but the most time-consuming and effortful attempts to get it out. As an additional benefit, NAC has a variety of anti-cancer (both prevention and treatment) effects, including scavenging free radicals—especially in the liver and lungs. *Bromelain*—a proteolytic enzyme derived from pineapple—aids the digestive breakdown of whatever it accompanies, which improves absorption through the intestines and thus increases effectiveness. Taken along with NAC, for example, it amplifies the mucolytic effects. And Mr. Yance finds that taking it along with an antibiotic doubles its effectiveness without increasing side effects. Recent research on bromelain also points to anti-cancer effects. Bromelain is widely available, unlike *serraflazyme*—his first-choice proteolytic enzyme. This is made by *Cardiovascular Research* and is found only in top-of-the-line health food stores.

Dosage: NAC is available in health food stores in capsule or tablet form. The capsules contain from 500–600 mg. The total dosage is anywhere from 1,000–3,000 mg daily, taken either 500 mg or 1,000 mg at a time, 2–3 times a day. Start with 500 mg, and if you don't experience significant benefits after a week or so, begin increasing it. Bromelain is taken in 500 mg doses, 2–4 times a day.

Mr. Yance also recommends foods that can help thin mucus. *Horseradish* is one, and it also has potent activity against germs that can infect the respiratory tract (more on fighting infection later in this chapter). The suggested amount is about 1 gram, 3–4 times a week. *Ginger* is another, either 1–3 grams of fresh ginger root added to raw or cooked food, or 2–6 capsules of dried ginger.

Lobelia tops the list of herbs that function well as expectorants, helping to rid your lungs of this excess—and now more liquefied—mucus. (It also has a side benefit of relaxing the airways.) Lobelia is also a gastrointestinal irritant. Although in large doses it causes nausea and vomiting, *small doses* are enough to get airway mucus moving, but not enough to cause stomach discomfort. If by some chance it causes a bit of queasiness, take a stomach-soothing herb along with it: *chamomile* or *licorice* (the herb, not the candy!) is excellent. (If you have high blood pressure, make sure to get deglycyrrhizined licorice, also called DGL.) A fringe benefit of lobelia for anyone with constipation problems is enhanced stomach and bowel motility. And a fringe benefit of licorice is enhanced immune response. *Do not go beyond the upper dosage indicated here for lobelia under any circumstances!* Larger doses can make you quite sick, and also risk severe breathing depression—something a COPD patient must avoid.

Dosage: The range for a 1:5 tincture for lobelia is .3–1 ml 3 times a day (just before you sit down to eat). Chamomile is available as a tea. And licorice/DGL is taken in capsule form: 175–325 mg 2–3 times a day.

Preventing Infection

Garlic—very high on the shopping list here—goes right to your lungs. The fact that its volatile oils—which are its therapeutic compounds—make our breath smell illustrates why this member of the onion family is so helpful. The volatile oils are absorbed into our bloodstream, and from there are taken into the alveoli of our lungs. When we exhale, the oils are expelled on our breath—hence, that telltale aroma. But before they are exhaled, these therapeutic volatile oils are washing our lungs. The critical aspect of taking garlic therapeutically is that it must be crushed—mechanically or by eating—to release the enzyme that initiates the breakdown process that terminates in the presence of sulfur compounds—

which give garlic its characteristic odor *and* its medicinal effects. These volatile oils are extremely antiseptic, with potent action against bacteria, viruses, and fungal organisms.

Garlic can be taken raw, lightly steamed, or added to the last 5 minutes of cooking. Chop half a clove, put it in some olive oil, and toss that on your salad or a cooked vegetable. Dr. Low Dog finds that some patients like to put chopped garlic in honey and let it sit for 6 weeks. If you prefer taking garlic capsules, remember that quality varies widely. Look for one of the brands recommended at the end of this chapter.

Dosage: the equivalent of one clove a day.

Garlic also has a number of important fringe benefits for your health: it helps to control cholesterol levels, reduces the formation of fatty deposits in blood vessels, helps normalize blood pressure, and has a mild anticoagulation effect just as aspirin does. And if you like to combine your garlic with olive oil, remember that olive oil belongs to the group of healthy fats that actually improve cardiovascular health—in moderate amounts, of course!

In terms of edibles, *horseradish* is also highly antiseptic—even more so than garlic, Mr. Yance points out. Garlic is a lot more versatile, both for use in food and in availability in capsules, but adding horseradish to your diet provides variety—and helps with your mucus as well.

Propolis is one of Mr. Yance's favorite infection fighters, potent in warding off bacterial, fungal, and viral infections. Propolis is a black, gummy, resin-like substance that bees take from trees and use in the hive as glue, and as an antiseptic. Propolis turns the hive into a virtually germ-free environment. Propolis is so resinous that it's not water-soluble, and only comes in extract form. It can be used as a preventive—during the flu season, for example, or when you suspect something might be brewing—and to assist your antibiotic if you actually contract an infection.

Dosage: As a preventive, take 10–25 drops, 2–3 times a day. For actual treatment, increase that amount to 5–6 times daily.

For help with an infection that is just beginning, *echinacea*—taken in the right way—can make a dramatic difference, especially with a viral infection. The extract of echinacea root has a proven effect on stimulating the white blood cells that fight these microbes. There are two rules: *start without delay*, and *take a lot of it.* The moment you feel something brewing—whether it's a hint of a scratch in your throat, a runny nose, a feeling in your eyes and sinuses, or a general feeling of malaise that isn't typical for you—reach for your echinacea. Take it frequently during the first 2 days—every 2 hours is not too much—and then taper off for the next 3. Do the same if someone you live or work with comes down with a cold or the flu.

Dosage: 2–3 ml every 2–4 hours for the first 48 hours; then half that dose every 2–4 hours for another 3 days.

Mr. Yance finds value in combining propolis and echinacea, and perhaps adding *wild indigo* (also called *baptesia*) to the mixture. It increases echinacea's activity, and historically these two plants were typically used together. If using wild indigo, Dr. Low Dog cautions that a large dose—such as a cup of strong tea made from this herb—can cause nausea and vomiting. When it is combined with echinacea, the *maximum* dose for wild indigo should not exceed 1 ml every 4 hours.

As Dr. Low Dog emphasizes, if—despite your best efforts at clearing your lungs of mucus, using food and herbs that kill infectious microbes, and getting your flu and pneumonia shots—you do get sick, let your doctor know immediately so that you can begin antibiotic therapy. And once you're finished with the antibiotics, remember to take an *acidophilus* supplement for the following 2 weeks to repopulate your gut with beneficial flora as quickly as possible.

Coping with Cough

A chronic uncontrollable cough is annoying and irritating. It needs to be controlled—but not *over*controlled. Because coughing is a healthy, protective mechanism when it functions appropriately—to clear mucus and irritants from our lungs—COPD patients are especially in need of a responsive cough reflex. The cough you want to get rid of comes from an irritated mechanoreceptor in the throat. The cough you want to keep is governed by the cough center up in the brain. So you want an antitussive that leaves the cough center alone. Codeine, for example, is an excellent cough suppressant, but it works by damping down the brain's cough center.

Dr. Low Dog emphasizes that anything that coats your throat functions as an effective antitussive for COPD patients. *Wild cherry bark* has been used for a very long time. Mucilaginous plants—which have to be prepared as a tea—will coat your throat *and* your stomach, which can be an excellent choice if you are taking lobelia to bring your mucus up. *Marshmallow*—both root and leaves—is extremely mucilaginous, and a very gentle plant. The root has the higher mucilage content, making it more effective but also making it gel up as the tea is prepared. Taken just 1 tbs at a time, it's like a thick syrup going down. But some people find the texture of a full cup of the tea too much like raw oyster. Because the leaf produces a nice sweet drink without the sliminess, many find it a lot easier to tolerate. The tea is made by steeping 1 tbs of root or leaf in 1 cup of boiling water for 5–10 minutes, then straining it. *Slippery elm* is another helpful herb in this context.

Vitamins and Minerals for COPD

Vitamin A is very important to the health of epithelial tissue—the kind of tissue that lines our lungs—and so should be taken regularly whenever the epithelium needs to be healed. Dr. Low Dog prescribes a beta-carotene supplement, which is transformed into vitamin A when it is digested. She prefers to stay on the conservative end of dosing, running counter to the tendency these days to boost beta-carotene intake. She disagrees with those who advocate 100,000 IU and up, and finds it wisest to stick with a dose of 25,000 IU. Many multivitamins nowadays include around 10,000 IU of beta-carotene anyway, so her dosage level leaves room for this additional source. Mr. Yance uses any of four possibilities: a full-spectrum carotenoid supplement called *Betaplex;* mycelized vitamin A—an emulsified form that does not require breakdown by the liver and gall bladder; purified shark liver oil—which also includes vitamin D and the healthful omega-3 fatty acids EPA (eicosapentaenoic acid) and DHA (docosahexaenoic acid); or Eskimo Oil—a fish oil preparation from *Tyler Encapsulations.* He also advises patients to take advantage of winter vegetables when the season comes around—sweet potatoes, orange and yellow squashes—all of which get their color from their *carotene* content.

As a fringe benefit of omega-3-containing fish oils, Dr. Low Dog points to their proven anti-inflammatory actions. This makes them helpful in any disease involving a significant inflammatory component, whether it's in the airways, the gastrointestinal system, or the joints.

An increasing number of health care professionals place fundamental importance on recent research indicating the importance of *vitamin C* for respiratory health in people with hyperresponsive airways. Many COPD patients eventually develop a hyperreactivity to histamine released by mast cells in their airways, and indications are that vitamin C plays a role in reducing elevated histamine levels in the respiratory tract. Eric Gershwin, M.D., at the University of California-Davis—who directs a multi-faceted research program to identify effective nutritional aids in treating asthma and allergies—told us that vitamin C is one of the compounds he is particularly excited about. One study has been published, with a much larger one now in progress. Dr. Low Dog adds that vitamin C also enhances the activity of infection-fighting white blood cells, giving it antiviral and antibacterial qualities as well. So she finds high-dose vitamin C an important addition for people with chronic lung disease who are also prone to respiratory infections. She recommends the highest dosage that a given patient can tolerate, but not going above 3,000–5,000 mg a day because it is likely to be of no use. Divide your overall daily dose so that you take it in segments every 4 hours. It should be taken in a buffered form, which is the kindest to the gastrointestinal tract, and is most bioactive when taken along with an equal amount of bioflavonoids. When taking a buffered form of vitamin C, make sure to avoid one with a high calcium/magnesium content or you risk upset stomach and diarrhea. Dr. Low Dog finds the buffered vitamin C crystals helpful for people at the high end of dosing. A half-teaspoon contains about 1,100 mg of vitamin C along with about 225 mg of calcium and a little less of magnesium.

Zinc also helps in maintaining the health of epithelial tissue—and thus the lungs—and is important in promoting wound healing and moderating allergic responses. Dr. Low Dog recommends 50–75 mg daily in the form of *zinc picolinate*. The picolinic acid is what enables the zinc to be absorbed across the intestinal wall. A possible role in prostate health is a potential fringe benefit for male COPD patients.

Miscellaneous Supplements

Dr. Low Dog recommends *ginseng* for any of her patients who periodically require oral or inhaled steroids. The concern with pharmaceutical steroids is their potential for suppressing the adrenal glands' own production of these hormones. Ginseng helps to prevent this outcome because it stimulates production of ACTH—adrenocorticotropic hormone—by the pituitary gland, which is the body's messenger for turning on the adrenals. There are several kinds of ginseng, all of which include the term *Panax* in their botanical name—*Panax ginseng* (from China and Korea) and *Panax quinquefolium* (from the United States), for example. Please note that Siberian ginseng is not a Panax species. It possesses some similar activity, but lacks the basic compound thought to be responsible for much of the *Panax* species' effects. (Siberian ginseng, though, does help rejuvenate people convalescing from an illness, as well as those with a chronic illness.) Dr. Low Dog offers cautionary advice on what kind of product to buy, because ginseng is so commonly adulterated with cheaper herbs to lower the price. Unless you know without a doubt that your tincture comes from a reputable manufacturer, she recommends that patients buy the standardized extract. This will be in tablet or capsule form, and state clearly on the container that it is standardized to a specified content of ginsenosides.

Dosage: For Panax ginseng, a 1:5 tincture should be taken twice a day, with each dose 3–5 ml. The standardized extract should be taken in a dose that provides 100–200 mg of ginsenosides a day. Anyone taking ginseng on a long-term basis should alternate on-off periods: 60–90 days on followed by 60–90 days off.

Quercetin, which is found abundantly in such foods as onions and broccoli, as well as in eucalyptus and licorice, is a supplement that Mr. Yance relies on for its potent anti-allergy and anti-inflammatory effects. He finds that combining it with both NAC and bromelain—and taking the mix daily, 15–20 minutes before each meal—is very helpful for COPD. He prefers using a tablet prepared by *Source Naturals,* which combines the right amount of quercetin and bromelain along with vitamin C, and adding the NAC.

Dosage: He recommends 1–2 tablets 2–3 times a day, going for the low end of this range (1 tablet twice daily) during more stable intervals, going as high as 2 tablets 3 times daily when airways are more hyperreactive. *Fringe benefits:* Quercetin is a potent antioxidant and cancer preventive, and so has a variety of health benefits.

Mr. Yance also recommends *chlorophyll*—preferring either whole foods or a food-derived supplement—to improve lung health. Nettles—the stinging plant—are an excellent source, and have been used by herbalists for their anti-allergy effect. He suggests that people with a garden try growing them, and cook them like spinach or make a tea. And freeze-dried nettles are available from *MediHerb* in 500 mg capsules, to be taken, 1–6 a day, on a regular basis. The benefits appear only gradually, so you have to take it for a while before you can be aware of them. The next best chlorophyll sources are algae supplements.

Anxiety

Periodic panic attacks and a general underlying sense of anxiety are a common part of life for many COPD patients. "When you can't breathe, that's a very understandable reaction," Dr. Low Dog says. Although taking the best care of your lungs and your general health that you can, exercising, and learning to use your energy efficiently will all help your breathing and your morale, many patients find their panic and anxiety reduced but not eliminated. Dr. Low Dog makes several recommendations.

She finds *hypnosis* an extremely valuable tool. Most people, unfortunately, have a distorted, Hollywood-influenced "look into my eyes" or "watch the swinging pendulum" image of hypnosis and hypnotists, which does the profession—and those who stand to benefit from it—a great disservice. Evidence indicates that hypnosis has been in use for at least several thousand years, and it is increasingly substantiated by research studies for its ability to give patients the tools for bringing pain or disruptive behaviors under control. "Panic and anxiety attacks are a kind of uncontrollable hyperresponsiveness of the autonomic nervous system—that 'fight or flight' adrenaline reaction when you're afraid that you may not be able to get enough air," she says. "And a good hypnotherapist is trained to work on the autonomic nervous system."

The hypnotist is able to induce a state of very deep relaxation, then help you image how you will respond to your initial signs of rising panic, then help you develop the ability to call on this positive response whenever you need to. It may not sound like much when you read this description, but "it is a very powerful treatment," Dr. Low Dog observes. Working at this deep level can have astonishing results that are impossible to achieve simply by thinking and talking about it. And an important side effect of this newfound reliable ability to control your panic is the overall sense of mastery and confidence it engenders.

Two national associations—the American Society of Clinical Hypnosis and the Society for Clinical and Experimental Hypnosis—will provide the names of accredited hypnotherapists in your area (see the end of this chapter for contact information).

Dr. Low Dog finds that *valerian* is an excellent herb for providing gentle anxiety reduction. Those of us at all familiar with this herb think of it in terms of a sleep aid, but that involves a relatively high dose. When doses are very small, the effect of this interesting herb is quite different. It doesn't put you to sleep at all. Instead it functions as an *anxiolytic*—it simply settles your stomach and has a general calming effect. *Make sure* to get the right type of valerian, one that uses *Valerian officianalis*. (The other two types, *Valerian edulis* and *Valerian walichii*, actually contain stimulants.)

Dosage: "Low dose" means 1 ml of a 1:5 tincture before each meal, or 180 mg in capsule form (often preferred because the liquid has a very difficult taste).

Lemon balm is an herb that Dr. Low Dog finds excellent for nervous tension and anxiety because it calms the limbic system, the part of the brain that interfaces with the autonomic nervous system—central in the "fight-or-flight" response. Because lemon balm is also a digestive aid, a mild expectorant, and helps to reduce mucus production in the respiratory tract, it provides several benefits simultaneously to COPD patients. (The one caution: Patients who also have thyroid disease must avoid large doses of lemon balm because it can slow thyroid function.)

Dosage: Drink 2–3 cups of tea as needed throughout the day, or 3–5 ml of tincture 2–3 times daily.

But Dr. Low Dog's favorite herb for anxiety and panic is *kava*. It soothes and calms, and she points out that German physicians prescribe it as an *anxiolytic* in the same way that doctors in the United States prescribe benzodiazepines (Valium, for example). Use either a standardized extract (standardized to 30–35% kavalactones) or a 1:5 tincture.

Dosage: 100 mg of the standardized extract 3 times a day; 2–3 ml of the tincture 3 times a day.

Depression

Dr. Low Dog notes two primary possibilities for easing mild to moderate depression, and neither of them will interfere with your breathing. One is the plant *St. John's Wort*, which has been in the news a great deal as an antidote to mild depression that helps a significant number of people and acts without the side effects that accompany antidepressant drugs. The other is *SAMe* (S-adenosyl-L-methionine) supplements, which are a concentrated version of a compound that we naturally manufacture in our bodies. It also appears to achieve its antidepressant action without unpleasant side effects, and its anti-inflammatory effects can provide a fringe benefit for arthritis pain. Dr. Low Dog recommends that they be used together.

Dosage: For St. John's Wort, start with 300 mg of the standardized tablets or capsules 3 times a day. If you don't experience adequate relief after the first 4 weeks, double the dose to 600 mg 3 times daily. For SAMe, take 400 mg 2–3 times a day.

Miscellaneous

Aromatherapy uses essential oils, such as eucalyptus, pine, thyme, rosemary, lavender, nutmeg, lemon balm, or some combination of these. They are available at health food stores. You may even find some already combined and indicated for respiratory problems. Mr. Yance instructs you to place 5–10 drops in a bowl in which you have just poured freshly boiled water, then hold your head over the bowl and drape it with a towel to prevent the steam from escaping. These oils can help to ease some of your symptoms, and additionally—the steam releases antimicrobial agents in these oils, and you breathe them directly into your lungs.

Another way to benefit from hot water and herbs is with a *whole body bath*. A bit before bedtime, make a tea from herbs that you find beneficial, take a warm bath right after you drink it, then go to bed. The warm bath facilitates the speed with which these herbal compounds reach your lungs, where they will work their benefits while you sleep and give you a more comfortable night.

Mr. Yance recommends an old-fashioned *poultice*—a mustard plaster—to improve circulation in the chest area. Mix 1 tsp dried mustard powder with 2 tsp flour and add boiling water to make a paste that you wrap in an old dish towel or cloth diaper. Put Vaseline or another light cloth on your chest to prevent your skin from being burned, and then the poultice. Let it sit for 20–25 minutes. You can expect to feel, very suddenly, a tremendous amount of heat in that area, and then your chest tightness easing significantly.

Dr. Low Dog agrees with the substantial value of mustard plasters. She adds that onion plasters also work quite well—and are very inexpensive. An advantage for the elderly—whose skin typically has become quite thin—is that an onion plaster is less likely to burn their skin compared to the effects of mustard. The one caution is to guard against excessive heat when the plaster is initially applied to the chest. Prepare the plaster by sauteing a large chopped onion until it becomes transparent, then wrap it in a cloth that you place on your chest and cover with a towel to help retain heat. Leave in place for 15–20 minutes.

Resources

Herbs

Cardiovascular Research: Call their distributor, Emerson Ecologics, Inc. at 800-654-4432 to find out which health food stores in your area sell these products.

Enzymatic Therapy
No mail order, but their website (*www.enzy.com*) describes their products and indicates health food stores across the country that carry them. You can also learn of the health food store nearest you by calling them at 800-783-2286.

HerbPharm: for tinctures
541-846-6262: Call them for a price list enabling you to order by mail or phone, or to find which health food stores in your area sell their products.

Nature's Herbs Inc. (part of Twin Labs)
600 Quality Drive
American Ford, UT 84003
801-763-0700; *www.twinlab.com*
Their products are available in many health food stores. They also
have a catalog for mail order.

Prevail
800-248-0885: You can call for a catalog, or to find out which
health food stores in your area sell their products.

Source Naturals: Call their distributor, Threshold Enterprises, Ltd,
at 800-777-5677.

Hypnosis

American Society of Clinical Hypnosis
33 W. Grand Avenue, Suite 402
Chicago, IL 60610
312-645-9810; fax: 312-645-9818
The society will provide a list of local professionals who use clinical
hypnosis in their practices if the request is in writing and accompanied by a stamped, self-addressed envelope. They do have a website
(*www.healthfinder.gov/test/orgs/hr0302.htm*), but it contains only the
above information.

The Society for Clinical and Experimental Hypnosis
2201 Haeder Road
Pullman, WA 99163
509-332-7555; fax: 509-332-5907; *sceh@pullman.com*
Call for the names of qualified hypnotists in your area, or send a
letter.

12

Oxygen Therapy

A critical turning point in treating COPD patients has been the availability of oxygen equipment for use outside the hospital. First came the large oxygen containers with long tubes that enable advanced COPD patients to move around their homes while breathing supplemental oxygen. Then came portable units that opened the outside world for them.

Each advance in providing regular adequate oxygen represents a major improvement in health and lifestyle for these patients. Body and brain function far more effectively and the heart is healthier. They also restore a critical degree of self-sufficiency and independence by allowing these patients to resume basic self-care and home-care responsibilities and involvement in valued activities outside their home. In sum, these advances improve the length and quality of their future.

Portable oxygen equipment—allowing the patient to move about (ambulate) freely—has substantially extended the limits of medical care available to advanced COPD patients. Two major conferences published this statement: "The exercise occasioned by *ambulation* for all daily activities both in and out of the home is a *major component in the standard of care and rehabilitation* (our emphasis) for patients with advanced chronic obstructive pulmonary disease."

The problem as of the writing of this book is that the wonderful potential of oxygen has been diluted—moderately or dramatically—for many patients because a great deal of power has been allowed to accumulate in the hands of the *durable medical equipment companies*—called *DMEs*—the companies that provide oxygen supplies to patients at home. The bottom line is whether coverage is provided by Medicare or by an HMO. Roughly 1 million patients in the United States require oxygen at home, and the great bulk of them are covered by one or the other of these health care coverage structures.

Many HMOs contract out to the DME with the lowest bid. Because bidding low without hurting profits requires minimizing costs, a significant number of DMEs substitute a less costly method of oxygen delivery than prescribed. The most portable units are the most expensive to provide, so many patients who can remain on the go with portable oxygen are forced to remain homebound by these DMEs.

Before we describe the equipment alternatives—and the current barriers to making full use of them—it's helpful to take a brief look at how our current understanding of oxygen's function and value evolved.

Understanding Oxygen

Combustion—the process by which fire burns—and *respiration* in our cells are similar processes. *They both burn oxygen to produce energy.* Combustion's energy takes the form of heat. Cellular respiration's energy is the vital force that powers life. Awareness of this similarity has been part of mankind's knowledge since ancient times. Efforts to understand its basis eventually unlocked the door to understanding how and why breathing keeps us alive.

The early Romans were the first to write of the relationship between fire and breathing. Vitruvius, ancient architect and engineer, described how deep-well diggers used fire's need for oxygen to see if a well shaft contained enough fresh air for safety. If a lamp lowered to the bottom continued to burn, they knew it was safe to descend. Galen, the Roman Empire's foremost physician, directly compared respiration to a flame. Our language has handed down this analogy between respiration and combustion with such phrases as "flame of life," "fire of life," and "vital flame."

When seventeenth-century scientist finally began to understand why they are so similar, the accurate understanding of breathing became possible. John Mayow, born in London in 1643 and a graduate of Oxford University, made perhaps the most important of these early contributions. Others had already shown that something in the air is essential for combustion, but it was Mayow who first theorized that the *air* we breathe contains something specific—a "nitro-aereal spirit"—essential to both fire and respiration.

He demonstrated this by placing each of two animals in separate airtight glass containers. To one he also added a fire-burning lamp. The animal in the container always died first. He wrote:

> . . . Let any animals be enclosed in a glass vessel along with a lamp so that the entrance of (outside) air . . . is prevented . . . . We shall soon see the ani-

mal will not long survive the fatal torch. For I have ascertained by experiment that an animal enclosed in a glass vessel along with a lamp will not breathe much longer than half the time it would otherwise have lived.

. . . Since the air enclosed in the glass is in part deprived of its nitro-aereal particles by the burning of the lamp . . . it cannot support long the breathing of the animal, hence not only the lamp but also the animal soon expires for want of nitro-aereal particles.

Mayow made his glass containers airtight by placing the opening over water, which creates a vacuum seal. He didn't know the water was also absorbing carbon dioxide, the by-product of oxygen use. But this explains why Mayow always found substantially less air in a container after the flame went out and the animal died. He had clearly demonstrated that something from the air was used during these two processes, even though he did not understand what his "nitro-aereal particles" really were.

This "something" turned out to be oxygen. It was first identified—independently—by Dr. Joseph Priestly of England and Dr. Carl Wilhelm Scheele of Sweden. But it was the French scientist Antoine Laurent Lavoisier who named it, and put together the pieces to explain the true nature of respiration and combustion. Lavoisier summarized his two basic findings: "(1) Respiration affects only the respirable air; the rest of the air [nitrogen] . . . remains unchanged. (2) Animals shut up in a confined atmosphere succumb, so soon as they have absorbed or converted into 'aeriform calcic acid' [carbon dioxide] the greater part of the respirable portion of the atmosphere, leaving the remainder." The fact that using this "eminently respirable air" produced acid led Lavoiseir to name the gas *oxygine.* Typical for his time, he had turned to ancient Greek, combining the words for "acid" and "beget" (or "produce").

Then everyone jumped on the bandwagon. Oxygen was hailed as a panacea, and indiscriminately prescribed to cure every problem from infertility to hysteria. Because its frequent inappropriate use led to many apparent "failures," oxygen was eventually branded a hoax. By the end of the nineteenth century, it had fallen into clinical disrepute.

But that soon changed dramatically, all because the airplane—invented early in the twentieth century—became a highly successful fighting instrument. Pilots in both world wars were venturing up into an environment where available oxygen was often inadequate. The sometimes profound impact on their thoughts, abilities, and temperament touched off a research explosion, with growth of a solid, extensive body of knowledge concerning the effects of oxygen—and its lack.

The two-pronged conclusion with basic consequences for medical treatment was that: (1) reducing the oxygen we normally breathe impairs us physically, mentally, and emotionally; and (2) these harmful consequences can be reversed by carefully adding oxygen to the environment.

The first major medical success for oxygen was in treating pneumonia. In the second decade of our century, doctors learned that the pneumonia symptoms reflecting low oxygen—cyanosis (bluish tint to lips and nails), tachycardia (racing heart rate), delirium, and coma—frequently disappeared within just a few hours after beginning oxygen therapy. Before long they also realized that patients on supplemental oxygen—which relieved them of the burden of inadequate oxygen—had a much better chance of surviving their pneumonia. In 1921, an expert in treating pneumonia wrote that oxygen therapy to prevent hypoxia " . . . is perhaps the most important factor in the treatment of pneumonia, apart from the specific cure of the infection. . . . "

Dr. Alvan Barach of New York City pioneered the broader use of oxygen in medicine, going from lobar pneumonia to *cor pulmonale*. In 1936, he wrote that "oxygen therapy in suitable cases [of *cor pulmonale*] relieves difficult breathing, restores strength and helps reduce the swelling of the patient's legs and back. "He noted, too, that oxygen helped relieve these patients' dyspnea during activity.

Modern Use

In the 1950s, intensive research on oxygen therapy for COPD patients was carried out on both sides of the Atlantic. These early studies showed that certain COPD patients seemed to improve in many ways—especially in their exercise tolerance—when they breathed pure oxygen instead of room air. But for some time, researchers could not find evidence of actual physiological change underlying these apparent benefits.

Two studies in the mid-1960s—one in Denver, Colorado, and one in Birmingham, England—placed the use of oxygen on more scientifically solid ground. They found that:

1. Physiologic exercise tolerance increases.

2. Constriction of the lungs' blood vessels caused by chronically low oxygen disappears, taking a great load off the heart, which then functions more effectively.

3. Performance improves on a variety of neuropsychiatric tasks, for example: attention span, verbal ability, abstract ability, simple sensory and motor skills, complex perceptual and motor skills, and memory. In other words, the brain works better.

Oxygen had obviously improved the level of functioning of the patients who had been tested. But several important questions remained to be answered. First: in these two studies, each patient's responses to added oxygen were compared with his earlier responses, instead of with a similar patient who was not getting extra oxygen. Researchers could not know if some—or most—of their improved exercise tolerance and neuropsychiatric performance were due to receiving the special attention research subjects get. These studies had to be repeated, using matching patient groups. They would receive that same attention and testing, but only one would be given extra oxygen to breathe—and none of the patients—or the testers—would know which patients were getting oxygen and which weren't. Second: how many hours should a patient spend on oxygen for maximum benefit? Third: since oxygen is a drug, and so cannot be totally free of side effects, how can we clearly identify those patients who need oxygen?

Development of easily portable oxygen containers in the late 1970s made possible the two large-scale, three-year studies that would answer these questions. The Nocturnal Oxygen Therapy Trial (NOTT) in the United States was supported by the National Institutes of Health. The British Medical Research Council supported a similar study in the United Kingdom. Patients chosen for these studies showed chronic symptoms of seriously inadequate oxygen (very low arterial blood oxygen, evidence of *cor pulmonale,* and/or too many red blood cells—polycythemia). Each study divided these hypoxic patients into two groups. In the American study, one group breathed extra oxygen only during sleep (because oxygen reaches its lowest levels then), while the other breathed it 24 hours a day. In the English study, one group breathed extra oxygen 15 hours a day. The other group had no extra oxygen at all.

The most striking conclusion was that extra oxygen improves survival. Remember that—at the start—all the participating patients had severe COPD. When the studies ended three years later: 75% of the patients getting oxygen 24 hours a day were still alive; 50% of the two part-time oxygen groups were still alive; and only 35% of those without any extra oxygen had not died.

Continuous extra oxygen is more effective than part-time use for at least two reasons. First, removing the burden of inadequate oxygen on the heart and lungs day and night—instead of only during sleep—more substantially prolongs the capacity of these organs to function reasonably well. Second, the availability of an easily portable daytime oxygen supply enables these patients to get around much more than they had been able to in quite some time. They resume activities at home and outside, including participation in a pulmonary rehabilitation program. Increased physical activity, plus the rehabilitation program, improve physical tone and stamina, overall health and productivity, and are emotionally and psychologically rewarding.

Using Oxygen at Home

Is It Inevitable?

No. Some COPD patients eventually need supplemental oxygen. Some never do. If you reach the point where adding oxygen to the air you breathe will help you, your doctor will let you know.

In the group of patients requiring supplemental oxygen, needs differ. Some benefit only during strenuous activity, some need it only at night (when ventilation normally diminishes), some need it both times. And some need extra oxygen continuously, meaning all day and night. How much extra oxygen is added to a patient's air at any given moment depends on the oxygen demands of what he is doing then.

How Does Your Doctor Know If You Need It?

In most cases, the criteria that guide your doctor's decision about prescribing supplemental oxygen are very clear-cut. They depend on the amount of oxygen in your arterial blood. If this concentration falls below a specific point, or if it falls within a middle range *and* you also have *cor pulmonale*, he will want you to have oxygen therapy. (Medicare—which presently covers 80% of all patients on oxygen therapy—ties its reimbursement criteria to these same guidelines. If your doctor strays from these criteria, you will not be reimbursed.)

What Changes Will You Experience?

You will have more energy, generally feel better, and be sharper mentally. You will be able to resume activities that had become too strenuous for you. And you will have the stamina to participate in a rehabilitation program designed especially for COPD patients, which is critically important in helping you get the most you can out of your life despite your disease. (The following chapters detail this program.) If you have developed pulmonary hypertension—meaning that the blood vessels in your lungs have become narrowed—the added oxygen will relax these vessels. Because the blood passing through your lungs then circulates much more freely, your heart no longer has to strain to push it through.

Some Patients Refuse Oxygen Therapy

Before we discuss the different kinds of oxygen equipment for home use, we want to underline the importance of hanging onto a well-balanced perspective when your doctor tells you he wants you to use oxygen regularly at home. Many patients try to turn a deaf ear, even when they hear the statistics providing they will live longer, far more comfortably, and in better health if they add oxygen to their "diet."

One objection has to do with how they fear other people will react to them. Will people find them unattractive with their oxygen equipment? Will they be regarded as an invalid? Will any of this make them unacceptable to others?

The other objection has to do with how they see themselves. People with a chronic, progressive illness often deny its seriousness in that very human attempt to turn a blind eye to their own mortality. Accepting his doctor's determination that he needs extra oxygen during his daily activities forces a COPD patient to acknowledge—if he hasn't yet done so—the inroads his illness has made on his health. Ironically, refusing supplemental oxygen will bring about the very thing he is trying to avoid. We don't want to beat around the bush. If your doctor advises oxygen therapy and you refuse, you will probably die sooner, and the time left you will be far more restricted and uncomfortable.

If you find yourself intent on avoiding your confrontation with reality, we hope you will agree to a one-month trial run. In any case, it is recommended that COPD patients starting oxygen therapy be retested after four weeks of oxygen use. Some patients turn out to need only this temporary "zap." After four weeks their oxygen level is adequate, and remains so for some time. If you agree to a trial, then find you still need supplemental oxygen after that month, we hope your taste of oxygen's benefits will have helped you disentangle your anxieties from this profoundly helpful treatment.

Oxygen Equipment for Home Use

Oxygen equipment has two basic components. One is the container that holds the oxygen. The other is the means for getting the oxygen from that container into your lungs. There are alternatives for each. (See Table 12.1 summarizing advantages and disadvantages.)

The Oxygen Container

If you begin—or are already on—oxygen therapy, you should have two types of oxygen sources. One is a large stationary unit you use in your home. The other is a small portable unit that goes everywhere with you when you leave your home. Three oxygen-supplying systems are currently available in the United States: high pressure compressed gas cylinders, liquid oxygen storage flasks, and oxygen concentrators (Figure 12.1). Some are easily portable, some are not.

The *high pressure compressed gas cylinder*—large, green, and ugly—was the first home oxygen system. Although currently inexpensive and the most easily available system, these tall green cylinders have drawbacks. Both the home and portable cylinders (called E-cylinders) run out of gas fairy quickly. And the portable gas cylinders are both heavier than would be ideal, and dangerous to refill (or "transfill," as the lingo goes) at home from the large cylinders. So for the stationary and portable cylinders, you need either the room to keep an ample supply on hand, or you need frequent replacement deliveries.

Liquid oxygen storage flasks hold oxygen in its liquid—rather than its gaseous—state. (Whether a particular element is in its solid, liquid, or gaseous form depends on the temperature of its environment. The most familiar example is water, which freezes at 32°F, becomes steam at 180°F, and is liquid between the two.) Extreme cold is needed to condense oxygen into liquid. Stationary and portable storage units, which resemble

Table 12.1	ADVANTAGES AND DISADVANTAGES OF HOME OXYGEN SYSTEMS	
Type	**Advantages**	**Disadvantages**
Liquid	Valuable in pulmonary rehabilitation and active lifestyles because the portable unit is lightweight and allows for long-range ambulation	More expensive generally Not available in small or rural communities
Concentrators	Lower cost Convenient for home use Attractive equipment Widely available	Electricity required and can be expensive Need tank back-up system Not portable Noisy
Compressed gas	Lowest cost (except when used continuously at high flows)	Not as effective as liquid oxygen for pulmonary rehabilitation or active lifestyles because multiple tanks or transfilling system needed for long or repeated ambulation periods Relatively low volume of even the large tanks means frequent home deliveries Tanks are heavy and unsightly

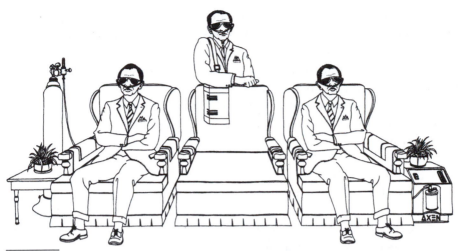

Figure 12.1   Home oxygen storage systems. *Left:* The patient is breathing from a large, H-size oxygen tank. *Middle:* The patient is carrying a portable liquid oxygen reservoir. *Right:* The patient is using an oxygen concentrator.

giant and extra-large thermoses, respectively, maintain the super-cold temperature needed to liquefy oxygen. As the liquid is drawn out it meets room air, which warms it, returning it to its gaseous state so it can be breathed.

These liquid storage flasks have two advantages over gas tanks. First, because you get the same amount of oxygen in a much smaller, lighter container, the stationary unit takes up less space and the portable unit is much easier to carry around. (The same volume of oxygen takes up significantly less space as a liquid than as a gas, so it needs a smaller, less weighty container. And since liquid oxygen doesn't build up the pressure that a gas does, the container doesn't need to be as strong. This makes it lighter still.)

Second, refilling your portable flask from the large one is safe and easy. Your DME dealer refills this large tank at regular intervals. You can breathe directly from it when you are at home and reserve your portable unit for your time away. Or you can use your portable unit full-time, treating the large tank simply as your storage facility.

These advantages make liquid oxygen particularly suitable for patients who go to work every day, and those whose desire to be on the go a lot takes them away from their stationary oxygen source for prolonged periods of time. *In fact, these small units revolutionized the lives of advanced COPD patients by enabling them to participate in activities outside the home.* There are devices to help you carry or wheel it around with you.

Continued improvements in both design (minimizing oxygen waste) and materials (making flasks lighter and stronger) have made the portable units even more mobile. The current state of the art is the new HELiOS oxygen system manufactured by Mallinckrodt. It features a portable oxygen unit weighing less than 3.4 lbs.—worn on a waist belt or shoulder strap or in a backpack—and provides 10 hours of use (at the standard flow rate of 2 liters/minute) between fillings. Filling is easily accomplished from your home reservoir in about 40 seconds, and the reservoir itself needs only 8 to 10 refills a year. Health care professionals who work with COPD patients are unusually excited about this system, which is expected to become available as we go to print.

But the liquid oxygen is not perfect. Like a pressure cooker, the storage flasks need a built-in leak to prevent buildup of explosive pressures, so some oxygen is lost from the tank when the patient isn't using it. A bigger problem—particularly if you travel out of town—is that none of the several brands of liquid oxygen are compatible. You cannot refill your flask from a larger container of a different brand. Also, liquid oxygen is typically more expensive than compressed gas oxygen. But all these disadvantages are usually outweighed by the ease of mobility liquid oxygen provides. If you are going to use liquid oxygen, *it is essential that your doctor specify it in your oxygen prescription.*

If you choose an *oxygen concentrator,* your DME dealer will provide you with equipment only. This electrically powered machine makes its own oxygen supply by separating it out of the surrounding air. It is cheaper and more convenient than compressed gas and liquid oxygen systems. More than 20 different devices currently exist for filtering oxygen out of room air. The major drawback of all these commercially available concentrators is their reliance on electricity. For starters, this means that patients using a concentrator must also keep a compressed gas system on hand in case the power fails. The need for electricity also precludes portability. And since a portable liquid gas flask cannot be refilled from a concentrator, the portable alternative is usually one of the precautionarily stored compressed gas canisters. Finally, although a concentrator's rental is subsidized by medical insurance, the cost of the electricity that runs it is not. Yet it increases the typical oxygen user's monthly electric bill an average of $40. The heavy user pays an average of $120 more per month.

The one caution with concentrators is their need for regular servicing to assure proper oxygen purity and flow rate. Do not consider renting an oxygen concentrator from a DME dealer who will not include an adequate servicing arrangement in your contract. Purchasing your own concentrator rather than renting doesn't seem to solve any problems, while it can add the burden of responsibility for repairs further complicated by a serious lack of service facilities.

Although little significant progress has been made in developing portable concentrators, a *cryocooler* system now in prototype form is being developed by InX for home use. The system—which will function as a middleman between your oxygen concentrator and whatever portable liquid oxygen system you use—is designed to divert a liter of oxygen per minute from any concentrator to the cryocooler, where it is cooled sufficiently to change from gas to liquid. This system will generate 0.8 lbs. of liquid oxygen daily in your home, enough to give you 8 to 10 hours away from home—depending, of course, on the rate of flow you require and whether or not you use a conserving system. If the engineering challenges presented by some of its components are solved, this equipment will dramatically reduce the need for oxygen deliveries and thus produce huge savings to suppliers. Dr. Tom Petty, one of the longtime leading lights in working for improved care and quality of life for COPD patients, suspects that "only regular preventive management will be required. And," he adds, "I see a role for the respiratory care practitioner coming into the home to help trouble-shoot and instruct patients in using this unit." He calls it "an exciting new development."

We hope that portable oxygen concentrators will be commercially available in the not too distant future. A prototype battery-powered concentrator was demonstrated at the 1987 World Congress on Oxygen Therapy held in Denver. Because a concentrator is not dependent on a preset oxygen supply, a portable device would provide unlimited freedom—as long as you have a battery supply on hand. A patient could, for example, go on vacation without needing to establish a network of oxygen suppliers.

Getting Oxygen from the Container to Your Lungs

The Initial Continuous Flow Device   The most common connection between you and your oxygen source delivers it continuously though your nose. (First came the *mask*, fitting over mouth and nose. This is infrequently used now because it is cumbersome and makes speaking difficult.) The *nasal cannula* is a piece of plastic tubing connected to the oxygen container that ends in two small prongs which rest in your nostrils. The tubing leading to your nostrils rests on your ears (Figure 12.2). It does away with the mask's difficulties, but some patients find it irritates their ears and/or nose.

But delivering oxygen continuously throughout the respiratory cycle is wasteful. You are paying for a substantial amount of oxygen you never get to use. During exhalation, the extra oxygen joins the stale air leaving your lungs. Oxygen delivered during the second half of inspiration never goes beyond the dead space. Only oxygen taken in during the start of inspiration actually reaches the alveoli to participate in gas exchange. Recognition of this problem has led to alternative solutions. Laboratory studies indicate that these newer, more efficient techniques achieve the same oxygenation while using substantially less oxygen, and work well for the majority of patients.

Transtracheal Oxygen Delivery   This technique—the most innovative and perhaps most important refinement in oxygen therapy—maintains continuous flow but moves the delivery site below the dead-space area. Permanently inserting a catheter (a thin plastic tube) into the patient's trachea to bypass dead space (Figure 12.2) was the brainchild of Dr. Henry Heimlich—the same person who developed the "Heimlich maneuver" for choking victims. Much more of the supplemental oxygen reaches the alveoli because little is wasted in dead space, oxygen is lost only at the start of expiration, and the oxygen accumulating in the trachea during the rest of expiration can go right to the air sacs when inspiration starts. Patients switching to this technique drop their oxygen consumption by one-half to two-thirds.

Patients switching from a nasal cannula also spontaneously lower their ventilation (the amount of air they breathe in each minute), which reduces the effort they put into their breathing. This means less stress on

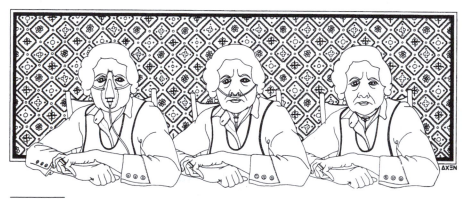

Figure 12.2   Oxygen delivery systems. *Left:* The oxygen mask is usually used in a hospital setting, but may be used at home to relieve irritations from a nasal cannula. *Middle:* The nasal cannula is the most popular method of oxygen delivery. *Right:* Transtracheal oxygenation, a new technique. Early research suggests that it may be more effective than either the mask or nasal cannula. It is certainly less obtrusive to wear and more aesthetic.

their respiratory system, and frees for other muscles the additional oxygen the respiratory muscles would otherwise be using. There are also indications that switching results in less dyspnea. There are other advantages. The tracheal catheter is less noticeable (in fact, it can be completely covered) and more comfortable than tubing that crisscrosses the middle of your face. And it is less likely to become disconnected during sleep.

Reservoir Cannulas Oxygen flows continuously from the container, but enters the nasal cannula only during inhalation. A tiny oxygen reservoir—either coupled to the nasal prongs or worn as a neck pendant—stores the oxygen during exhalation. Then it joins the start of inhalation. Patients adding such a reservoir to the standard nasal cannula drop their oxygen consumption by one-half to three-fourths.

Electronic Demand Devices Also called conserving devices, these electronic devices can sense the start of inspiration, and rapidly deliver a short burst of oxygen during that phase of the breathing cycle. Avoiding dead space and exhalation means it should all go to the alveoli. So far these devices have been used with a nasal cannula rather than a tracheal catheter. In general, oxygen consumption with these electronic devices is one-half to one-fifth what it would be on continuous flow oxygen. Because a relatively small amount of gas can be stretched over a relatively long time period, this setup is much less costly than liquid oxygen.

The *caution* is that these electronic conserving devices are not appropriate or safe for all patients. *Not all patients can use them safely during activity requiring an effort.* Patients with severe disease, patients with end-stage disease—even patients who do not have good breathing technique—will not maintain a high enough level of oxygen in their blood when they exercise or carry out an activity that—for them—is relatively strenuous. The DMEs favor conserving devices along with gas canisters because this increases their profit. The problem is that any supply company considering a conserving device along with a gas canister for a particular patient is supposed to make sure that his oxygen level remains safe—yet too many them do not do this. Rehabilitation personnel estimate that roughly one-third of patients do not oxygenate adequately with conserving devices and need to be on continuous flow. (The few small studies confirming this observation need to be supported by a definitive study involving a large number of patients in different pulmonary rehabilitation programs across the country.) It is very important not to let your DME insist that you use a conserving device unless you have been properly evaluated and *know* that this gives you enough oxygen regardless of what you are doing. If the DME persists in providing you with a conserving device despite it being wrong for you, ask your doctor and your rehabilitation professionals to put their weight behind you.

We have encountered only one problem with electronic demand systems when used by certain patients in our closely supervised laboratory *while they exercise*. These are patients who either talk while they exercise, or breathe through their mouths. During exercise, the oxygen level in their blood falls. One of our patients in this category has a portable unit that can be set for either "continuous" or "demand" delivery. Normally he uses it on the "demand" setting, and changes it to "continuous" only when he is exercising.

Cosmetic Improvements

As we said in an earlier section, the tracheal catheter is much less noticeable than tubes crisscrossing a patient's face. It can even be completely covered up.

Insurance Reimbursement

Note: The status of appropriate and adequate insurance-covered oxygen availability for COPD patients needing this supplement is in flux. The situation presented here describes the lay of the land at the time this book entered the printing process. Because advocacy efforts may well have produced significant improvement since then, what you read here may already be out of date. If you have any questions or concerns, you can check the appropriate websites or contact PERF, *The Pulmonary Paper*, and/or NHOPA (National Home Oxygen Patients Association) for up-to-the-minute news. If you subscribe to *The Pulmonary Paper* or PERF's *Second Wind*, these newsletters will automatically keep you abreast of any important changes.

Oxygen used at home for long periods is expensive whether the pocket paying for it belongs to the patient, a private insurer, or a government agency. But this cost must be weighed against the far greater economic impact from loss of employment, repeated hospitalizations, and eventual full-time health care at home or in an institution.

But as too often happens these days, insurance payments have been complicated by legislation. Despite overwhelming acceptance of oxygen's benefits for patients with chronic hypoxia, government regulations—in the form of Health Care Financing Administration requirements introduced in 1986—permit doctors little flexibility in prescribing oxygen therapy for patients who need insurance reimbursement. In brief, they allow home oxygen only for severe lung disease associated with these significant symptoms and signs of hypoxia: pulmonary hypertension, congestive right heart failure from *cor pulmonale*, polycythemia, impaired neuropsychiatric function, nocturnal restlessness, and morning headaches.

The doctor's prescription must list the diagnosis, acceptable laboratory evidence of hypoxia (current criteria are a stable oxygen tension of 55 mmMg or less or a blood saturation level of 88% or less), required oxygen flow (for example, 2 liters/minute), estimated frequency, and duration of oxygen use. And because reimbursement is not tightly tied to this prescribed amount (calculated on a monthly basis), patients who find themselves needing more must pay the difference themselves until their doctor writes them a new prescription.

Prescriptions for portable oxygen must also be carefully worded. They must be for the therapeutic purpose of promoting exercise and muscle conditioning, with concretely specified goals (for example, to participate in a pulmonary rehabilitation program, or to increase activities of daily living). Otherwise, portable oxygen will not be reimbursed.

Since the first edition of this book, the changing economics of health care have seriously cut into the adequacy of home oxygen for those who need it. A spokesman for the Pulmonary Education and Research Foundation (PERF) explains what has happened. First we'll describe the difficulties that have developed as a consequence of cuts in Medicare reimbursement, then we'll touch on the impact that HMOs now have.

Many of the DMEs had become rather unscrupulous, profiting quite lavishly on supplying home medical equipment of all kinds and, as a result, building a very negative reputation in Congress. Congress attempted to restrain this excess by passing a bill enacting a substantial two-part cut across the board in Medicare reimbursement. The problem is that the politicians drafting this bill were unaware that home oxygen users would be needlessly penalized by the fallout—that the DMEs would attempt to compensate for these cuts by picking on a highly vulnerable group of patients. COPD patients are so concerned with getting enough air to breathe that they are not easily roused to noisy protest, and the fear of those who did realize the potential consequences was that the typical DME would ignore the specifics of a physician's prescription and uniformly give clients the cheapest service.

Unfortunately, notice of the bill and the upcoming vote on it had been so sudden that spokesmen for home oxygen users had only a few days to prepare their case, and that was not enough time to gather the kind of data needed to respond to this threat. Because they had no opportunity to show Congress that home oxygen must be exempt from these cuts in order to preserve patients' access to the air they need for conducting their lives, the bill was signed as written. Medicare reimbursement for all home medical equipment was cut by 25% beginning January 1998, and by an additional 5% in January 1999.

The consequence is that oxygen is reimbursed at a flat rate that is 30% less than it had been before January 1998. So the less a DME spends for home oxygen equipment, the more they profit from Medicare reimbursement. Concentrators and gas canisters are cheap; liquid oxygen is not. And what was predicted has now come to pass. PERF points to the recent survey by the Government Accounting Office (GAO) that found 80% of home oxygen users are now relegated to E-cylinders. Although the GAO views E-cylinders as portable, they are not. When full, and with the cart needed to transport them, they weigh up to 30 pounds and run for a maximum of 4 hours at 2 liters/minute. A canister of liquid oxygen weighs just 5 pounds, and the eagerly anticipated HELiOS system weighs even less. Set for the same flow rate, it will last for 8 hours. This spells freedom. The E-cylinder does not.

(To be fair in portraying the overall fallout from this bill, DMEs were financially devastated by these cuts. Many went out of business, while others are still struggling to survive.)

Phil Porte, Executive Director of the patient advocacy group NHOPA (National Home Oxygen Patients Association), emphasizes that these problems are compounded by the fact that Medicare—unusually—does not require the supplier to follow the physician's prescription. "A physician can write a prescription for an oxygen concentrator for nighttime use, plus an ambulatory liquid system set for three or four liters/minute during exercise, and so on," he explains, "yet the company filling this prescription is permitted to say: 'All we supply are oxygen concentrators.' This is unheard of in any other area," Mr. Porte comments. "When was the last time you went to the pharmacy with a prescription and the pharmacist insisted that you had to accept something different and not as satisfactory!" One way in which some of the DMEs try to reduce their costs is by providing a conserving device along with E-cylinders, insisting that increasing the usage time makes them more portable. But these cylinders are just as heavy and difficult to maneuver, and the companies that do this tend not to make sure that this setup goes only to patients who can maintain their oxygen levels with it.

Phil Porte also notes that the supplier industry defeated a strong attempt in 1997 to gain home oxygen reimbursement that is modality-specific, a change that would have removed any profit-based incentive to supply the cheapest type of oxygen. "And patients are getting short-changed. Availability of liquid oxygen has decreased and the use of concentrators has gone up—just as the physician community predicted," he adds. He is advocating for reimbursement tied to modality, and for a law requiring DMEs to provide for each patient they service the modality the physician ordered.

We cannot stress enough that your doctor *must* specify liquid oxygen in your oxygen prescription if portability will enable you to leave your home. But the process may not end there. Some DMEs require so many letters of need documenting a hardship for the patient on an E-cylinder that even the most persistent of physicians may be tempted to give up. If nothing seems to work in getting liquid oxygen from the DME that you have to deal with, you might want to follow the lead of a very frustrated patient we heard of. She got her liquid system after threatening to contact the local investigative TV reporter, and has had no further problems with delivery.

As for the HMOs, if their overriding concern is the financial bottom line, it can significantly compromise what COPD patients receive. We were told of one HMO that always chose the lowest-bidding DME for providing home oxygen. This tended to be a small company that could only meet this low price by *not* providing adequate service. This meant no oxygen deliveries on a regular basis; not providing items that normally are part of the setup—like oxygen tubing and conservation devices; and limiting patients to 3 or 4 E-cylinders a month rather than giving them as many refills as needed and/or placing them on a more portable system. And such DMEs do not monitor patients on conserving devices to make sure that their oxygen level doesn't fall during exercise. Although active complaints at the highest level of government have improved this particular local problem, the danger still currently exists.

So for COPD patients, pressures affecting home oxygen adequacy are coming from several directions at once. *Advocacy is crucial—by you as well as by those who have made it their job to speak out on your behalf.* Patients and their families are advised to write to their senators and congressman whenever a relevant issue is coming up for a vote. Joining NHOPA and PERF is important, to add strength to their growing numbers. And they will also keep you informed about timing for writing letters and making phone calls. For specific reimbursement or HMO problems, your local office of the Health Insurance Counseling and Advocacy Program or the Medicare Advocacy Program *may* be able to help. We are told that they vary tremendously in effectiveness, but it's worth a try. Sometimes they are truly helpful.

Pulmonary Education and Research Foundation
P.O. Box 1133
Lomita, CA 90717-5133
310-539-8390; *perf@packbell.net*
www.Perf2ndwind.org

National Home Oxygen Patients Association
888-NHOPA44

A final note: A group that may make life a little easier when you travel, whether it's for business or pleasure, is *Freedom Link*, a service provided by the VGM Group, an independent buying alliance for DMEs. Find out if your DME belongs to the VGM Group. If they do, tell them of your travel plans—location and dates—and they will request the VGM Group to locate an appropriate oxygen supplier at your destination and make all the necessary arrangements for you to be properly supplied.

Some basic information on air travel can be found on the web at *www.access-able.com/tips/oxy.html*, and the group providing this—*Access-Able Travel Source*—can be reached at 303-232-2979. Then there is *The Oxygen Traveler*, a travel agency specializing in securing—for a fee—whatever is necessary for oxygen-bound patients on the go: 937-848-7100; *www.oxygentravel.net*; *oxygen0202@aol.com*.

13

Physical Therapies for COPD

Physical therapy was first developed to rehabilitate muscles that were injured or paralyzed. Today it covers much more—including training the heart and lungs to supply oxygenated blood to the body much more efficiently than they could before. Sometimes this is necessary after an acute health problem, such as a heart attack. Rehabilitation should also follow illness requiring prolonged bedrest. *It is of major importance during a chronic condition, such as emphysema or chronic bronchitis.* That is the focus of this chapter.

First we will talk about the more traditional aspects of pulmonary physical therapy, that is: relaxation techniques, exercises for breathing more effectively with hyperinflated lungs and obstructed airways, postural drainage to clear the airways of tenacious mucus, and an effective way to cough. Then we will describe the newly developed technique for actually strengthening the respiratory muscles. The remainder of this chapter is devoted to the importance of physical fitness.

Goal Setting

Before actually beginning a program, you will get the most out of it if you, your physical therapist, and your doctor spend a little bit of time identifying your particular goals—what *you* want to get out of the program. This will also facilitate the partnership between the three of you that is an essential ingredient in maximizing your success. In addition, the three of you in cooperation will produce the most realistic set of goals for *you*. And knowing that your needs have received central attention in structuring your program will be a powerful motivator in helping you stick to it.

Relaxation Techniques

Muscle relaxation techniques include four overlapping approaches: (1) working directly with the muscles; (2) music; (3) different forms of meditation; and (4) biofeedback. Physical therapists often combine several to get optimum results. (In some hospitals, meditation and biofeedback are carried out by a department other than physical therapy.)

Muscle Relaxation

Jacobson's relaxation technique, the most widely used of the many relaxation methods, bears the name of the man who developed it in the early 1920s. Edmond Jacobson was a Chicago physician and physiologist who theorized that muscle relaxation and psychological stress cannot coexist. A growing body of evidence now suggests that muscle relaxation causes physiological changes that are the mirror opposite of those occurring with stress and anxiety. Taken together, these changes are called the *relaxation response.*

In theory, if stress cannot exist in a relaxed body, then improving your ability to relax your muscles at will should eliminate whatever role anxiety plays in worsening your condition. Research with asthmatics, for example, indicates that the regular use of a muscle relaxation technique reduces the intensity of attacks.

Jacobson's technique is a prescribed sequence of quiet muscle exercises that alternately tense and relax all of the major muscle groups. While one group is being focused on, all of the others are to remain as relaxed as possible. A few sessions with a physical therapist are usually all that is needed to learn this technique of progressive relaxation.

Initially the exercises should be done while lying down in a quiet, dimly lit room (Figure 13.1). Loosen all restrictive clothing and remove your shoes. Once the technique is mastered, it can be done while sitting in a comfortable chair, or even at work. Start at the head or toes, focusing on each part of the body in order until the end of the sequence is reached. The sequence progresses over seven areas: (1) ankles, shins, calves, knees, thighs, buttocks, lower back; (2) stomach; (3) neck, chest, shoulders; (4) jaws, lips, head; (5) eyes; (6) forehead, biceps, elbows; (7) fingers, hands, forearms, upper arms.

Within an area, each muscle site is tensed individually for 5 to 10 seconds, then relaxed for about 30 seconds. This is repeated several times before continuing to the next group of muscles. With each muscle, the person concentrates on how the contraction makes it feel, and how it feels when it relaxes. The entire procedure takes about 30 minutes. Several ses-

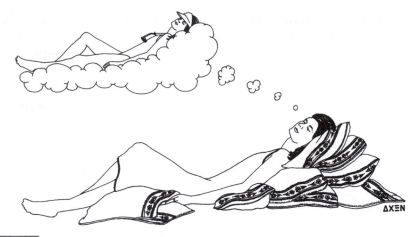

Figure 13.1   Supported positioning for facilitating relaxation.

sions gradually produce a clear memory of what relaxation feels like, and the ability to control it. You will get out of this program what you put into it, which means that it can work only if you are committed to doing it regularly. Ideally, a specific time each day should be set aside for these relaxation exercises.

Music

Music influences our brain's rhythms, which in turn affects some of our bodily responses. Because the right kind of soft, slow music tends to calm physiologic responses, it can provide a soothing, helpful background for learning and practicing relaxation exercises.

We know that instrumental music is more calming than vocal music, and classical music is more calming than either jazz or rock 'n' roll. Since very rhythmic compositions can actually bring the listener's breathing and heart rates into synchrony with it, a slow, strong rhythm especially promotes deeper and more efficient relaxation. So selecting slow—particularly rhythmic—movements from classical pieces is most appropriate for aiding your muscle relaxation work. But if music is not to your liking, recordings of gentle rain, sounds of the sea, and bird songs also stimulate relaxation responses.

Meditation

The effects of meditation are very real on a physical level. Successful use of a meditation technique actually means that the person has learned to control certain aspects of his central nervous system. This is another way to achieve the relaxation response.

Transcendental meditation (TM) has been studied extensively, perhaps because of the sudden popularity it attained during the 1960s. TM definitely lowers oxygen use, ventilation, and heart rate. An experiment specifically with asthmatics found TM to lower airway resistance by half, and increase air flow by a small but meaningful amount. But the long-term relation of meditation techniques to mysticism—because of their historical roots in Eastern and Western religions—has kept them from the mainstream of therapy.

The meditator's goal is to empty his mind, remaining totally passive in mind and body for the duration of his meditating time. TM gives an excellent illustration of the basic meditation technique. The environment is quiet, and as free of stimulation as possible. To lessen his chances of being distracted, the meditator learns to repeat a specific word continuously without concentrating on it, and also learns to ignore any thoughts that still do intrude.

Biofeedback

Biofeedback uses a learning situation to change the nature of a physiological response (heart rate, for example). Electronic or mechanical equipment continuously measures and displays (for the eye and/or ear) this physiological behavior, so that the patient can see what happens when he attempts to change it. In this way he learns how to achieve this change. Biofeedback has been used with COPD to facilitate relaxation training.

For relaxation training, the electrical activity of the muscles supplies the feedback that helps the patient do a more effective job of reducing his muscle tone. Electrical activity diminishes as the muscles relax. During training sessions the patient sits by himself in a quiet room, which helps him in his relaxation effort.

Any of several muscles may be monitored, but some consider facial muscle tone to be particularly important. Relaxing the forehead muscle automatically relaxes the scalp, neck, and upper body. The mechanism behind this connection is presently a mystery, but the implications for relaxation training—particularly in COPD—are clear.

Biofeedback will not be successful for the patient who cannot make the commitment to practice his newly learned skill at home. It takes diligent practice to produce this reflexive response so that it can easily be called up in everyday stress situations.

Breathing Exercises

Breathing exercises—based on the substantial voluntary control we have over our respiratory muscles—are probably the most widely used of all respiratory physical therapy techniques. COPD patients can use this control to improve their respiration by learning the most effective way to breathe with hyperinflated lungs and narrowed airways.

What Needs to Be Changed About the Way You Breathe?

First, remember that you are short of breath in part because your diaphragm—your primary inspiratory muscle—is no longer working properly, and your accessory inspiratory muscles are not able to give much help. (We're going to summarize a few relevant facts brought out in Chapter 2. With the amount of ground covered in the intervening chapters, this brief refresher will be very helpful for many readers.)

Your diaphragm is the dome-shaped muscle separating your chest and abdominal cavities. With healthy lungs it contracts during inspiration, pulling the dome down flat into the abdominal area. But the COPD patient's diaphragm remains flattened because his permanently distended lungs continuously press down upon it. It can no longer contract. Over-inflated lungs also shorten the accessory inspiratory muscles between the ribs, so they, too, remain in an inspiratory position before inspiration even begins. This limited inspiratory muscle movement allows only very small breaths. The consequence: patients become so anxious for air, they no longer finish exhaling before starting their next breath. So the air trapping that caused the hyperinflation gets even worse.

Second, remember that the faster you try to force air through airways narrowed by mucus and inflammation, the more resistance the air encounters and the harder your respiratory muscles have to work. Some patients naturally adopt a slow style of breathing. Others, perhaps from greater anxiety about their disease, breathe much more rapidly than they need to. Because this makes their breathing far more difficult, they become even more distressed and anxious.

What Can Breathing Exercises Do?

The basic breathing exercises—*diaphragmatic breathing* and *pursed-lip expiration*—were developed with two goals in mind. They teach you to breathe more *effectively*, meaning they improve your ventilation. They teach you to breathe more *efficiently*, meaning you use less effort. This happens by helping your diaphragm function more effectively, and slowing down your breathing rate to ensure complete exhalation and minimize resistance. These breathing techniques may also help keep the airways open. (Because these exercises relax the abdominal muscles, they also help reinforce the results of the relaxation techniques that we discussed earlier in this chapter.)

Note: Although both components of the breathing exercises are simple to learn and do on your own, it is a good idea to learn them from a physical therapist to make sure that you are doing them properly.

How to Do the Breathing Exercises

Since Figure 13.2 illustrates the breathing exercise variations, referring to it as you read this section will be helpful.

Lie flat on your back with a pillow under your knees, because this position exaggerates abdominal movement. First preference is a carpeted floor, second preference is a firm bed. Keep your mouth closed so that you always breathe through your nose. Rest one hand on the middle of your chest at about your nipple level. Place the other hand on your abdomen, thumb just below your navel. Since your abdomen—not your chest—should move as you breathe, the hand that moves tells you whether or not you are doing the exercise properly.

First, concentrate on letting your abdominal muscles relax. As you breathe, you should feel the hand on your abdomen rise and fall while the hand on your chest remains still. When you are ready to add pursed-lip expiration to diaphragmatic breathing, inhale slowly and smoothly through your nose, then purse your lips (like you're getting ready to whistle) and breathe out slowly. Your lips should be tight enough so that the air comes out with a soft hissing sound. You should feel your abdomen moving inward, with no movement in your chest. Keep relaxed, and avoid straining with the upper part of your chest and your neck muscles.

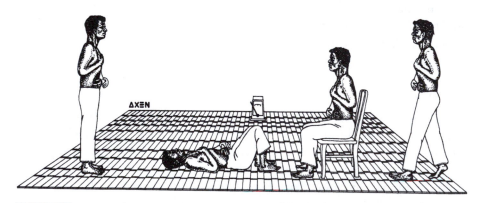

Figure 13.2 Breathing exercises should be performed in each stationary position, and then while walking. Expiration should take twice as long as inspiration. A metronome can be a helpful timing device. Set it to a one-second beat, then count out three beats for inspiration, for example, and six beats for breathing out. Breathe in through your nose and expire through pursed lips.

Make your expirations twice as long as your inspirations. Some people find that a two-second inspiration and four-second expiration work well. Others prefer three seconds "in" and six seconds "out." A loud clock or a metronome can help to pace your breathing. (Aim at keeping your breathing rate between 10 and 15 breaths per minute.)

Once your breathing feels relaxed, practice taking deeper breaths. The deeper the breath, the more you have to concentrate on keeping your upper chest relaxed. To exhale properly, pull in your lower ribs as well as contracting your abdominal muscles. Periodically do four or five of these deep breaths, then return to your natural rhythm.

Practice this exercise combination for 20 minutes a day. When it has become quite effortless, do the exercise sitting up instead of lying down. Once this becomes very easy, graduate to a standing position, and then finally do it while you walk. (Your breathing rate may increase slightly to make up for the added oxygen demands of walking.)

Why Do These Exercises Work?

Everyone agrees on the benefits of the slow, relaxed breathing that diaphragmatic breathing and pursed-lip expiration foster. Discussion continues, though, as to what underlies these benefits. One school of thought claims that making breathing slower allows it to become more coordinated. The other feels that the pressure developed by expiring through pursed lips actually keeps the airways open. There is also controversy as to the best method for achieving slow, relaxed breathing: Is it diaphragmatic plus pursed-lip breathing, yoga, Zen meditation, or learning to play a wind instrument (such as flute or recorder)? Our feeling is that none of these techniques is harmful, and anything that increases a patient's sensitivity to what his respiratory system is doing must be helpful.

Recovering from Shortness of Breath

An important aim of breathing exercises is learning the positions and breathing patterns that will enable you to regain control of your breathing if you suddenly become short of breath. You've probably already discovered on your own that sitting straighter while also bending forward slightly at the waist is very helpful. There is logic behind this: bending forward causes your abdomen to push your diaphragm up into a more efficient position, and lengthening your spine gives your better-placed diaphragm more room to move. Figure 13.3 shows some sample positions.

The first point is to find a place to sit down if at all possible. Then stabilize your arms—either rest your elbows on your knees or place your forearms on a table in front of you. Use pursed-lip expiration along with

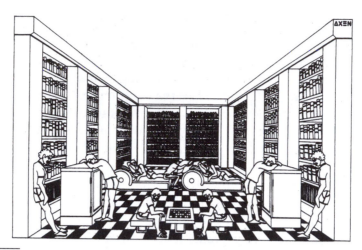

Figure 13.3   Temporary relaxation positions help you catch your breath by briefly lowering your energy demands and easing your breathing.

a breathing rate that feels comfortable to you. Don't worry if this is quite rapid at first. Try to gently prolong expiration in a 1:2 inspiratory-to-expiratory ratio, meaning that your expirations are twice as long as your inspirations. As you feel your breathing coming under control, try gradually slowing your breathing rate and at the same time breathe more deeply.

If sitting isn't an option, don't panic. These same principles can be practiced standing up. The important point is to support yourself while you bend forward at the waist to raise your diaphragm to an easier breathing position. Face the nearest wall or ledge and stabilize yourself with your hands or forearms against it while you bend forward. Or lean back against the wall or ledge, and bend forward while you support yourself by placing your hands above your slightly bent knees.

During the physical therapy session, it will be extremely helpful for your therapist to try recreating the situations that typically make you short of breath. The safety of the physical therapy setting will give you the sense of freedom to take some "risks" in trying coping strategies to find what works best for you. And this will have an immeasurable impact on your confidence in your ability to handle these situations on your own. Some of the activities you might want to practice include walking up inclines, climbing stairs, rushing to answer the phone, and grooming activities that require repetitive arm movements.

Postural Drainage

The patient whose mucus is so tenacious that coughing does not bring it up can benefit from a technique called *postural* or *gravity drainage*. As the name implies, this technique uses gravity to help drain mucus that has been loosened by clapping (technically called *percussing*), and then vibrating, the patient's chest and back. This is done in a variety of postures for a maximum of 30 minutes. (Although 12 postures exist, only 9 are commonly used.) Someone else usually does the clapping and vibrating. Most often this is a physical therapist or nurse, but the technique is so easy that a family member—or even the patient himself—can learn it from one of these professionals in just a few sessions.

Twelve different positions exist for drainage because the bronchial tree branches in many directions. Figure 13.4 illustrates the 12 common positions in which clapping and vibration must be applied to drain each section of the lungs.

Postural drainage needs to be done only when a great deal of tenacious mucus is being produced. For some patients this means daily, and for others it is only periodic. Not all patients need to use all 12 positions for effective mucus drainage. If postural drainage is included in your rehabilitation program, make sure to get a written list of the positions you and your partner are being taught. It's too easy to forget one once you're on your own.

A large glass of water is taken before doing postural drainage. (COPD sufferers should always be well hydrated, which means having an ample amount of fluid in your system. This is especially important for patients with tenacious mucus. Drink 6 to 8 glasses of water every day—unless you have a heart or kidney condition that can't sustain this amount of fluid.) Although a slant board is most convenient for the positions lying down, you can also use your bed. Stack several large pillows on the floor, close to your bedside, so they end about 18 inches below your bed. Hang over the edge of your bed so you can rest your forearms on the pillow stack. (If you want to use a slant board, your physical therapist can tell you where to purchase one.)

Each position should be held for 2 or 3 minutes while clapping and vibration are done. Clapping is done with a cupped hand to produce a hollow—not sharp—sound. Vibrating is done during expiration by quickly shaking the hand on the designated area. Mucus doesn't always come up immediately. So if you don't cough sputum up right away in a particular position, hold it up to 15 minutes.

Precaution: Many elderly people have fragile bones, especially if they have been on steroids for a long time. An elderly person with this problem risks rib fracture from the clapping. If there is the slightest question about this possibility, consult your doctor.

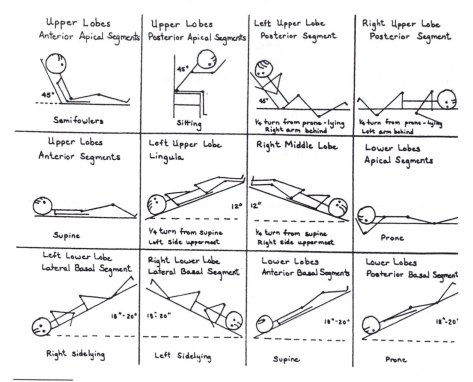

Figure 13.4   Typical postural or bronchial drainage positions for ensuring that each segment of the lungs is drained.

Source: Reproduced with permission from S. L. Garritan, Chest physical therapy treatment of the patient with chronic obstructive pulmonary disease. In F. Haas and K. Axen (eds.), *Pulmonary Therapy and Rehabilitation: Principles and Practices,* 2nd edition (Baltimore: Williams & Wilkins, 1991), p. 226.

Hints for Thinning Mucus Before Drainage

1. Use an ultrasonic nebulizer or aerosol treatment.
2. Take a hot, steamy shower.
3. Drink hot liquids, such as tea.
4. Use a bronchodilator 20 minutes beforehand if bronchospasm is one of your symptoms.

See Chapter 11, on Complementary Therapies, for herbs that are also helpful in thinning and bringing up excess mucus.

Timing of Postural Drainage

Patients who produce large amounts of mucus generally get the most out of postural drainage by doing it in the morning before eating breakfast.

This helps to reduce coughing during the day. If postural drainage needs to be repeated several times during the day, avoid doing it right after eating and disturbing your digestion—and it can be helpful to emphasize a different set of positions each time. The patient who is frequently awakened during the night by coughing often finds it helpful to have a postural drainage session about 1 to 2 hours before going to bed.

But in *all* cases—whatever the timing—remember that it may take up to an hour *after* the actual drainage procedure for the mucus to move to a point at which you can clear it. So relax—and give yourself time.

Relearning to Cough

An effective cough is supremely important in heading off respiratory infections and preventing air sac collapse—termed *atelectasis*. It helps steer clear of respiratory infections by clearing bacteria-collecting secretions out of the airways. No one is yet quite sure how a good cough prevents atelectasis, but we suspect that—similar to pursed-lip breathing—it creates a back pressure that keeps vulnerable air sacs from deflating.

Despite the particular importance of an effective cough for COPD patients, people with advanced COPD have a particularly difficult time producing one. The severe damage to their lungs produces coughing that is excessive, exhausting, and ineffective. But the typical vigorous cough of a healthy person would be just as dangerous for them. In a severe COPD patient, such a cough collapses the airways and so prevents removal of mucus. These patients need to learn *huffing* to help bring up their sputum, because it requires less energy, is still strong enough to push secretions along, and avoids airway collapse—which would otherwise trap mucus.

How do you huff? Take as full a breath as you can, then breathe out sharply, pushing out the air with your abdominal muscles while your vocal cords stay open. Its sound is "breathy" rather than the explosive sound of a typical cough.

Ironically, huffing's gentle nature is also a drawback. Our physical therapists report that many of the advanced COPD patients they work with don't believe anything so gentle can be effective. So they often ignore it—to their detriment. *Don't be fooled by the fact that huffing doesn't feel or sound high-energy. It works!*

Huffing can also provide postsurgical help to COPD patients who still have their normal strong cough. Because it is less painful than regular coughing after abdominal or chest surgery, this low-energy, effective technique for removing airway mucus is temporarily useful in these situations.

Respiratory Muscle Strengthening

Once the amount of work required of a muscle goes beyond its fatigue threshold, that muscle's endurance quickly declines. In severe COPD, the respiratory muscles are working at their limit during resting breathing. So any increase in ventilatory demand—which in turn increases their workload—fatigues these muscles and so contributes to respiratory insufficiency. Exercise raises that fatigue level.

Until recently, it was thought that the respiratory muscles couldn't benefit from exercise. But current research has repeatedly shown them to be no different than the muscles elsewhere in our body. Their strength and endurance can be increased by appropriate exercises.

The standard technique uses a small, inexpensive device (there are several on the market) consisting of a plastic tube capable of adjustment to a variety of inspiratory resistances. The resistance can be progressively increased as needed. Expiration is through a low-resistance flap. Breathing through this device is done for 15 minutes twice a day. Both the initial resistance setting and the rate of your progression through the resistance levels are decided by your doctor.

Physical Fitness

If exercise substantially increases dyspnea for so many COPD patients, why are we encouraging you to exercise? In part, it is for the same reason that we encourage most people to exercise. The overwhelming weight of the evidence is that exercise is good for you. And in addition, it has been shown that patients with respiratory problems who continue to be physically active are in better health and function more effectively than their sedentary counterparts.

Part of the benefit we all get from regular exercise is that our muscles "learn" to use oxygen more efficiently. They do more work with less oxygen. (We call these muscles "trained" or "conditioned.") For COPD patients, this ability to do more with less oxygen is critical.

And it enables them to avoid a critical pitfall—the typical COPD vicious cycle of deconditioning described in Chapter 1. At the end of this vicious cycle, the typical patient reaches a point at which deconditioning has eroded his physical capacities well beyond what his pulmonary function tests indicate they should be. He finds even basic daily activities of self-care too demanding, and accepts the passive lifestyle of a respiratory cripple. *The aim of a physical fitness program is either to prevent this cycle from taking hold, or to reverse it when it already has.*

How Does Exercise "Teach" Our Muscles?

Our body—in particular, our cardiovascular system—adapts to exercise. The kind of exercise we are talking about is "aerobic" exercise, which means that the muscles get their energy from oxygen-fueled metabolism. "Training" is the term given to the cardiovascular adaptation process.

During any given bout of aerobic exercise, our exercising muscles need more and more oxygen. Our heart helps by pumping faster, increasing both the amount of blood circulating through our lungs to pick up oxygen and the amount of oxygen-rich blood carried to the muscles. The rest of the job belongs to our respiratory system, which must make more oxygen available for the increased volume of blood now traveling through the lungs. Our respiratory muscles work harder to breathe deeper and faster.

What happens when this exercise is repeated on a routine (meaning at least three-times-a-week) basis? Training takes place. This does not mean that the heart or lungs become better at their job. It is the muscle tissue that becomes much more efficient at taking oxygen out of the blood circulating through it. As the muscles "learn" to use a much greater proportion of the oxygen available to them, the heart no longer has to pump as much additional blood, and the respiratory muscles do not have to help the lungs bring in as much additional air.

Because the exercise level is unchanged, even though the heart and respiratory system are no longer working as hard, the person's maximum exercise capacity is now greater than it was. This means that reaching the maximum effort his heart and lungs are capable of will require more intense exercise than it did before. This is another way of saying that training has occurred.

We aren't suggesting that every COPD patient can achieve the same level of exercise training as healthy people (and even some patients with cardiovascular disease). Though they may never run a marathon, *exercise conditioning unquestionably provides significant benefits for most COPD patients.* Many studies demonstrate their improved work capacity, greater sense of well-being, and increased participation in activities of daily living. Statistics show that these "in-shape" patients are much more likely to remain productive members of society.

Questions About Exercise

When it comes to exercise, you're obviously going to have more questions than someone with healthy lungs, and ask them with greater concern. Every patient wants to know:

☐ What kind of exercise is best for me? Should I swim, walk, get an exercise bicycle?

☐ How long should my exercise periods be?

☐ How hard should I exercise?

Here are some answers.

What Kind?   Although any kind of exercise you enjoy will improve your fitness, we specifically recommend walking for COPD patients. There are three reasons. Because walking is something you do every day, improving your walking speed and endurance directly improves your daily life. Because you walk every day, it is easy to fit into your daily routine. Last of all—once you have a comfortable pair of shoes—it doesn't cost anything!

How Long and How Often?   Experiments tell us that 20 to 30 minutes of sufficiently intense exercise done three times a week greatly improves exercise capacity. Below this minimum, results are substantially less gratifying.

What Is "Sufficiently Intense?"   Intensity of effort is the single most important criterion for identifying effective exercise, but determining it—especially for more severe COPD patients—is not straightforward. Each person must find what is appropriate for him.

Under normal circumstances, heart rate is the typical indicator of how hard someone works during exercise. That's because—for people without severe respiratory problems—it's usually the heart that limits the amount of strenuous work he can do. This limit is expressed as his *maximum heart rate*, which is how fast his heart is pumping when he suddenly becomes too tired to maintain the set pace. *The ideal exercise increases your heart rate to somewhere between 60 and 70% of your maximum.* Then comes the question: How do you find out your maximum heart rate and then what your upper limit for exercising should be?

Finding your upper limit heart rate for exercising if you have mild to moderate COPD   For COPD patients in this category—as well as for healthy people—it's nothing fancy. Since your heart sets the limit, and that relationship is affected by age, we can safely estimate your maximum heart rate with a simple formula: 220 minus Age equals HRmax (subtract your age from the typical youthful maximum heart rate of 220 to get your current maximum). So a 50-year-old COPD patient with only moderate disease would do exercise to maintain his heart rate at an upper limit somewhere between 102 to 119 beats per minute: $220 - 50 = 170$; $.60 \times 170 = 102 / .70 \times 170 = 119$.

Finding your upper limit heart rate for exercising if you have advanced COPD   But we can't use this formula for advanced COPD patients, because your respiratory system—not your heart—is setting the limit on your exercise tolerance, and this limit is lower than what your heart would otherwise set. If you are debilitated, your exercise tolerance is lower still. How much lower depends on how deconditioned you are. So the advanced COPD patient's "maximum" heart rate is simply how fast his heart is beating when he is working as hard as he can—however much or little that may be. Then a percentage of this maximum, plus the extent of both his disease and his debilitation, determine the heart rate he shoots for when he first begins exercising.

We can't safely estimate an advanced COPD patient's "maximum" heart rate. Instead, it is measured during a stress test under a doctor's supervision. Don't let the word *stress* scare your from reading further. A stress test is not designed to overwork or exhaust you, but simply to provide the information needed to prescribe a safe and effective exercise program. We prefer calling it an "exercise test." (Figure 6.4, in Chapter 6, illustrates the typical exercise testing apparatus.)

As you walk at a comfortable speed on the treadmill, we learn the level of physical activity you can comfortably—and safely—carry out, and how long you can comfortably—and safely—do it. Measuring exactly how hard you are breathing and how fast your heart is pumping when you eventually start to become short of breath pinpoints your exercise tolerance. If this level is less than what your overall medical profile says you should be able to do, we know you are debilitated and to what degree. Compiling all this information then tells us by what reconditioning schedule your exercise tolerance may be safely extended.

Then during your reconditioning program, a repeat exercise test every so often shows us—and you—your progress. And the amount of progress indicates when—and by how much—you can increase your exercise intensity.

Supplemental Oxygen? An exercise test also lets us see if a patient with adequate oxygen and carbon dioxide levels at rest become underoxygenated during exercise. These patients, and those whose oxygen level is always low, return for a second exercise test that they take while breathing supplemental oxygen. We want to identify those patients who are able to exercise longer when they use it. When supplemental oxygen does have that effect, we know it is important in that particular patient's treatment program.

How and Where to Exercise

Despite consistently impressive research results, the traditional fear—from both doctors and patients—of combining exercise and serious lung disease takes a long time to disappear. So—although exercise training facilities are now commonplace for healthy people and routine in cardiac rehabilitation programs—structured exercise training programs for COPD patients remain uncommon.

But that doesn't have to stop you. In the same way that healthy people don't have to join a health spa or gym to exercise, COPD patients also have more than one option. With your doctor's advice, you can devise a routine exercise program to do at home. *The core of this program should be a daily 20- to 30-minute walk, with 10 to 15 minutes of warm-up exercise before, and 10 to 15 minutes of cool-down exercise after.* Your walk can be around the house, around the block, or in a local shopping mall.

But talk to your doctor before starting, no matter how mild your symptoms are. The formula we described for determining your ideal exercising heart rate is a guideline, not a prescription. Make the actual decision together with your doctor. He may feel an exercise test is important first so he can advise you reliably on a safe exercise level to begin with.

When you are ready to begin, how will you know when you have reached the heart rate you need for your walk to be effective exercise? At the beginning, take your pulse every five minutes. (We describe the technique below, after outlining the exercise program in our laboratory. Your doctor or the physical therapist you work with can go over it with you if it gives you any difficulty.) You will quickly become aware of the amount of energy you need to put into your exercise to reach your heart rate target quickly. Then you only need check yourself twice—halfway through, and just as you finish. (If you and your doctor decide at any point that you can raise your target heart rate, you'll probably need to check more frequently again at first.)

Despite reassurances, some patients still feel too vulnerable and apprehensive to begin an exercise program on their own. If this applies to you, then it makes sense to search for an organized program, perhaps at a YMCA/YMHA or a hospital accessible to you. Call your local Lung Association, and the National Jewish Center for Immunological and Respiratory Medicine's Lung-Line. If this isn't helpful, call your local hospitals for information on cardiac rehabilitation programs in your area, then call these programs to see if they have added—or plan to add—a pulmonary component.

Advantages of a Formal Program   Over the past several decades, we have evolved a pulmonary exercise program in the laboratory here at New York University Medical Centers' Rusk Institute. Such a program does make the job easier for patients. The discipline of maintaining a schedule and not giving up is easier when exercise is done on a formal basis amid a highly supportive group of people. And doing the exercise in a group setting lends itself to satisfying social interactions. Exercising here also relieves a lot of anxiety because each person's heart rate is continuously monitored, and medical help—should it ever be needed—is instantly at hand.

Our Exercise Program

Patients who join the program come in for two-hour sessions three times a week for 12 weeks. They work in groups of four. Each group is led by a physical therapist. Postural drainage, for those who need it, is done shortly before the exercise "class" begins.

Warm-up Every class starts off with a 10- to 15-minute warm-up, which includes the breathing exercises described early in the chapter, plus exercises to stretch and strengthen the neck, arms and shoulders, trunk and legs. (Figure 13.5 illustrates some typical warm-up exercises.) A thorough warm-up helps the muscles work more efficiently by increasing circulation (which gets more oxygen to the muscles), improving flexibility, and slightly raising body temperature. A warm-up also reduces the chance of muscle injury.

Building Endurance After the warm-up, the patient goes to one of six conditioning exercise stations. Severely debilitated patients work lying down on a mat until they are strong enough to use the equipment. The other patients exercise on three different stations (occasionally two), with a 5-minute rest between each one. The majority combine 20 minutes on the treadmill with 15 minutes each on the stationary bicycle and/or upper extremity (hands, arms, shoulders) trainer. Patients capable of more strenuous exercise also have the rowing machine and cross-country ski machine as options.

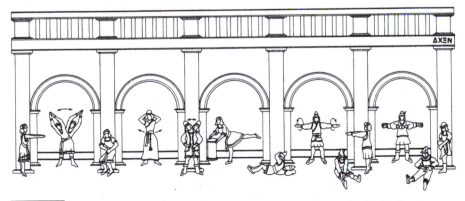

Figure 13.5 The purpose of warm-up exercises is to prepare the body for more strenuous exercise by improving circulation to the muscles, increasing flexibility, and raising body temperature.

Building Strength   Until recently, exercise for COPD patients was designated strictly to improve aerobic endurance. But it's recently become obvious that prolonged inactivity not only deconditions the cardiopulmonary system, it also weakens the skeletal muscles. Many patients eventually complain about the increasing difficulty of getting up out of a chair or putting groceries away in high cabinets. To counteract this tendency, we have introduced the use of light weights (2 to 10 lbs.) into the program to build up arm and back strength (Figure 13.6). In addition to improved strength, a growing body of research points compellingly to broader health gains. Stronger muscles are associated with a more responsive immune system, with better testosterone and estrogen levels, with improved cardiovascular health, and with reduced depression.

Other Activities   Let's face it—walking on a treadmill or riding a bicycle can become boring. To break up this monotony, we have introduced aerobic dancing and tai chi into the routine. Endurance benefits substantially, coordination and balance improve—and it is *fun*.

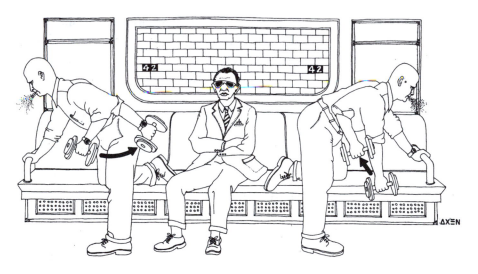

Figure 13.6   Here are two examples of resistive exercises to strengthen the back of the upper arm, the shoulder, and the back. *Left:* In the "triceps extension," the upper arm is held against the side while the forearm slowly opens from a right angle to a straight position, then returns to the starting position. *Right:* In the "one-hand row," the elbow is slowly pulled back from a straight-arm position to bring the weight up to the hip, then the weight is lowered back to the starting position. In the program at the N.Y.U. Medical Centers, these particular exercises are performed with 2- to 5-lb. weights and repeated from 10 to 15 times. A complete exercise program can be designed by a physical therapist or exercises physiologist in consultation with a physiatrist, a physician whose specialty is rehabilitation.

Cool Down   Training exercise is *always* followed by a 10- to 15-minute cool-down period to allow the metabolic waste products from exercise to be removed, and energy reserves to replenished. This can't happen if the exercise-produced circulation increase returns to normal too quickly. But a light workout for 10 to 15 minutes after exercising keeps blood flowing fast enough.

Oxygen Supplement   Two types of patients need supplemental oxygen when they exercise. One is on supplemental oxygen full-time. In that case, our job is to adjust their oxygen flow to maintain the proper amount of oxygen in their blood. The other type needs extra oxygen only during the early phase of their exercise program. We wean them from this supplement once their muscles begin using oxygen more efficiently.

Workout Intensity   Each patient's exercise intensity—and occasionally, duration—is chosen to produce the exercising heart rate we determined from his preliminary exercise test. At this heart rate, his body consumes 60% of the amount of oxygen it used when he exercised to his maximum. To find this target heart rate, we subtract his resting heart rate from his "maximum," multiply this difference by .60, then add the result to his resting heart rate. (For example, if your heart rate is 70 at rest and peaks at 120, your training heart rate should be 100 beats/minute: $120 - 70 = 50$; $50 \times .60 = 30$; $30 + 70 = 100$.)

As a patient's strength and endurance increase during the program, his exercise intensity and/or duration are increased appropriately to maintain his training level of exercise. When his 12 weeks are over, we work out a home exercise program for him based on the final training heart rate he has achieved. Depending on how much room still remains for improvement, this program is designed to maintain or improve this new exercise level.

Taking Your Own Pulse

There are several pulse meters on the market, but we find that most people can count their heartbeats accurately without special equipment. You need nothing more than a stopwatch, or a clock or watch with a sweep second hand.

The best place to take your pulse is at the side of your wrist slightly below your thumb (called the *radial pulse*). Figure 13.7 helps you locate it more precisely. Keep two cautions in mind. First, never use you thumb to take your pulse. Its own strong pulse obscures what you're looking for. Second, you may hear or read about another spot, the *carotid pulse*, in your neck. Although the pulse there tends to be stronger, and so easier to find, *it can be dangerous for a COPD patient to use.* If improperly done, pressure on the carotid artery can cause heart rate to drop suddenly.

Count your heartbeats for 10, 15, or 20 seconds. To convert your result to beats per minute, multiply it either by six (6 × 10 sec. = 60 sec.), four (4 × 15 sec. = 60 sec.), or three (3 × 20 sec. = 60 sec.). Or you can make a conversion table to keep handy. Table 13.1, which converts 10 seconds of heartbeats into heart rates per minute, is an example. Because heart rate slows rapidly once you stop exercising, take your pulse *immediately* upon stopping and do it as quickly as possible. We suggest using a 10-second interval.

The method is as follows:

- □ Start the stopwatch on the first detectable beat, but don't count that beat.

- □ Stop counting at the prescribed number of seconds.

- □ Convert the number of beats you just counted into a minute's heart rate.

Table 13.1 CONVERTING 10-SECOND HEART RATES TO 1-MINUTE HEART RATES

10-Second Count	Heartbeats/Min	10-Second Count	Heartbeats/Min
8	48	19	114
9	54	20	120
10	60	21	126
11	66	22	132
12	72	23	138
13	78	24	144
14	84	25	150
15	90	26	156
16	96	27	162
17	102	28	168
18	108	29	174
		30	180

Medication Adjustments

You will probably find exercising much easier and more pleasurable if you are breathing at your best before you start. Many COPD patients benefit from taking a bronchodilator 15 to 30 minutes before they begin exercising. Pre-exercise medication or, as it is usually called, *premedication,* is

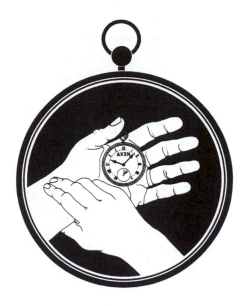

Figure 13.7 Finding your pulse. Palm up, place two fingers on the inside of your wrist. Count your pulse for a convenient period—10 to 20 seconds—and convert this number to heartbeats/minute (multiply it by six if you counted for 10 seconds; multiply it by three if you counted for 20 seconds).

always needed when severe obstruction exists before exercise even starts. It should be tried by patients whose disease is less severe to see if it helps.

The bronchodilator that seems particularly effective in protecting against exercise-induced bronchoconstriction and premature dyspnea in obstructed airways is *salbutamol* (also called *albuterol*), marketed under the names Proventil and Ventolin.

For those of you who normally use continuous supplemental oxygen, remember that exercise increases your body's oxygen needs. Talk with your doctor about increasing your oxygen flow during exercise to compensate.

One Exerciser's Experience

Leon Lewis—in his mid-70s—participated in the outpatient Pulmonary Rehabilitation Program here at the N.Y.U. Medical Centers. He learned—twice—that his moderate COPD became disabling for him unless he kept physically fit. When he learned we were writing a book for other patients with his disease, he asked if he could share his experience with them.

> I started smoking cigarettes when I was eight or nine. I don't remember why, but I guess smoking was an important part of the image I was holding up for people to see. Most candy stores and soda fountains sold them for a penny each. I bought them when I had the money, and begged them from friends and strangers when I didn't. That was par for kids who moved in my circle.

When I reached the point where I could support my habit, I was smoking a pack every two days, then every day. Then I become a radio disc jockey in Albany, New York. Something happened, and I found myself smoking the better part of two packs a day. Then as sales manager at an Albany radio and TV station, I was dipping into three packs a day. And by the time I got to New York City doing a telephone talk show from midnight until 6 A.M., I was well into four packs a day.

Working at night, I had a good part of the day to myself. The jogging craze was setting in, and I wanted to jog, but I couldn't. So I began a walking program. I was soon walking a couple of miles day, and for the first time I began to experience the "high" that exercise produces. I soon found that smoking was interfering with my walking, and so I did the impossible, the thing I'd had no urge or inclination to do for years. I stopped smoking. I just woke up one morning and didn't light a cigarette. But, oddly enough, my problems began after I stopped smoking.

I pushed myself hard because I still had this dream about jogging. I thought when I got in shape, I would be able to do it. I don't remember exactly when it was that I developed a cough. The doctor said I had chronic bronchitis. He gave me some antibiotics and a cough syrup, and it went away. In time I learned that when the stuff I coughed up was yellow or green, I had an infection which meant antibiotics and cough syrup. The treatment always relieved the condition, but the condition itself remained.

However, my walking program continued. On my bad days when I couldn't walk up the hill, I took the bus up and walked down.

I left my job in radio for the Community Film Workshop, helping train women and minority group people for entry-level jobs in TV news. It was fascinating and successful work (many of our students found jobs in TV stations all over the country, several with the networks right here in New York), but the old building we had converted into a newsroom, studios, and classrooms was the last place on earth I should have been. It was dusty, drafty, and often cold. And the hours were such that I virtually abandoned my exercise program.

In a little over a year, I left for a job with a public relations firm. It was part-time, but I never got back to my exercise program. At that point it was an effort for me to walk up the stairs form the subway. The cough and the infections began to plague me again.

In my search for more competent medical care, I came up with a Park Avenue doctor I thought was the answer to my prayers. He introduced me to anti-flu shots, anti-pneumonia shots, and a monthly intake of antibiotics he called a "flush." The last time I saw him, he listened to my chest and said I seemed a little congested. He sent me home. I didn't feel too well, but I didn't make too much of it until I went to lie down that night. I found I couldn't. I couldn't breathe. I thought I was living the last hours of my life.

The most comfortable position I could find was standing up and leaning on our grand piano. I was still there when my wife discovered me in the morning. I told her I was dying. She suggested I call Columbia Presbyterian Hospital to see if they could help me. The answer was "Yes, but you have to get here." Breathing was a real struggle, but my wife and I got a cab, and we made it. I was in the emergency room roughly four hours before I began to think I might live.

I never went back to my Park Avenue doctor. I began seeing an internist in private practice at Columbia Presbyterian Hospital. She put me on Theodur and the Proventil Inhaler. I thought I was out of the woods. But one evening after dinner at a friend's house, I had an attack and ended up back at Columbia Presbyterian's emergency room. I was not so frightened this time, because I knew what they could do.

They also got in touch with my doctor, who wanted me admitted. While I was waiting, I met another man who had already survived one such attack and was also waiting to be admitted. In one hour I learned more about my disease from him than I had learned from all the doctors I had seen. Maybe that isn't quite right. Let's say I learned more about how to take care of myself than anyone else had taught me till then. And he told me that Columbia Presbyterian had a Chest Clinic and a Chest Physiotherapy Department. I learned about percussion and vibration, the way they thump the chest to loosen up mucus.

Shortly after I left the hospital, a friend saw a news story about an experimental exercise program for pulmonary patients at New York University's Rusk Institute. They needed volunteers. I applied. I was eventually accepted. It was the turning point of my life.

I was put on an aerobic exercise program, a half-hour three days a week, and I began to feel like a human being again. This program set me free. I no longer had to plan ahead to make a trip to the bank, or keep a business appointment. I no longer had to avoid hills, stairs, and any unnecessary exertion.

Then, wonder of wonders, I was offered a job opportunity on the island of Jamaica. It was both exciting and frightening. I was afraid to be that far away from the N.Y.U. program, but I was intrigued with the idea of living in Jamaica. For years I had dreamed of living in another country, learning another culture and language.

I talked it over with the people directing my program at Rusk. They didn't foresee any problems as long as I took my medicine on schedule and continued my exercise program. I wasn't so sure, but I closed my eyes and jumped. I lived nearly five years in Jamaica with, as prescribed, regular medicine and exercise and no problems.

Three days a week I got up at 5:30 A.M. and drove up to the Mona Reservoir in Kingston. It was a popular place to be that early in the morning. Jamaica's Prime Minister was often there, joining many of the city's professional and business people. The walk around the reservoir is 1.7 miles. Normally, I made it around in just under 30 minutes. I wasn't trying to set any records. I simply needed 30 minutes of aerobic exercise. And at that hour, just before dawn, with the moonlight shining on the water and the stars burning brightly in the sky, it was almost a spiritual experience.

When I returned to New York, I went back to N.Y.U.'s program immediately. I credit it with saving my life. I haven't had a single attack since I began. I have learned a great deal about my problem, and a great deal about how to take care of myself.

I owe an enormous debt to the man I met in the emergency room at Columbia Presbyterian Hospital. He has since died, but even in death he taught me a lesson. He died because he didn't get to an emergency room quickly enough. The lesson is, if you have a problem—even if you only *think* you have a problem—get to an emergency room.

Medicare Coverage

Medicare coverage for pulmonary rehabilitation is an uncertain, patchwork affair at this point. Because there is no national policy on coverage, it is left up to the individual state and the carrier that processes reimbursement. Florida is among the few states that has an official history of reimbursement directly for pulmonary rehabilitation, although each of these states has a different set of rules and regulations. Of the remainder, some states provide only partial coverage, and others provide none at all. New York State is typical of the latter. What rehab facilities tend to do in this kind of situation is break their program down into its component parts and bill each separately, specifying that the patient is being treated for "disuse atrophy"—indicating muscle-wasting due to lack of use. The fact that pulmonary impairment has prevented their use does not make it into the official paperwork. Even physical therapy cannot always be designated as intended for chronic pulmonary disease.

The irony of this need for subterfuge is that cardiac rehabilitation—also a multi-component approach involving exercise, physical therapy, education, and support for improving both health and quality of life of patients with a chronic disease—is officially covered (and includes 32 sessions). So the Cardiac Rehab program submits each patient's claims to Medicare as a clearly named entity. And the Pulmonary Rehab facility next door has to edge in through the back door to gain reimbursement for providing the same kinds of services in a conceptually similar situation.

This piecemeal approach, though, is often far from getting the job done. Noah Greenspan, PT, founder and Program Director of the Pulmonary Wellness Center in New York City, emphasizes that the key to a successful program is its comprehensiveness. "It must combine physical therapy, exercise, education, and psychosocial support. But education is not a covered modality, and support groups are not always covered. And many programs will not provide a service for which they won't be reimbursed." He goes on to talk about the importance of a maintenance program for retaining the exercise gains made during rehabilitation, and the coverage limitations suffered here as well. Medicare usually pays for a maximum of 15 sessions, enough to achieve significant gains. But we all know what happens once we stop exercising and return to our sedentary ways. And many rehab programs either lack a maintenance component altogether, or price it in the neighborhood of $150 per session—the same rate as the more complete and more intensive initial rehab phase. "And not many people can afford to pay $150 twice a week to come in for exercise," Mr. Greenspan points out.

A ray of hope, however, may be shining from the state of California. As of November 1, 1999, the agency governing Medicare reimbursement began allowing reimbursement directly for pulmonary rehabilitation. Patient advocates who have been fighting for it there consider this a major victory. The federal officials involved with Medicare reimbursement policy have indicated that they plan to keep an eye on the situation that evolves in California. The hope is that the anticipated success there will result in the appearance of national, uniform coverage for all of the elements required for successful pulmonary rehabilitation—finally catching up to the situation that has existed for cardiac rehabilitation for some time now.

14

Conquering the Emotional and Psychological Consequences of COPD

As you already know from living with it, COPD is a serious chronic disease. Serious illness affects us emotionally as well as physically. COPD pressures your emotional resources from several directions:

1. Your health is not what it was, which is depressing and anxiety-provoking. The profound uncertainties and sense of helplessness that beset COPD-uneducated patients create deep anxiety. Frequent dyspnea is very frightening for them.

2. These health changes are not going to disappear. They are with you for life. Depression and withdrawal—which also typify many COPD patients—are a fairly common response to living with a chronic disease.

3. If your COPD becomes severe enough to change your blood gases (*hypoxia*, or insufficient oxygen; *hypercapnia*, or excessive carbon dioxide) and increase the carbonic acid in your blood (also from high carbon dioxide), these biochemical changes directly affect your mood and mental functioning.

4. If your COPD has also forced you to stop working, there are additional strong emotional consequences to deal with. (We treat this separately in Chapter 16, which outlines the rehabilitation resources available to help you deal with these consequences as well as find satisfying, health-friendly work.)

As a consequence: paralyzed by anxiety and depression, the typical COPD patient who has not benefited from a well-rounded rehabilitation program is convinced that his life is basically over. He sees only a severely limited, fear-filled existence devoid of any real pleasure. He is unaware that the destructive emotions identified above are causing much of his misery. Yet he has been living at their mercy, as they prevent him from regaining control of his life.

What Can You Do?

Plenty! *COPD is not a dead end!* This chapter focuses on coping directly with the profound emotional impact of COPD. (The remaining chapters discuss successful approaches to coping with other aspects of your life that may have been limited by your disease. And improving your mastery and satisfaction in these areas will improve your emotional health as well.)

First comes identifying and understanding the powerful emotional changes that affect people who live with COPD. After discussing these often paralyzing feelings, we spell out the variety of resources to help you and your family come to terms with them, *and go beyond them.* And because relaxation and optimism improve your breathing as well as your outlook, this chapter will help you breathe easier—in more ways than one.

Neuropsychological Changes in COPD

Neuropsychological changes in COPD patients involve the ways in which inadequate oxygen and excessive carbon dioxide hamper the responsiveness of your central nervous system. We already know from the vast amount of research the Air Force conducted on healthy people that even a temporary loss of adequate oxygen interferes significantly with our thought and coordination processes, and makes us irritable.

Much more recently—in the 1970s and 1980s—two large studies on hypoxic COPD patients each gathered patient data from a number of medical centers. They both showed that patients with too little oxygen are also neuropsychologically impaired. Just as with high-flying pilots who don't get enough oxygen in the air they breathe, in severe COPD the parts of the brain involved in various types of thinking and behavior don't get enough oxygen to function properly. It feels like you've become less intelligent. You're less able to grasp abstract concepts, to think flexibly and solve problems, and you have lost subtle physical coordination. Although hand–eye coordination and memory are only mildly affected at first, they worsen slowly as the disease progresses. Attention span is unaffected by mild hypoxia, but becomes shorter and shorter if hypoxia increases. (Word skills, at least, are relatively resistant to the effects of hypoxia.)

The issue was also examined from the other side. Several studies of severely hypoxic COPD patients who had not previously been on oxygen therapy showed that adding oxygen to their air produced a small but significant improvement in their neuropsychological performance. (Today, it has become standard procedure to place advanced COPD patients on supplemental oxygen for their general health, which benefits their brain function as well.)

Although we have not found research to document the effect of hypoxia and hypercapnia on mood in COPD patients, many professionals who have spent long careers working with them have observed that they produce a depressed person. Common sense indicates that some of this emotional change is probably directly due to these chemical changes, while some is a reaction to the loss of brain function we just described.

Emotional Effects
Mourning, and Its Resolution

Everyone—both patient and family—goes through a period of mourning after they first discover the presence of a permanent disability. The patient's health has abandoned him. His body has been irreversibly damaged, and his ego has had the rug pulled out from under. This loss of health has also destroyed the unconscious sense of physical and emotional invulnerability with which he had faced the world every day, and which shielded him from having to accept the inevitability of his own death.

Mourning is a dynamic, potentially healthy process that ideally progresses through five stages: shock, panic, denial, grief, then resolution. Achieving resolution—which translates to acceptance as you now are, not as you used to be—productively concludes the mourning process. Accepting this irrevocable loss frees you and your family to marshal your resources for coping with the disease and getting on with life.

Mourning in itself is not a problem. If it concludes with acceptance of what cannot be altered and a determination to master the disease as much as possible, then your experience has been a healthy one. The problem arises if you get stuck partway through the mourning process.

Some patients (and/or family members) never progress beyond panic, treating the disease as a burden out of all proportion to its actual severity. They overprotect themselves or their loved one to a degree that often creates problems in daily life. Some patients who cannot progress beyond the denial stage refuse to alter their ways. They won't cooperate in taking their medication and monitoring their symptoms, they continue smoking, they belittle rehabilitation exercises and energy-conserving ways of doing daily tasks. With others, denial is manifested as anger at their doctors. These people need someone to blame for their disease and its continuing presence, and doctors make a very handy target. They spend their time looking for new doctors or trying the latest nonmedical trends. Some patients (and sometimes family members) forever grieve over their loss, remaining passively sunk in self-pity.

The common denominator among all these patients (and/or family members) stuck in the mourning process is that they are unable to take an active role in their treatment. They cannot help themselves.

Fear and Anxiety

Even with a healthy conclusion to mourning, fear—and its companion, anxiety—are present in varying degrees and contexts from the first realization that you have COPD. Mastering your fear is a critical battle to win.

At the beginning, much of your fear stems from profound uncertainty: not yet understanding your disease adequately, not fully knowing what is going to happen next, having no idea how your disease is going to evolve over time. This sense of dire helplessness and uncertainty can be terrifying.

Then there are your diminished physical capacities and resilience. The physical activities you are no longer capable of (or can do only with great difficulty) and your susceptibility to difficult respiratory infections have probably made you feel fragile, vulnerable, and anxious. Frequent dyspnea, in particular, tends to produce spiraling anxiety. The initial intense anxiety worsens your blood gases, which intensifies your dyspnea, deepening your anxiety, etc., etc.

This happens because strong emotions (such as anxiety, anger, and elation) increase our energy expenditure. So when we are "worked up" for whatever reason, our body needs more oxygen and produces more carbon dioxide. Normally, this poses no problem. But for a person whose respiratory system is already seriously stressed, it is a poorly tolerated burden.

So when hypoxic COPD patients get excited, they start breathing so rapidly to try to take in more fresh air that they no longer have time to exhale fully after each breath. The vicious cycle begins. More air becomes trapped in their lungs, overdistending them and so making them less effective. Less effective lungs worsen these patients' dyspnea. Understandably, this makes them even more anxious and fearful. So the cycle continues.

The typical patient eventually becomes impatient and compulsive in response to this intense anxiety. But the strong emotions this involves exacerbate rather than ease his state.

Ultimately, many of the highly anxious COPD patients who cannot progress beyond this state become severely depressed. It is more intense and extensive than the subtle depression often accompanying chronic illness. Some doctors feel this overwhelming depression is in part self-protective because it shuts out the strong feelings that provoke their dyspnea. But it is self-defeating as well, because it also closes these patients off from their family and close friends, deepening the loneliness that chronic disease and physical limitations often cause.

The early fears and anxieties of COPD are normal. As with mourning, they become a problem only if they remain so overwhelming that they continue to dominate your vision, and you cannot see beyond them. Then these emotions will continue dictating how you handle your disease, which significantly limits your ability to cope well. Unmanageable fear and anxiety short-circuit your best intentions for treating COPD appropriately and helping yourself to the best quality of life available to you.

It is also very important to realize that—even with the most successful handling of the fear and anxiety that unavoidably mushroom when you realize your lungs can no longer provide enough oxygen for you to live as you used to—anxiety never fully disappears. After the intense anxiety eventually dissipates, a thread usually remains woven through the background of consciousness for both patient and family. It is always there, rising and falling, anticipating a possible setback no matter how well your lungs have been doing. Don't worry about it. It's simply part of living with this kind of disease.

Preexisting Emotional Problems

A COPD patient with any kind of preexisting emotional "problem" may be finding that it used to be a lot easier to handle than it is now. That's because his emotional resources are now fully occupied with the tremendous emotional pressures COPD involves. Some preexisting problems can exacerbate these pressures and interfere with effective treatment.

Hypochondria, a preexisting anxiety problem that has been part of the patient's personality for a long time, is a prime example. Because a hypochondriac is obsessively preoccupied with personal health and reacts with spasms of anxiety to meaningless changes, it can hamper a COPD patient's ability to deal effectively with his disease. The hypochondriac's excessive concern about every minute change in his health, plus his tendency to overmedicate himself, are counterproductive to controlling symptoms and improving quality of life.

Spouses and Family

We have been repeating the phrase *and/or family members* because the emotional fallout from COPD very definitely includes them in its circle. It can be very frightening when the person you've closely shared your life with for many years, and whom you depend on for basic emotional—and perhaps financial—support, can't always get enough air into his lungs. He can no longer undertake oxygen-demanding activities and responsibilities. You may now have to do things for him that he had always done for himself. The fear of dyspnea from strenuous activity has made sex a thing of the past. If your spouse feels less of a person—because he is limited and/or dependent and/or can't satisfy you sexually and/or can't work and/or feels you (and others) are pitying him—he has probably become some combination of depressed, withdrawn, and angry—and therefore very difficult to live with. Your relationship itself has become a source of stress.

You are probably very frightened—both for your spouse *and* for yourself—and you are probably very angry. You are angry at your spouse, which makes you feel terribly guilty, and you are angry at God or at the random cruelty of Fate, which makes you feel terribly helpless. You may feel that something is wrong with you for not finding it easy to be a saint in these trying circumstances. You're reluctant to share many of your feelings with your spouse because he has enough on his shoulders already, plus you're afraid he wouldn't understand your anger at him. You feel very much alone in your suffering. This was not the future of your dreams.

Emotional Recovery

It Starts with Your COPD Education

A thorough COPD education is the necessary first step in getting your emotions out of the driver's seat. (In fact, you have already started taking your first step by reading this book.)

The essential prerequisites are a knowledgeable, caring, and available physician, plus the pulmonary rehabilitation program he refers you to. A sympathetic, supportive doctor can alleviate a great deal of the average patient's anxiety by combining this nurturant character with a thorough, realistic COPD education for both patient and family concerning his disease and how to live with it most effectively. The education itself takes place gradually. Some of it is introduced during doctor visits. Some is gained by phone each time you call your doctor because of an "emergency."

Some of your education also results from directly learning to handle a variety of situations and problems. Some comes from the various rehabilitation professionals who will be working with you. And some of it comes from the confidence that eventually grows with the realization of how much you have learned about your disease and how much you are in control.

Four COPD newsletters are helpful supplements for keeping your

COPD education current and well founded. *Batting the Breeze* is published by Emphysema Anonymous, Inc., P.O. Box 3224, Seminole, FL 34642-0224; 813-391-9977. *Second Wind* is published by the Pulmonary Education and Research Foundation, P.O. Box 1133, Lomita, California 90717-5133. *The Pulmonary Paper* can be contacted by mail, phone, or e-mail: P.O. Box 977, Ormond Beach, Florida 32175; 904-673-5108; Belyea@aol.com. *Respiratory News & Views* is published by the Asthma/Emphysema Self-Help Group, 172 East Fourth Street, #11F, New York, NY 10009; 212-777-0486; *respiratorynews@aol.com.*

Dealing Directly with Stress and Anxiety

In addition to your COPD education, a variety of more direct stress- and anxiety-management techniques can aid patients with breathing disturbances. The list includes individual and group psychotherapy, relaxation techniques, hypnosis, and biofeedback. These techniques cannot harm you, and for many patients one or more of them offers substantial help. Technique and focus differ, but they all work toward the same goal: helping you share responsibility in your own treatment. In addition to helping you feel better about yourself, this also helps you cope more effectively with your disease.

Caution for Patients   These techniques most certainly can be useful additions to the essential basics—medication and the various physical rehabilitation modalities—of COPD treatment. The potential danger lies in deciding that if a particular technique helps you a lot, you can substitute it for your medication. You can manage your COPD most effectively by adding one or more of these techniques to your medical therapy. The goal is a balanced program integrating the benefits of medication, self-regulation of stress/anxiety, and exercise.

Caution for Doctors   Because the respiratory improvement gained from stress/anxiety management techniques is relatively small compared to the changes that result from drugs, some doctors feel that these techniques are not worth the time and effort. Their value, though, is not measured only by the numbers on pulmonary testing instruments. Even a very modest improvement, or just simply stabilizing a patient's pulmonary behavior, is of great clinical importance if it provides the edge that maintains his ability to function normally. And even if there are no direct pulmonary benefits, the ability to calm himself substantially decreases the fear and panic that often mushroom when respiratory distress suddenly occurs. As we all know, the calmer we are, the better we handle things.

Group or Individual Psychotherapy

"I Don't Need It"

Although the majority of COPD patients and their close family can benefit from some temporary form of emotional as well as physical therapy, many are very resistant to the whole idea. It is often much easier to recognize the value of help for physical difficulties—from strength and flexibility exercises after healing a sprained ankle or a broken arm, to physical rehabilitation after a stroke or the inroads of pulmonary disease—than for emotional difficulties.

Some people have always felt that needing emotional help means they are shamefully inadequate in some way. Other patients feel so precariously balanced that any prospect of change—particularly when it would be initiated by a "stranger"—seems threatening.

So they say "No" to counseling, to therapy, to a support group—to any attempt to help them modify their basic emotional response to their illness. Unfortunately, remaining in emotional handcuffs really limits the benefits that a COPD patient can get from his physical rehabilitation program.

It's crucial to remember two things about the powerful emotional consequences of COPD: (1) They are unavoidable. Your fear and depression are a very human reaction to the presence and nature of your illness. They reflect your humanity, not your weakness. (2) They are also changeable. Most of us have resources for growth that we are unaware of until we are forced to tap them. Emotional therapy helps us find and strengthen these resources so we can use them on our own. Then you can regain a sense of control over your life.

Individual Psychotherapy

Sometimes the treating physician needs to refer a patient to a psychiatrist or psychologist for treatment of a serious emotional problem he cannot help with. It might be severe depression associated with the disease, it might be hypochondria (or another unrelated, preexisting problem that is damaging his ability to cope with his COPD), or it might be the prolonged and debilitating stress from loss of a loved one. (A considerable problem with individual psychotherapy, though, is that its great financial expense makes it inaccessible to so many of the patients who could benefit from it.)

A Word of Warning   The referral must be to a therapist who understands the physical and emotional realities of COPD. It is often very difficult for the average (meaning "non-COPD trained") psychiatrist or psychologist to help a COPD patient, because they—in a subtle version of the patient's natural responses—exaggerate his physical problems. The patient, quick to pick this up (even if he isn't consciously aware of it), becomes more instead of less anxious. If patients also sense the personal anxiety behind the therapist's reaction, they label him as someone who does not understand their disease. Therapy hasn't a chance in these circumstances.

More Than Group Therapy: COPD Support for Patient and Family

Invaluable for COPD patients and those they live with is a *support group*—a group of people in your identical situation. It offers far more than standard group therapy, because you are together with other COPD patients and their spouses (or lovers and/or children). These patients are able to give you something that no physician can provide, no matter how caring he is and how thoroughly he educates his patients and their family.

Everyone in this group lives with COPD every day and every night. Each newcomer discovers a group of peers who know exactly what he is going through—the experiences facing him and the feelings he is struggling with—because they have all been through it themselves. New victims are no longer alone in this strange world they have suddenly been shifted to. And seeing the accomplishments of others who are much further along in the rehabilitation process helps you rebuild your confidence and create a positive sense of your place in the world.

In addition to ending the terrible sense of isolation most newly diagnosed COPD patients (and family) feel, the opportunity to talk out their experiences and feelings with others who understand them firsthand is irreplaceable. It makes their feelings human and acceptable, placing them in perspective. Reticent group members get the support and encouragement that help them bring their feelings out into the light of day. Members who have been unable to resolve the mourning process are helped to recognize this, and given the support they need to make their way through it.

The group is also an indispensable educational network, a rich source of effective practical advice in handling many aspects of COPD. Much of this information is otherwise not readily available, particularly for the layperson. A great deal of frustrating misinformation tends to fill this vacuum.

Any support group's composition changes gradually over time as "old" patients and family leave and "new" ones come. Even with these changes, the group retains a good mix of experienced and neophyte members. Experienced members provide support and information to newcomers, who are eventually able to give of themselves in this way too. Some concrete examples of the different kinds of needs that find support: getting through the initial realization; learning about the disease; dealing with—or leaving—an insensitive physician; generally defining and attaining one's rights within the medical establishment.

And everyone is able to share. They share their angers, fears, guilts, doubts, and joys; they share a great variety of experiences involving their lives; they share good and bad times with doctors, emergency rooms, friends, and relatives; they share good vacation spots, practical advice, equipment recommendations; etc.

Locating a Support Group   If there are no formal pulmonary rehabilitation facilities near you, you will need other sources for learning of local support groups. There is the American Lung Association, which is headquartered in New York City at 1740 Broadway, New York, NY 10019; 212-245-8000. Most states and large communities also have a local affiliate. You can locate your regional Lung Association in your telephone directory, or by calling the national office in New York City.

Then there is the National Jewish Medicine and Research Center's Lung-Line. The Center (in Denver, Colorado), one of the foremost institutions for lung disease treatment and research, provides a trained staff of registered nurses to answer general questions over the telephone about lung diseases. You can also request information on COPD support groups in your area. This free Lung-Line is in operation Monday through Friday from 8:30 A.M. to 5:00 P.M. Mountain time. Messages are taken at other times, and these calls are returned as soon as the Lung-Line reopens. The toll-free number if calling from outside Colorado is 800-222-LUNG; from within the state, call 303-398-1477.

No Nearby Support Group?   If there is no support group close enough for you to join, subscribing to *Batting the Breeze, Second Wind, The Pulmonary Paper,* and *Respiratory News & Views* will help lessen your isolation and provide practical advice. If you have Internet access, the *Second Wind* organization provides a chatroom four times a week for an hour each session. The schedule and instructions are available on their website: *www.2ndWind.org.* Click on the table of contents to locate their chatroom link.

You can also try starting a group in your area. Recruit members by posting notices in your doctor's office, other medical offices your doctor recommends, local churches and synagogues, and senior citizen centers. One of these facilities should also be a good place to hold meetings (unless you prefer rotating among members' homes). Your regional Lung Association should be able to give you guidance in getting started, and perhaps finding someone to lead your new group.

15

Daily Living

These next four chapters provide general information and advice to help you cope as successfully as you can with COPD's impact on your daily life. Obviously, the specific items relevant to you depend on the severity of your illness and the area(s) of your life that have been most vulnerable to its impact.

This chapter covers "taking care of myself" (preventing respiratory infections, diet, and dealing with the environment) and hints for daily living (energy-saving strategies). Chapter 16 talks about work and play, including what to do if you must give up your present occupation or primary avocation. Chapter 17 on sex gives advice and techniques for enjoying it despite limitations on strenuous activity. Chapter 18 combines travel tips that make the experience substantially easier and more comfortable.

Minimizing Airway Infections

COPD patients are more susceptible than most to respiratory infections, and especially vulnerable to severe consequences from them. Frequent uncontrolled lung infections accelerate pulmonary destruction, and in advanced COPD patients they precipitate life-threatening crises. So it is critical for COPD patients to protect themselves against airway infections. *Avoidance* measures make infections less frequent. *Control* measures minimize the impact of those airway infections that can't be prevented.

Keep Your Distance

One way to minimize respiratory infections is preventing your exposure to them. Winter is the obvious time for heightened caution. During this season of colds, avoid small, crowded places when possible. Always avoid close contact with anyone—child or adult—who you know is sick, or who looks/sounds as if they are. Cancel an appointment if necessary, with an honest explanation. Don't endanger your health because you fear hurt-

ing a friend's feelings. Anyone who cares for you will instantly understand, and welcome your honesty. Anyone who feels slighted has his own
ego, rather than your health, at heart.

Vaccinations

Vaccination protects us against a particular disease by providing us with
antibodies that destroy the causative microbe whenever it invades. Our
body normally produces antibodies after our first exposure to a microbe.
(That's why people don't usually get chicken pox or mumps twice.) Vaccination injects altered microbes into our body—they are dead, or greatly
weakened in some way—that will still cause antibody formation, yet
won't make us sick.

But there are still many microbes for which we lack a vaccine. For
some, the challenge is changing the microbe so as to maintain the antibody response without making the person seriously ill. For microbes that
come in large families (such as those that cause colds), vaccines are
impractical unless they protect against all family members at once.

Vaccine protection against respiratory infection extends so far to flu
and bacterial pneumonia. The flu vaccine is highly effective. Although
some doctors question the effectiveness of the pneumonia vaccine, we
know of no harmful effects. *Every COPD patient should have both these
vaccinations.*

Flu Shots   The flu (short for *influenza*) requires a yearly vaccination
because the influenza virus mutates—slightly alters its structure—very
rapidly. It changes just enough to go unrecognized by the flu antibodies
already in your system. Each year's flu vaccine is *polyvalent*, meaning that
it works against several viral strains simultaneously. Each year's new crop
of flu viruses follows a similar migratory pathway around the world, typically starting somewhere in Asia. (The geographic origin explains flu
nicknames, for example, *Hong Kong Flu.*) That gives vaccine specialists in
the West time to culture the newest strains and produce the new vaccine
before the altered microbes arrive.

Serious reactions to the flu vaccine are rare, and the benefit to you far
outweighs this unlikely hazard. The worst to expect after a flu shot is a
few days of mild fever, malaise, and other flu-like symptoms. The only
words of warning are for people allergic to eggs. Because the flu vaccine
is grown on egg proteins, people with an egg allergy cannot use it. In
those patients, *amantadine* and *rimantadine* (antiviral drugs) given by
mouth are effective alternatives. To be effective, though, they must be
started early—as soon as you know you have been exposed to someone
who has the flu.

Pneumonia Shot   Pneumonia can be caused by viruses—for which there is no vaccination—or by bacteria—for which there is. Luckily, it is the bacterial pneumonias that are more virulent. The polyvalent vaccination, directed against the several strains of pneumococcal bacteria, is a once-in-a-lifetime affair. Although its effectiveness is still somewhat controversial, current evidence suggests that it does offer some protection against this kind of lung infection, and it does no harm.

Antibiotics

Arrival of the chest infection that couldn't be prevented is always heralded by warning signs: malaise, easier fatigability, worsening dyspnea, fever, nasal congestion, increased coughing combines with more difficult expectoration (clearing the mucus out) as the mucus becomes yellow or green or much more viscous. These infections are typically caused by certain bacteria (*Haemophilus influenza, Streptococcus pyogenes, Diplococcus pneumonia, Klebsiella pneumonia*) and/or viruses (*influenza, adenovirus, respiratory syncytial virus*).

Because these airway infections are a major cause of exacerbated symptoms for CODP patients—especially those with substantial chronic bronchitis—it is critical to control them, and to do so quickly. Call your doctor the moment you notice any of the warning signs.

Environment

In addition to avoiding respiratory infections, respiratory irritants should also be avoided. Although completely avoiding respiratory irritants is clearly the best state of affairs, it is often impractical or impossible to accomplish. In that case even partial avoidance is helpful.

Indoor Avoidance/Elimination of Triggers

Although many of the same indoor respiratory irritants—the most common are cigarette smoke, house dust, and odors—are found both at home and in the work place, avoidance and elimination techniques are usually easiest to implement at home. So your house is where efforts should start. If you write down a step-by-step irritant elimination plan for each room, you will minimize the chance of missing something important. Start your efforts in the bedroom, since this is where people spend the large majority of their household time.

If you do not live alone, then this process has to be a cooperative effort. Remember that everyone in the family must share in eliminating respiratory irritants from your home.

House Dust House dust is made up of natural and synthetic fibers, plant material, fungi and bacteria, dried flakes of human skin, pulverized food remnants, inorganic debris, dust mites, and sometimes animal dander and/or cockroach and other insect parts and feces. House dust is everywhere, but it causes the greatest difficulty at night for patients who sleep with their heads buried in dust-laden pillows, mattresses, and blankets.

How you clean is more important than how vigorously you do it. It is best done with a damp cloth rather than vacuuming. Vacuuming should be kept to a minimum because it stirs up dust. A particular focus for dust-cleaning efforts are the baseboard and molding behind the bed, and the floor underneath it.

Household Rules *Certain general rules should be adopted for the house.* No smoking. No fires in the fireplace. No strong odors, such as perfume. Use a kitchen exhaust fan whenever anyone cooks. Do not use aerosol or spray cans. Do not vacuum while the COPD patient is in the house, and do not let him return until the vacuuming dust settles. Keep the temperature between 65 and 70°F.

Miscellaneous Charcoal filters for odors may be helpful. Air conditioners with effective filters can reduce the indoor level of airborne particulate matter from outdoors. Baseboard electrical heating is much better than forced air, oil, gas, or coal furnaces. It attracts and spreads much less dust than a furnace does, and is much cleaner in terms of the possible irritant by-products of combustion (nitrogen dioxide and carbon monoxide). In the same vein, electric stoves are cleaner than gas appliances.

A source of pollution in the home that cannot be easily eliminated, and which can be particularly irritating to the airways, is *formaldehyde*. Formaldehyde is released from plywood, from particleboard, and from urea-formaldehyde foam (which is used in insulation).

Air Cleaners No matter how well the above controls have been carried out, some patients will be affected by particles still left in the environment. If this happens, it is time to consider buying an electrical air cleaner. The "Air Cleaning and Purifying" section of your telephone directory lists local dealers. Choose one that both rents and sells air cleaners, so that you can try out the machine you are considering before you buy. If the machine that seemed right does not do the job you need, try out a different one.

The best of the electrical air cleaners is the *high efficiency particulate air (HEPA) filter.* It removes close to 100% of airborne particles. It is more effective than the best of the electrostatic air cleaners, which remove only

70 to 90%. Both kinds of air cleaners are expensive, but the electrostatic cleaner also requires high-voltage safeguards and produces ozone, a potential irritant.

A number of small, inexpensive tabletop air cleaners became available in response to public concern about smoke pollution. Manufacturers claim that these devices eliminate all particulate matter in the air, plus odors and bacteria. A large quantity of air, though, must circulate through a machine that can filter the air in an entire room effectively. This requires a large motor, and large motors are expensive to buy and operate (as with vacuum cleaners and air conditioners). So a small, inexpensive unit is unlikely to do a thorough job.

You need two types of information to help you decide on an air cleaner. One is how quickly a particular machine does its cleaning job, indicated by the number of times an hour it will change the air in your room. The other is how efficiently the machine does its job, which is its ability to remove the particles that irritate your airways.

To determine how rapidly a machine will clean your room, you must know how much air circulates through the machine every minute (its cubic feet/minute displacement—or CFM—rating), and the amount of air (in cubic feet) contained in the room where the air cleaner will be used. You can learn the CFM from a salesperson or sales brochure. To get your room's volume of air, multiply its length by its width by its height. Then multiply the CFM by 60 to get the amount of air the machine cleans in one hour. Dividing this hourly total by the cubic room size tells you how many times an hour a particular machine will clean the air in this room. This can all be written in a simple formula to carry with you when you go shopping:

$$\frac{\text{Amount of air cleaned in 1 hr (CFM} \times 60)}{\text{Amount of air in room (Room L} \times \text{W} \times \text{H)}} = \frac{\text{no. of air}}{\text{changes/hr}}$$

Two air changes an hour is the minimum rate acceptable. Four is considered significantly more effective, but going much beyond this rate will not make a real difference. Ten air changes an hour is regarded as overkill.

An air cleaning machine's efficiency rating tells you how well it cleans. The best source for this information is the machine's manufacturer, who will send you (on request) a graph that shows how completely—or not—the machine cleans different types of particles from the air. Because this graph provides much greater detail than any sales brochure can, you will know how efficiently the air cleaner removes the specific particles that exacerbate your COPD symptoms.

If you find that your local dealer cannot answer all you questions, several companies that specialize in equipment and supplies for people with respiratory problems provide help by phone and on their web sites. You may also want to buy your air cleaner from one of these sources, as their prices are competitive. EasyBreathe is at 1781 Kingsdale Center, Suite 125, Columbus, Ohio 43221. Their toll-free number for questions, help with product selections, and orders is 800-735-4772. Go on-line at *www.easybreathe.com,* click on "Great Products" and then "True HEPA Air Cleaners" for information and details on True and Honeywell products. BreatheFree.com can be reached toll-free at 877-374-0344, or at 562-921-9756, with questions in either English or Spanish. Go on-line at *www.breathefree.com,* click on the option "Not sure what air purifier to buy? Visit our air purifier buying guide" for a variety of facts and a descriptive menu of the products they carry.

Humidifiers and Dehumidifiers   The effect of humidity on COPD patients seems to be a very individual matter. Some do better in humid weather, while others find themselves more comfortable in drier conditions. The best indoor humidity range seems to be between 35 and 50%. If the humidity level in your home is not at a comfortable point for you, a humidifier or dehumidifier should solve this problem. The comfort gained from a humidifier, though, must be balanced against two potentially important disadvantages. Both dust mites and molds prefer—and thrive in—humid environments.

There are three types of humidifiers: reservoir, evaporator, and jet spray. The one most appropriate for you depends on the size and design of your house, the kind of heating system you have, and the climate of your area. Whatever you choose must be cleaned regularly and treated with a mold inhibitor to minimize the chance of contaminating the air with bacteria or mold.

A dehumidifier will do away with excess humidity. But before buying an expensive machine, there are much cheaper measures to try that may reduce the humidity as much as you need. Installing a venting fan in the kitchen and bathroom(s) reduces humidity in these areas. If you have a clothes dryer, make sure that it is vented to the outside. Wrap cold water pipes in insulation to stop them from sweating. Putting plastic sheeting over a dirt basement floor and over crawl spaces reduces the moisture entering the house from outside.

Outdoor Avoidance/Elimination of Irritants

Some Major Outdoor Irritants   The amount of *air pollution* in an area at any particular time results from two factors. One is the amount of fuel-burning activity (as from power plants, factories, automobiles) that produces the pollutants. The other is existing atmospheric conditions, which determine how quickly or slowly fresh air is replacing the polluted air. So it is a combination of how much pollution is produced, and how quickly it dissipates.

Burning any type of fuel (except for nuclear fuel, which has its own set of problems) produces carbon monoxide and nitric oxide. Nitric oxide converts to *nitrogen dioxide*, which can be highly irritating to the airways. In addition to this, when small hydrocarbons (residue from burning fossil fuels) and strong sunlight come together, ozone and other photochemical products are formed. If there are no winds to disperse them, the result is *photochemical smog*, also called *Los Angeles smog* after the city where it is best known.

Then there is *London smog*, named for the killer smog that caused 3,500 to 4,000 premature deaths in that city in just four days in December 1952. London smog can occur when coal, or oil high in sulfur, is burned in a power plant. This releases *sulfur dioxide* (in addition to carbon monoxide and nitric oxide), which combines with both oxygen and moisture in the air to form *sulfuric acid*, which then combines with ammonia in the air to produce particles of *sulfate salts*. All these sulfur by-products are potent airway irritants. In December 1952, they stagnated over London in substantial amounts during four windless, foggy days.

When similar pollution and atmospheric conditions existed in 1948 over Donora, Pennsylvania (population 14,000), there were 18 smog-related deaths. Ninety percent of the town's asthmatics got significantly worse during the smog, and 40% of the nonasthmatic population complained of respiratory problems.

In addition to *weather's* role in creating smog, weather changes of any kind can produce an unpleasant reaction in COPD patients. The humidity and temperature changes that affect them indoors have the same affect outdoors. The weather change that seems particularly difficult for COPD patients is rapid temperature drop.

Relocating　Physicians are often asked if there are places to live that take the edge off a COPD patient's symptoms. The answer is "Yes."

Low-altitude spots with a mild climate and low pollution level are normally best. The area bordering the Gulf of Mexico from Florida to Texas, the Southwest region, and the West Coast cities of San Diego and Palm Beach have become popular because of their minimal pollution and temperate climate. Unfortunately, the large number of immigrant northeasterners there who planted the trees, flowers, and grass they loved at home has transformed these areas into centers of asthmogenic pollen. For the patient with COPD alone, there is no problem, but patients with both COPD and asthma should avoid these places.

Anyone considering such a dramatic approach to coping with COPD symptoms should first take an extended vacation (3 to 6 weeks) in the area he is considering relocating to. If this possibility remains appealing, there are some cautions to keep in mind when making the big decision. Although the medical condition may improve substantially after such a move, experience suggests that these benefits must be balanced against the unavoidable financial, psychological, and social stresses of a major move. The ideal solution—for the few who can afford it—is to keep two places, moving to sun country for the winter and returning home for the milder months.

Protecting Yourself at Home   If you are without such financial resources, or are simply unwilling to undertake a major move twice each year, there are several ways to protect yourself from outdoor irritants. The simplest is to stay inside while you keep pollution outside. The best way to keep it there is with a central air conditioning unit—even in winter—fitted with air purification filters. Combining a regular air conditioner with a HEPA air cleaner is much less expensive, and still does a reasonably good job.

During air pollution alerts, be especially disciplined in carrying out your normal daily precautions. Avoid any unnecessary physical activity outdoors. Be especially careful to stay out of rooms filled with smoke or other irritants, and stay away from anyone with a cold or other respiratory infection. Call your doctor to see if you should temporarily increase any of your medications. (Remember that he will probably be busier than usual, and so harder to contact.) Make sure that you have all emergency telephone numbers close at hand. If the high pollution is expected to continue for several days and you can afford to leave the area during this time, that is obviously the ideal solution.

Nutrition

Good nutrition is always important. We have more energy and we feel better when we eat enough of the foods our body needs most for energy production, tissue repair, and general functioning. But good nutrition becomes especially important when our innate physical resources have diminished. Then we need to take advantage of every support we can find to help us function as best we can in the face of this loss. In addition, there are several ways in which what—and how much—COPD patients eat has a very specific impact on their daily function and on their mortality. Since Chapter 11—which describes aspects of complementary medicine that can be helpful for COPD patients—includes nutritional elements, you may want to review it and incorporate some of the items discussed there into the dietary changes you make.

Weight Problems and COPD

About one-half of the patients with moderate to severe COPD eventually lose a significant amount of weight without any apparent reason. This weight loss comes from both fat and muscles. Why they lose too much weight is another of COPD's mysteries.

Some scientists think the energy these patients use for breathing becomes so great that their normal calorie intake cannot fill the need. Others believe that COPD patients become uncomfortably short of breath when they eat, and so tend to eat less and less at meals. Still others suggest that the problem is actual loss of appetite related to the severe psychological depression a fair number of these patients develop. Then there are the scientists who think this weight loss is due to subtle, as yet unidentified, biochemical changes that come along with the disease.

Whatever the cause, the fact is that underweight (which translates to *undernourished*) patients don't live as long as those whose body weight stays close to normal. Their poorer survival statistics are attributed to loss of muscle protein, further weakening the already overstressed respiratory muscles. Muscle protein is lost because that's where the undernourished body turns in an attempt to meet its energy needs. Because the already weakened respiratory muscles are not spared this cannibalistic process, they atrophy and impair breathing still further. A vicious cycle is sometimes established of weight loss—respiratory muscle-wasting—worsening lung function. Malnourishment can also impair the body's infection-fighting defenses.

Obese COPD patients are a far less common sight, but no less serious a problem. Their substantial added weight aggravates symptoms in two ways. First, their gas exchange needs are substantially increased. All of their extra bulk needs oxygen, and adds to the amount of excess carbon dioxide that must be removed. These needs fall on an already greatly stressed respiratory system. Second, as the weight of chest and stomach increases, the respiratory muscles work harder and harder. It becomes increasingly difficult to expand the chest wall, and for the diaphragm to contract against the weight of the stomach.

It's a problem finding sound guidelines on diet and nutrition at your local bookstore or library. The popular literature is filled with nutritional misinformation—inadequately researched "facts" and a lot of pet theories that have never been tested. Just as you wouldn't take drugs that haven't been properly tested and evaluated, it makes no sense to follow untested (or improperly tested) instructions in choosing the foods you put into your body.

The rest of this section contains reliable, sensible advice to make it a little easier for patients to maintain a good weight and eat healthily. And whenever something is still more theory than fact, we let you know.

Background

Most foods combine each of the three basic elements in varying proportions. These elements are: carbohydrates (sugars and starches); proteins (made up of amino acids, which break down and become the building blocks of all our bodily proteins); and fats (from animal sources, such as butter; from vegetable sources, such as olives and corn). And foods contain various mineral and vitamins, also necessary for continued good health. The ideal diet is *balanced*, meaning it includes the appropriate amount of each substance.

Recommendations

Foods to Avoid?   The goal for COPD patients—just as for everyone else—is a balanced diet. There are no foods that need to be avoided unless there's a good medical reason for doing so, or the food is upsetting for one reason or another. Some people, for example, find that milk or milk products increase their mucus production. Despite the lack of objective proof that this happens, those who discover that dairy products increase their mucus should cut them out of their diet. In the same vein, cut out cold drinks if they increase coughing and mucus.

If foods with gas-causing potential (such as beans and fibrous raw vegetables) have that effect on you, and so distend your abdomen, they may well be aggravating your symptoms. A distended abdomen limits abdominal muscle relaxation, which then limits the diaphragm's movement.

Small, Frequent Meals   Similarly, because large meals distend your stomach—limiting your diaphragm's descent—eat a number of small meals during the day instead of three large ones. And there's another good reason to become a nibbler: digestion takes energy. The larger your meal, the more energy you need to digest it.

More Fat, Less Sugar? In recent years, debate has developed about COPD patients possibly increasing fats in their diet and reducing carbohydrates. Those advocating it base their argument on the fact that carbohydrates are less "cost effective" than fats are in COPD. Although all foods are eventually metabolized to water and carbon dioxide, an ounce of carbohydrate produces less energy and more carbon dioxide than an ounce of fat. Since advanced COPD patients often have difficulty getting rid of excess carbon dioxide, these scientists reason that eating less of the high carbon dioxide–producing foods would reduce the carbon dioxide load in these patients. To this end, special nutritional supplements high in fats and low in carbohydrates have recently been developed. But their benefits remain unproven, and they may well increase risk factors in COPD patients with cardiovascular disease.

Fluid Needs COPD patients must be careful to avoid the extremes of fluid intake. A common tendency is to drink very little to avoid the unpleasantness of a distended abdomen. But drinking too little will dehydrate you, and that will permit your airway secretions to thicken. So adequate hydration is important in keeping your airways clear. Drink frequently but in small amounts, just as we recommend for meals.

Overdoing fluids in the other direction is also harmful. Then you will tend to retain fluid in your tissues, and this could permit fluid to build up in your lungs. This is especially likely to happen if you have problems with either high carbon dioxide levels or cardiac failure. So avoid both excessive fluid and salt intake. The easiest way to cut down on salt is simply to stop using it when you cook, and to stop putting it on the table at mealtimes. You'll be surprised at how quickly you'll lose your taste for the amount of salt you've been used to!

Alcohol What about COPD patients and alcohol? In sufficient amounts, alcohol can adversely affect your heart, muscles, and lungs, and it can be a powerful respiratory depressant. But in small amounts—1 ounce of hard liquor, 4 ounces of wine, 12 ounces of beer—alcohol does no harm, and it may actually do some good. It may act as an appetite stimulant, and it certainly provides extra calories—without adding much salt—for patients who have to regain lost weight. A 12-ounce can of regular beer, for example, represents a low-salt addition of 130 to 170 calories.

Vitamins and Minerals A balanced diet should, in theory, provide all the necessary vitamins and minerals we need. But in fact, a truly balanced diet is often difficult to achieve. And there's an additional problem: as we get older, our ability to absorb many nutrients decreases, so that even an adequate diet can no longer fully provide the full range of vitamins and minerals that we need for optimum health. This makes a good vitamin and mineral supplement essential. Twin Labs and New Chapter are among the companies that make a very reliable high-quality product.

Energy-Saving Strategies

Everything we do—even sitting and doing nothing—requires energy. (Table 15.1 lists the energy costs of a variety of things we do often or every day.) And this is the crux of COPD's impact.

The net effect of COPD is that it significantly reduces the amount of physical energy available to you. To get the most out of this limited energy, you need to adopt two kinds of strategies. One is learning new ways to do things, ways that get the job done using less of your energy. The other is improving the effectiveness of your breathing to raise your energy limit.

Although a multi-topic book such as this one can't go into the lengthy detail available for energy-saving strategies, we are providing the general guidelines you will find useful in devising your own energy conservation techniques. (We have chosen "homemaking" as our focus because many of these tasks have a counterpart in the workplace.)

Once you read through these hints, you'll realize that most are based on common sense rather than sophisticated physiological principles. Your own common sense will extend these principles to your own activities.

If you wish, you can also get more information on specific energy-saving techniques and devices from both physical and occupational therapy departments at large hospital centers with rehabilitation services.

1. *Always be aware of how you are breathing.* First, incorporate pursed-lip and diaphragmatic breathing into your daily life if you haven't yet done so. If you have been in a rehabilitation program, you have already learned these breathing exercises, If not, try practicing them from our instructions in Chapter 13 (and perhaps ask your doctor to watch you and give you feedback).

   Second, try to coordinate your breathing rhythm with what you are doing. Breathe in during the less strenuous phase of a motion, and/or when movement goes away from your body. Breathe out with the strenuous phase of a motion, and/or when movement is towards your body or to gravity. Some examples: exhale as you bend down, inhale as you come up; inhale as you reach into the cabinet, exhale as you carry the object back towards you; inhale as you take the broom to you, exhale as you take a sweeping stroke.

2. *Sit for as many activities as possible.* Standing always takes more energy than sitting. Do food preparation at the table instead of the counter. (You can even shower sitting down, which we talk more about later in this chapter.) Don't feel embarrassed to ask for a seat on the bus if one isn't immediately available. If you must stand at a counter, remember to keep your body as straight as possible. Try to get a counter that's the right height for you—two and one half inches below your bent elbow.

3. *There are certain general rules for moving.*

   □ When you bend, lower your body by bending your knees, not your waist.

Table 15.1 RELATIVE ENERGY COSTS[a] OF A VARIETY OF DAILY ACTIVITIES

Activities of Daily Living		Housework	
Activity	Cost[b]	Activity	Cost
Sleeping	0.7	Sewing	1.0–1.5
Lying quietly	0.8	Sweeping	1.5–1.8
Standing	1.0	Shining shoes	1.5–2.8
Eating	1.4	Polishing	2.5–5.0
Conversation	1.4	Scrubbing	3.0–7.0
Dressing	2.0–3.5	Window cleaning	3.0–4.0
Undressing	2.0–3.5	Hand washing	3.0–5.0
Washing	2.5	Ironing	4.0–4.5
Brushing hair	2.5	Making beds	4.0–5.5
Showering	3.5	Mopping	4.0–6.0
Walking @ 2 mph	2.0–3.0		
Walking @ 3 mph	3.0–5.0		
Walking @ 4 mph	3.5–7.0		
Climbing stairs	10.0–14.0		

[a] The energy cost of a particular activity is rated by comparing the amount of oxygen it uses to how much is consumed when we sit quietly at rest (which equals 1).
[b] One energy cost figure for an item in the table means either that only one study was published, or that all the studies done came up with the same average energy cost. A range of figures reflects variation between different studies.

- ☐ Come back up by straightening your legs. Use leg power, not your back and shoulders.
- ☐ Arm lifting is high energy. Avoid raising your arms if there is an adequate substitute.
- ☐ Don't overreach. If you can't get to something easily, use a stepstool or have someone else get it for you.
- ☐ When you can, slide heavy items (like large pots and pans) instead of lifting them.

4. *In general, use the largest number of muscles to do a job.* The greater the amount of muscle used to do something, the less effort is felt in doing it. If you must carry something, for example, use both arms and hold the item close to your body.

5. *Easy does it.* Slow, smooth movements consume less energy than quick, jerky motions. And above all, *don't rush.*

6. *Rest.* Fatigue increases dyspnea. Resting between tasks is not laziness. It's wonderfully good sense.

   Resting is also an essential aid whenever your breathing becomes uncomfortable, or verges on going out of control. Rest immediately, choosing the position that best suits the situation you find yourself in—sitting on a bed or chair, standing, etc.

7. *Evaluate chores that are very frequent or lengthy.* For frequent chores, see what steps can be combined or eliminated. Example: instead of scrubbing each dish and piece of silverware, then rinsing, put everything to soak in soapy water for a while. Then most items will only need rinsing. And instead of lifting each piece of silverware to the dish drain, collect it all in the clean side of the sink so you can pick up a handful at once, minimizing the number of times you have to lift your arm. For lengthy chores—such as laundry—break them up into small units (transporting clothes to laundry area, sorting them, loading the machine, etc.) and rest in between each one. Once you develop a pattern that is easiest for you, use it every time. As your nerves and muscles become more proficient—which they do with repetition—they become more efficient.

8. *Organize.* This applies to both your activities and work space.

Activities

- ☐ Spread your more energy-demanding tasks over the week. (Don't wash the floor, do the laundry, and cook for a dinner party all on the same day.)

- ☐ Within each day, alternate harder tasks and easier ones. (After clearing the dinner table, sit down and write letters.)
- ☐ Schedule your day's most difficult activities for the time of day when you normally feel your best. This "peak time" differs from person to person.
- ☐ Organize your chores by location when you can, to avoid making multiple trips.

Space

- ☐ Keep the things you use most often closest at hand.
- ☐ Keep heavier items on shelves or hooks close to waist height to minimize reaching and lifting. Don't store your large cast-iron frying pan on the highest shelf!
- ☐ Keep your supplies as close to your work surface as you can to minimize getting up and down, and reaching.

9. *Use a rolling cart to transport multiple items.* A cart on wheels can be a good friend indeed. It helps a lot in reducing the number of trips you have to make. If you're cooking, for example, you can get everything you need from the refrigerator, then stop at your utensil drawers and cabinets and return to your work area in just one trip.

10. *Use the lightest tools for the job.* Aluminum cookware is much lighter than enamel, for example.

11. *For fixed source supplemental oxygen, don't be afraid to use long tubing.* We know someone who has enough tubing to reach every part of his apartment from his oxygen tank. (Keep in mind, though, that such tubing can be tripped on.)

12. *Hints for personal hygiene and dressing.* Feeling clean and well groomed helps us feel better about ourselves. But it isn't always easy for COPD patients—especially if their disease becomes severe—to maintain their accustomed efforts. We don't realize how much energy—and therefore oxygen—it takes to bathe, dress, shave, comb our hair, and so on, until our pulmonary reserves leave us little to spare.

One of the male COPD patients we used to see in the Department of Pulmonary Rehabilitation at New York University Medical Centers is normally meticulous about his appearance. Yet every so often he used to stop showering and shaving. "Why?" we wondered. We learned from him that it happened whenever he was especially depressed or dyspneic, because at those times it took too much energy, even for him.

He's right. A series of landmark studies in the 1950s determined the amount of energy used in carrying out a variety of ordinary daily tasks. And a shower requires more energy than walking at 2.5 mph! We taught our patient how to get the same results with much less energy.

Showering: Remember our advice above to sit instead of stand whenever you can? Do it when you shower, too, whether you have a stall shower or tub shower. Keep a stool in there. And with a tub shower, the stool can also facilitate getting in and out for patients who may find this difficult. A stall shower reduces this difficulty, but it is not often feasible to replace a tub with a stall.

Dressing: First, organize the different aspects of getting yourself dressed. Ideally, your dresser and closet should be next to each other. Use a small rolling cart to collect all of your needs in one trip. Because you will sit on the edge of your bed to dress, lay everything out on the bed within arm's reach of this spot.

Since dressing the lower part of your body takes the most energy, do that part first. Shoes and socks are the most difficult of all. To use less energy putting on your socks or stockings, bring your feet up rather than bending down to them. Use a long-handled shoehorn for your shoes. Wear shirts and sweaters that button all the way down the front, to avoid the energy cost of pulling clothes on over your head. Suspenders are more comfortable than belts because they don't constrict your abdomen.

The overall key is working s-l-o-w-l-y.

Shaving and Combing: For both, use your head instead of raising your arm. Sit at a table with a mirror standing on it, with your right or left elbow—whichever hand you prefer—resting on the table. When shaving, the hand holding the razor remains in that position. Move your cheeks and chin against the razor. When combing and brushing your hair, use the same technique.

How One Patient Manages

Ted Schneider began participating in the Pulmonary Rehabilitation program here at the N.Y.U. Medical Centers during his sixties. He had learned that he had COPD—primarily emphysema—in his early fifties. He began supplemental oxygen 24 hours a day at age 75. He successfully lived alone, and told us how he accomplished this.

I discovered that I had emphysema when I was 52. I had smoked for 40 years. I remember sneaking out with friends during my Bar Mitzvah celebration, going to the bathroom for a cigarette! I started with half a pack a day, and went up to three to four packs a day plus cigars—which I inhaled. When my doctor told me I had emphysema, he also told me I'd be dead in 4 to 5 years if I continued smoking. So I stopped. Cold.

Now I live under the conditions that I imposed on myself by having smoked all those years. I can't move rapidly, or even slowly. Walking, cooking, shaving, relieving myself in the bathroom—no activity is easy for me to undertake. Everything has to be done in such a way that I don't expend energy. I have to rest every 15 to 20 feet when I walk. I sit on a chair in the shower. I sit on a chair in the bathroom to shave. I have organized things in my small apartment so that I can sit in one place and reach practically anything I need—newspapers, mail, typewriter, bathroom, kitchen. I have a cordless telephone that I take to bed with me so I don't have to get up to answer the phone or make a call. I have household help to clean once a week. I keep my apartment neat so I don't have to use energy straightening things up.

I have some advice for you if you have COPD. The first thing is—*If you're smoking, stop!* Second, if you're active, *don't stop being active.* Just learn how to conserve your energy. Third, *exercise regularly* so your muscles can do their best. And last, *try to live as normally as you can,* which is what I do within the limits of my ability to cope with my disease.

Improving Your Sleep

A common complaint among COPD patients is poor sleep—but this complaint rarely makes it to the doctor's office. Doctors typically don't ask their patients about the adequacy of their sleep, and patients tend to think that it's not a legitimate medical problem to bring to their doctor. Yet good sleep is an essential ingredient to staying as healthy as we can, to maintaining our emotional equilibrium, and to rising to our best energy level.

Sleeping pills can depress your breathing, so they are to be avoided. But there are a number of small steps to take that can add up to a significant improvement—the rules of sleep hygiene. Do not drink caffeinated beverages except early in the day—and that includes no soda with dinner. Do not eat at all during the 2 to 3 hours before bedtime. Exercise daily for at least 15 minutes. Avoid excessive alcohol consumption, meaning no more than one beer or one glass of wine with dinner. Even though more than that may make you sleepy enough to fall asleep easily, you will tend to waken during the night and have a difficult time falling back to sleep. Your bed should be reserved for sleeping—no reading or watching TV there. Do those things in the living room or den! Because a high magnesium intake helps sleep, if you're taking a separate calcium-magnesium supplement, make sure to take it at night. Maintain a very regular schedule, going to bed at the same time every night and setting your alarm—and getting out of bed—at the same time each morning.

An important research study was just published documenting the ability of a warm bedtime bath to improve sleep significantly among older (65–83 years old) people. The warm bath involved soaking in water up to the neck for at least 10 minutes. Measuring equipment recorded much calmer sleep after a warm bath, and the enthusiastic reports from participants described greater ease falling asleep and feeling more rested on awakening. Several other research studies have found that a rapid drop in body temperature seems to be the signal our bodies need for falling asleep quickly and sleeping well. Since older people tend to be cooler to start with, it looks like they may benefit from warming up a bit before bedtime to restore the ability to cool down once they're in bed.

If these changes do not make enough of a difference, there are several herbs that are traditional sleep aids. (See Chapter 11 on "Complementary Therapies for COPD" for information about buying and taking herbs.) The really mild ones, such as chamomile and lemon balm, are very safe and effective even for small children, and should be the herbs that you try first. If they do not do the job, the next step is valerian—the sleep herb that's most well known and the most heavily studied. This old standard has been used since ancient times, and is recognized in almost every country worldwide as a useful sleeping aid. It shortens the amount of time to fall asleep and can reduce the number and duration of nighttime wakings. If you want to try it, first be sure that the preparation you buy is from the correct plant—you want *Valerian officianalis*, not *Valerian edulis* or *Valerian walichii*. The names may sound similar, but the effects are very different. Then once you have the right plant, Dr. Tieraona Low Dog—who uses this herb a great deal for patients with insomnia—explains that dosage is critical. You have to use enough of it, or it doesn't work. Most people prefer taking the dried root in capsule form, because this plant has an awful taste once it's been dried. People typically need 900 mg of the dried root—not the 150–300 mg frequently advised—and should take it 30 minutes before going to bed. If you wake during the night and don't fall back to sleep right away, then repeat this dose. Valerian will not leave you groggy, although some people may experience a headache and some restlessness if they have had to take several doses.

16

Work and Play

COPD often erodes the individual's ability to perform the work that has supported him over the years. Work in our society has value far beyond financial support, although one does not usually stop and think how important a long-term vocation is to one's psychological and social integrity until that work is no longer there.

Because COPD is a disease that progressively reduces the energy patients have available for work, many are eventually confronted with this frightening reality. Their profession makes energy demands their lungs can no longer fill. A particular job's energy demands usually determine at what stage of the disease this happens, and how profound the impact will be. The more strenuous the work, the earlier on the conflict arises, and the younger the patient is likely to be. The younger we are when disability forces us from our work, the greater the economic and psychological hardships.

Table 16.1 illustrates the relative energy costs of various vocations. Farming, for example, requires far more physical activity than a sedentary telephone operator's job. So a farmer faces the reality of job loss when his COPD is much less advanced, and he is much younger, than the telephone operator. The operator, in fact, will most likely be able to continue working until retirement age.

For those of you who want to continue at your job and workplace—but fear that there will be too many barriers—you do have certain legal protection. On July 26, 1990, former president George H. W. Bush signed the Americans with Disabilities Act (ADA) into law, landmark legislation that evolved from the civil rights movement of the mid-1960s. Briefly stated, its purpose is to provide a "clear and comprehensive national mandate for the elimination of discrimination against individuals with disabil-

232

ities." Covered impairments must limit a major life activity. Respiratory disorders are specifically noted in the approved list.

Title I of the ADA states that no business employing more than 15 people can discriminate against a qualified individual with a disability in regard to job application, hiring, training, advancement, compensation, discharge, and so on. In addition, employers are required to provide *reasonable accommodation*—unless this would place an undue hardship on the business. *Accommodation* includes job restructuring, modified work schedule, and acquisition of equipment or devices. From our reading of the text, we believe that this may include oxygen for COPD patients. In addition, state and local governments must make public transportation accessible to people in scooters or wheelchairs. And if you do think you are being discriminated against, you have legal recourse.

Restoring Your Ability to Work for a Living

Since Congress formally recognized the importance of rehabilitation services in 1920, they have considered regaining the ability to work as its primary goal. And the current Rehabilitation Services Act defines rehabilitation as the "rendering of a disabled person fit to engage in a remunerative occupation." This emphasis is appropriate.

When someone who has been economically self-supporting must relinquish this support prematurely, a profound economic and psychological impact ripples outward. The individual's sudden lifestyle limitations extend to his spouse, and an often shattered self-image seriously strains relationships with everyone—family and friends—in his close circle. Plus, the need for public assistance of some sort means money gone from the government's resources. COPD patients form one of the largest groups receiving federal disability payments.

A great many nonspecialized health care professionals don't realize that most of these patients still have the capacity to become self-supporting again—with the right help. It is part of the general mistaken attitude that rehabilitating someone with a progressive disease is a waste of time and money, because they are only going to get worse. Yet studies show, over and over again, how successful vocational rehabilitation is with seemingly "unemployable" COPD patients. Counseling and retraining have sent untold numbers of grateful patients successfully back into the world of work.

Table 16.1 RELATIVE ENERGY COSTS[a] OF A VARIETY OF VOCATIONAL AND
RECREATIONAL ACTIVITIES

Vocational Activities		Recreational Activities	
Activity	**Cost[b]**	**Activity**	**Cost**
Light		Walking @ 2 mph	2.0–3.0
Office work	1.5–2.0	Horseback riding	2.0–10.0
Taxi driver	1.5–2.0	Canoeing	2.0–7.0
Draftsman	1.5–2.5	Playing with children	2.5–10.0
Watch repair	1.5–2.5	Walking @ 3 mph	3.0–5.0
Printer	2.0–2.5	Walking @ 4 mph	3.5–7.0
Shoemaker	3.0–5.0	Dancing	4.5–7.5
Tailor	3.5–4.5	Gardening	4.5–10.0
Moderate		Golf	5.0
Housework[c]	1.5–7.0	Swimming	5.0–11.0
Bricklaying	3.5–4.5	Tennis	7.0–10.0
Plastering	4.0–5.0	Bicycling	7.0–20.0
Painting	4.0–5.0	X-country skiing	10.0–20.0
Carpentry	4.0–7.0		
Running @ 10 mph	19.0–20.0		
Tractor plowing	4.5		
Heavy			
Mining	3.0–10.5		
Mowing	6.0–10.0		
Steel mill work	7.0–16.0		
Sawing	7.0–20.0		
Axe work	9.0–20.0		
Shoveling	9.0–20.0		

[a]The energy cost of a particular activity is rated by comparing the amount of oxygen it uses to
how much is consumed when we sit quietly at rest (which equals 1).
[b]One energy cost figure for an item in the table means either that only one study was published,
or that all the studies done came up with the same average energy cost. A range of figures
reflects variation between different studies.
[c]"Housework" shows a broad energy cost range because it combines a variety of activities. Check
Table 15.1 for a detailed breakdown.

That is why vocational counseling is always an important part of any
comprehensive rehabilitation program. The vocational counselor on staff
provides two kinds of help. One is for patients who can resume their old
jobs once they learn where and how to reduce their energy consumption.
The other is for patients who need to choose and train for a different kind

of job, one commensurate with their skills and background yet still within the energy limits set by their respiratory system.

The Initial Decision

The first step in vocational counseling involves the big decision—is it possible and/or practical and/or wise to continue, or resume, your present occupation? Making this decision comes *after* you are medically stable, and have completed a reconditioning program bringing you to an optimum degree of fitness for the level of your disease has reached. Any attempt to jump the gun means you won't have all the major pieces of information you need to arrive at an accurate, satisfying conclusion.

Your vocational counselor is trained to evaluate information from medical, psychological, and vocational sources. Your pulmonary function test and exercise test tell a great deal about the adequacy of your respiratory reserves for carrying out a particular job. We say "a great deal" rather than "all" because of patients we see who continue successfully in their jobs for years after their pulmonary tests indicate they can't produce enough energy for it. The added ingredient is powerful motivation. So obviously, psychological factors—the intangibles—need assessment as well. This information is gathered during interviewing and appropriate testing. Added to the pot is relevant practical information, such as whether or not portable oxygen use—if it increases a patient's energy—is feasible in a particular job.

Based on assessment of tangibles and intangibles, you will be classified as either: (1) no vocational restrictions; (2) with some modification, can return to previous activity; (3) needs retraining in less energy-demanding work; (4) needs employment in a sheltered workshop; or (5) can't work outside the home. ("Sheltered workshops" are certified by the Federal or State Department of Labor to be beyond certain regulations, such as minimum-wage requirements and minimum quality of units of production per worker. So the workload is what each person *can* do rather than *must* do. These workshops are also equipped with supplemental oxygen facilities, and are geared to handle possible medical problems.)

Your classification incorporates two different aspects of the vocational limitations imposed by your disease. "Impairment" looks at what you can no longer accomplish. "Disability" determines whether or not this impairment prevents your from continuing—or resuming—your job. We discuss this more fully in a later section.

What Am I Going to Be?

The prospect of giving up a vocation that one has practiced for 25 or 40 years is not initially a cheerful or easy prospect, even less so if you really enjoyed your work. Circumstances beyond your control have forced you into a kind of identity crisis. But at least you have the best support possible in your vocational counselor. These counselors are specially trained to help you make the best choice you can for a new career.

First, your counselor adds a great deal more information to what has already been gathered. Through interviewing, standard intelligence tests, and paper-and-pencil tests (questionnaires), he learns about your education, skills, interests, intelligence, and personality.

Where you stand on a variety of standardized performance skills is gauged by work sampling tests. One example is the *Philadelphia Jewish Employment and Vocational Service Work Sample System* (*JEVS*), developed under the sponsorship of the U.S. Department of Labor, and designed to evaluate various work traits that collectively constitute performance skills. There are 26 different work samples that test such work characteristics as handling, sorting, manipulating, inspecting, and drafting. The test creates a realistic work atmosphere, and takes six to seven days to complete.

Once all your tests are completed, your counselor evaluates them with you in the framework of your pulmonary resources. In trying to identify appropriate job possibilities—work that satisfies your interests, abilities, personality, and intelligence, yet doesn't tax your energy—remember to set realistic goals. Too high, and you set yourself up for failure. Too low, and you won't find the satisfaction and gratification of working up to your potential.

Keep two other points in mind as well while you are going through this decision time. One is practical, the other concerns the light at the end of the tunnel. In practical terms, it makes sense to avoid work alternatives for which the job market is poor. All your excitement, motivation, and good training will be quite useless if you cannot find a job,

The other is to remind yourself, when things feel bumpy and bleak, just how valuable change can be. It's part of human nature to thrive on meeting challenges, however much we may also fear them. Just as we have found new, satisfying aspects of ourselves over the years by studying with new teachers, meeting new friends, and doing new activities, so those of us who are forced to change our professional lives midstream will eventually be able to look back and take pleasure in what this challenge, too, has brought out in us. It's called "growth."

Putting It into Action

Once you have taken that giant step, sucked in your breath, and said: "This is what I am going to do!," submit an application to the office in your state that provides vocational education support for people with disabilities. If you are in a comprehensive COPD rehabilitation program, your counselor will give you the application materials and instructions. If you do not have access to a counselor who can guide you, the first thing to do is locate the local office of your state agency. Most states call it the Office or Department or Division of Rehabilitation or Rehabilitation Services. Some specifically have a Division of Vocational Rehabilitation. New York State has VESID: Vocational Education Services for Individuals with Disabilities. The *National Clearinghouse of Rehabilitation Training Materials* website provides a full listing by state as well as a comprehensive treasure trove of other information and resources: *www.nchrtm.okstate.edu/index_3.html.* The Clearinghouse—funded by the federal Rehabilitation Services Administration—also publishes a regular newsletter that can be sent by e-mail or snail mail. An application for either format can be made from their website, or you can call 1-800-223-5219 to add your name to the mailing list.

The U.S. Department of Veteran's Affairs also has a website detailing benefits, programs, and services: *www.va.gov.*

Impairment vs. Disability

Once you are diagnosed as suffering from COPD, the severity of your symptoms may need assessment for legal—relating to *disability*—as well as medical purposes. More and more often, physicians are asked to determine medical impairment for disability evaluation hearings. The growing number of these hearings both from recent legislation entitling people to compensation whether or not their disability is work related, and from society's increasingly less negative attitude toward impairment and the receipt of compensation for it.

Although *impairment* and *disability* both refer to what the patient's disease prevents him from doing, the purpose—and therefore focus—of each is different.

Impairment

Impairment is a medical term pointing to an anatomic or functional abnormality. For COPD it means that abnormal respiratory function persists despite appropriate treatment; it is unlikely to be reversed; it interferes significantly with the patient's normal activities.

Degree of impairment is central to tailoring a fitting COPD treatment and physical therapy program. It also provides a helpful framework for vocational evaluation. Based on medical limitations, job impairment varies from "mild to moderate"—which precludes some types of work but not others, to "severe"—which precludes any type of gainful employment.

For the patient with an income-producing job, comparing his job impairment to his work determines whether or not he needs vocational rehabilitation, and therefore whether or not he is disabled.

Disability

Disability concerns the inability—which can be partial or total—to carry out a specific task or type of work. In other words, "disability" is the "impairment's" impact on specific aspects of the patient's life. It is usually evaluated in a job context. Obviously, degree of impairment and disability are not always the same. A mild or moderate COPD impairment can result in partial or total disability for a mail carrier, for example, but not for someone with a desk job.

Accurate disability assessment requires far more than just a good knowledge of the medical impairment's degree and impact. It must include awareness of the patient's age, sex, education, and socioeconomic status, and of his job's energy and skill requirements and possible exposure to toxic substances.

Evaluation Methodology

How COPD patients are evaluated for impairment and disability depends on where their application is being submitted. Will benefits be paid from the Social Security Administration (the SSA), or from the Veterans Administration (the VA), or from a private insurer? Each group defines disability with a different set of criteria. This in turn requires evaluation methodologies.

Sometimes disability is determined strictly by the patient's history and clinical examination. The other extreme requires only a cardiopulmonary profile. The most common approach is to create a profile based on degree of dyspnea, the physical examination, chest X-ray, and most importantly, the pulmonary function test.

The most frequently requested pulmonary function tests are vital capacity (for loss of lung volume), FEV_1 (for obstructed airflow), and either arterial blood gases or oxygen diffusion (for impaired gas exchange). Sometimes an exercise test is added to the menu.

Even if every compensation group used the same criterion tests, there is still the question of the cutoff points separating normal and disabled and distinguishing the different levels of disability. Numerical definitions are certainly necessary, but the lack of consistency from one agency to another can create injustices.

One system organizes cutoff points for vital capacity and FEV_1 only by height. Not taking sex and age into account means these criteria favor women of any age and elderly men, who normally have smaller vital capacities and lower FEV_1 values than young men of the same height. Another system appropriately compares impaired with healthy individuals of the same age and sex.

The American Medical Association's ad hoc committee on the medical rating of physical impairment was formed to try and put together a logical, reality-based set of evaluation categories. The respiratory impairment classification they issued in 1984 (Table 16.2) have also been endorsed by the American Thoracic Society. Although impairment classification criteria still vary from group to group, positive changes are occurring. The SSA, for example, recently changed its methodology and criteria significantly to be more in line with the American Medical Association's guidelines.

Who Pays Disability Benefits?

Social Security Disability Insurance (SSDI) is a federal program. Eligibility is based on medical proof of a disability lasting at least 12 months, and/or ending in death, plus the inability to earn a living. Benefit payments—which are determined by a multi-factor formula—begin six months after the disability has appeared. If SSDI is appropriate for you, your hospital's social work staff should be able to help get things started. If you have no such assistance, get in touch with your local Social Security Office by phone or use their website: *www.ssa.gov/SSA_Home.html.*

Public assistance is the term used for disability compensation from state and/or city sources. Monthly compensation can be either short- or long-term. Since local policies on qualifications and amounts vary, contact your state's Department of Social Services for information.

Some *employee* fringe benefits packages include provisions for short- and/or long-term *disability insurance* and retirement pensions. In this case, your employer can direct you to the appropriate person or agency for information and follow-up.

Table 16.2 Classification of Respiratory Impairment

Based on Dyspnea

Class 1 0%; No Impairment	The subject may or may not have dyspnea. If it is present, it is for nonrespiratory reasons or it is consistent with the circumstances of activity.
Class 2 10%–25%; Mild Impairment	Dyspnea with fast walking on level ground or when walking up a hill. Patient can keep pace with persons of same age and body build on level ground, but not hills or stairs.
Class 3 30%–45%; Moderate Impairment	Dyspnea while walking on level ground with person of same age or walking up one flight of stairs. Patient can walk a mile at own pace without dyspnea, but cannot keep pace on level ground with others of same age and body build.
Class 4 50%–100%; Severe Impairment	Dyspnea after walking more than 100 meters at own pace on level ground. Patient is sometimes dyspneic with less exertion or even rest.

Based on Tests of Ventilatory Function (FVC, FEV_1, FEV_1/FVC)

Class 1	Above the lower limit of normal
Class 2	Greater than 60% of predicted value for tests
Class 3	Less than 60% of predicted values, but greater than 50% for FVC, 40% for FEV_1, and 40% actual value for FEV_1/FVC ratio
Class 4	Less than 50% of predicted for FVC, 40% for FEV_1, 40% actual value for FEV_1/FVC ratio, and 40% of predicted diffusion value

Based on Maximum Oxygen Consumption[a]

Class 1	Greater than 25 ml/kg/min
Class 2	Between 20 and 25 ml/kg/min
Class 3	Between 15 and 20 ml/kg/min
Class 4	Less than 15 ml/kg/min

[a]Expressed as milliliters (ml) of oxygen per kilogram (kg) of body weight per minute (min).

The *Veterans Administration* provides compensation and pensions to eligible veterans.

Recreation

As with work, many recreational activities can become off limits because of COPD's energy production losses. Table 16.1 indicates the typical energy requirements of some common activities.

Typical energy cost, though, is not necessarily the decisive factor in determining your involvement with a particular leisure activity. A variety of issues come into play. One is that people can pursue the same activity with very different degrees of vigor. Swimming, bowling, fishing, golf, dancing, gardening, etc., can all be enjoyed over a broad energy expenditure range from low to very high. COPD patients can continue participating in all of them as long as the energy they put out is toward the low end. And some activates include different versions, each with different energy demands. A female patient of ours, for example, an avid tennis player for years, finally had to admit that singles games took more energy that she could produce. Instead of giving up the game, she switched to doubles.

Another issue is the improved availability of portable oxygen, which now permits a number of COPD patients to continue any low- to moderate-level activity outside the home that doesn't prevent having their oxygen source constantly at hand. You can't swim with your oxygen at your side, but you can certainly golf and go museum and gallery hopping.

17

COPD and Sex

A person's sexual activity and how he feels about it are basic components of his identity and self-esteem. Unfortunately, people with sexual problems do not have an easy time in our society. Reverence for physical perfection has combined with the remnants of our Victorian heritage of shame and secrecy about sexual matters—especially sexual difficulties—to make honesty and a search for solutions extremely difficult.

COPD Often Produces Sexual Problems

COPD has a rich potential for messing up sex lives, because sex—regardless of your motivation—is a strenuous physical activity. It's equivalent to a brisk walk up a flight of stairs. For the typical symptomatic COPD patient, the breathlessness he experiences is not love's intoxication, but intense dyspnea. And dyspnea makes him very anxious.

Anxiety can make dyspnea much worse. It also robs sex of much of its fun, pleasure, and spontaneity. The anxiety—on the part of the patient or a partner—can also bring on sexual failure. Then come even greater apprehension, often with fear and humiliation. Sexual activity becomes such a negative experience that one or both partners start avoiding it altogether.

A contributing cause of sexual problems among COPD patients is the pervasive depression many experience. Male impotence and female inability to reach orgasm are classic behavioral expressions of long-term depression.

The medical profession acknowledges the high probability that sexual problems will begin plaguing a COPD patient at some point, yet there is little or no discussion of this critical issue with patients themselves. The doctor's silent awareness does little to help the patient whose sex life, self-esteem, and intimate relationship(s) are suffering.

If you have encountered sexual problems involving your disease, you are not alone. Hopefully, this fact in itself will provide some reassurance that nothing terrible or unchangeable is wrong with you.

For change to occur, these problems should be dealt with on several levels. The psychological level involves feelings and attitudes. The pharmaceutical concerns properly timed use of medication that aids breathing. The practical involves use of energy-conserving positions for making love. It's the same approach we have advocated for all the other areas of your life!

How Do I Start?

First, you and your partner need to talk—really talk—about your disease. For each of you, this includes your feelings about it and its effects on your activities—including sex. Then you and your partner must both have an accurate understanding of what COPD is, and what your physical limitations really are, and aren't. A support group is a wonderful place to help you get started on this, or to help out if you get stuck. And it's extremely educational—and reassuring—to hear from members who have already worked through this.

If you aren't able to locate a support group, consider a joint session with your doctor. You might also want to show your partner the sections in this book that were particularly helpful to you in understanding your condition more clearly. Counseling can help to explore and resolve any lingering conflicts.

For some people, getting started at talking about their sex lives is a very frightening prospect. The reason may be an attitude of shame and secrecy inherited from one's parents, and/or certainty that revealing one's sexual "inadequacies" can only be humiliating. You have to be brave enough to take that first step. People can support you, but they can't do it for you. Once you take the plunge, you'll discover your listener(s) reacting with respect rather than contempt. They realize what an intimidating barrier you're trying to overcome.

Sex Is More Than Intercourse

Through all of this, try not to focus just on the physical aspects of making love. Too many people confronted by sexual problems look only at what happens with their genitals and their endurance during intercourse. They forget that sexuality includes so much more than just intercourse and orgasm.

Holding and caressing each other, for example, are other very important parts of loving. COPD may be making orgasmic satisfaction difficult or impossible for you and your partner right now, but it hasn't lessened your ability to hug, kiss, and caress the person you care so deeply about. Not all stimulating interactions have to end in intercourse to be acceptable. Each step along the way can also be enjoyed as an end in itself. Achieving intimacy and feeling accepted is the ultimate point of it all. Snuggle, hug, take a bath or shower together, and don't feel pressured to consummate if, for this moment, you are feeling wonderfully close and contented.

Important Things to Know

Normal Age-Related Changes

Since most COPD patients are approaching, or have reached, senior citizen status, it's very important to be aware of normal changes in sexual function that occur as we get older. Some of what you see as "problems" may really be these normal, unavoidable changes. They are part of what we must accept in return for living beyond our middle age.

Men take longer to get an erection, and the erection may not be as hard as it was in their younger days. They often need more stimulation than previously to have an orgasm. And much more time may be needed after ejaculating before another erection can occur.

At some point during menopausal changes, women often experience similar changes in their clitoris. It takes longer to become erect, and no longer becomes as engorged with blood as it once did. Because of this, the time to reach orgasm may increase and the intensity diminish somewhat—but the overall pleasure remains deeply satisfying. Most important is that women who are not on hormone replacements, and some who are, need to supplement their dwindling production of natural lubrication to prevent intercourse from being painful. Happily, pharmaceutical companies are starting to acknowledge women's needs in this area. Now, in addition to the artificial and messy K-Y Jelly, there are lubricants that mimic a woman's natural secretions—such as Replens, which is applied only every several days—and comfortable water-based lubricants such as Astroglide. The section of your pharmacy that stocks menstrual supplies is where you will find a selection of lubricants. Experiment to find the one that works best for you.

Another recommendation is the topical use of vitamin E. Puncture a capsule and apply it with your finger inside the vaginal canal before bedtime. It not only lubricates, but is thought to restore some of the tissue thickness and natural mucus production that are lost in menopause. It combats itchiness, and generally helps people to feel a great deal more comfortable. Get a natural vitamin E product, as research has shown it to be significantly more effective than the synthetic kind. The container may say "natural" or "d-alpha-tocopherol." If you aren't sure, ask. If lubrication is still inadequate, speak with your gynecologist about using a local estrogen cream in the vaginal canal.

The Good News

A new move toward openness about sexual difficulties is starting to make it easier for men and women to talk with their doctors about the physical changes that interfere with their sexual pleasure. Men can take advantage of one of the safe approaches now available for erection difficulties, ranging from external mechanical devices to mechanical implants to injectable drugs. Some women are experimenting with herbal antidotes intended to restore that lost edge. One product—which has undergone clinical testing with very good results—combines extracts of plants from the Amazon rain forest. Called *Jaguara*, it was developed by Raintree Nutrition in Austin, TX: 800-780-5902; fax: 512-833-5414; *info@rain-tree.com*; *http://www.rain-tree.com*. The same company has developed two products for men, both of which have also performed well in clinical testing. One is *Muira Puama*, the other is *Male Plus*.

The most exciting pharmaceutical news these days is the drug *Viagra*, a small blue pill taken at least an hour before beginning lovemaking. It permits a very natural experience, promoting a more substantial erection during the stimulation of foreplay that is easily sustained for the duration of intercourse. A less tangible—but very potent—benefit of Viagra's support is its vast boost to self-confidence. Although most of the data have been gathered from men, a small but growing number of studies on women suggest that Viagra may be helpful for both sexes. The several pulmonologists we have spoken with about Viagra all tell us that they prescribe it to their male COPD patients with excellent results.

As with all drugs, Viagra has its side effects. They affect only about 2% of the men who use it. The common ones are temporary distortion of color perception, headache, and flushing. Although Viagra does not appear to conflict with most other medication, *it should not be taken by any cardiac patients who use nitrates*. (This also applies to women experimenting with this drug, not just to male users.) And to be on the cautious side, discuss Viagra with your doctor beforehand in the context of other drugs you take. As with any medication, people who metabolize drugs more slowly than the norm—people with kidney or liver problems, for example—should use a lower than normal dosage.

Although there are currently no disease contraindications for taking Viagra, there are certain patient groups this medication has *not* been tested in. We do not really know how safe or effective it is in people:

☐ With a resting blood pressure below 90/50 or higher than 170/110
☐ Who have had a heart attack, stroke, or life-threatening arrhythmia within the past 6 months
☐ Who are in cardiac failure or have unstable angina
☐ Who have an eye condition called *retinitis pigmentosa*

Medication Can Affect Sexual Desire and Performance

Many of us are becoming more aware of some of the less publicized side effects that medications can have, particularly when we must take them on a long-term basis. Medicines are very helpful, but when they also produce an undesirable side effect, the help they give must be weighed against this difficulty. Table 17.1 lists a great variety of drugs that have possible side effects in the sexual arena. Although most medications COPD patients commonly use don't directly cause sexual problems, some of them can make existing problems worse.

If you suspect—after reading this section—that a medication you are taking may be dampening your desire or your capacity to achieve an orgasm, talk with your doctor. If your suspicions are accurate, the two of you need to discuss effective alternatives that are less likely to harm your sex life.

Bronchodilators Inhaled bronchodilators aid breathing, but can also cause shakiness and a racing heart when a patient first starts using one. Both these sensations tend to increase one's sense of anxiety, which can intensify existing sexual problems. But once these side effects disappear— after just a few weeks—the greater ease of breathing makes sex easier and more pleasurable. Another potential side effect of some inhaled bronchodilators is urinary retention, which can interfere with sexual arousal. Theophylline causes no problems as long as the blood level does not rise above the therapeutic range. But if it does, the nausea, shakiness, and headaches described in Chapter 9 become a problem affecting sex as well as other behaviors.

Steroids Steroids can cause weight gain. Being overweight often provokes very negative feelings about oneself, and consequent withdrawal from sexual involvement—especially where negative or ambivalent feelings about sex already exist. Steroids can also create a diabetic condition, which is known for its potential to interfere with erection capabilities. Steroids can also swing mood dramatically up or down. Both extremes— depression and hyperactivity—can decrease sexual desire.

Table 17.1 Drugs with Known or Suspected Links to Sexual Dysfunction

Use	Drug Category	Effects[a]
Anticoagulant	Heparin	Priapism
Antiglaucoma	Beta-blockers (Timolol)[b]	Impotence
Antigout	Colchicine	Libido
Antiulcer	Cimetidine (Tagamet)	Impotence
Anti-inflammatory	Naproxen (Naproxen)	Ejaculation, impotence
Cardiovascular:		
Antiarrhythmia	Dysopyramide (Norpace)	Sexual dysfunction
	Flecainide (Tambocor)	Sexual dysfunction
Antihypertensive	Guanethidine (Esimil)	Ejaculation, impotence
	Phenoxybenzamine (Dibenzyline)	Ejaculation
	Hydralazine (Apresazide)	Impotence
	Clonidine (Catapres)	Impotence, sexual dysfunction
	Methyldopa (Aldomet)	Libido, impotence
Diuretic	Acetozolamide (Diamox)	Impotence
	Spironolactone (Spironolactone)	Impotence, libido, sexual dysfunction
	Thiazides (Diuril)	Impotence, sexual dysfunction

Use	Drug Category	Effects[a]
Lipid-reducing	Clofibrate (Atromid)	Impotence
General cardiac medications	Beta-blockers (Inderal)	Sexual dysfunction
	Digitalis glycosides (Digoxin)	Sexual dysfunction
Neurologic:		
Anticonvulsant	Carbamazepine (Tegretol)	Impotence, sexual dysfunction
Parkinson	Levodopa (Larodopa)	Libido
Psychiatric:		
Antidepressant	Tricyclic drugs[c]	Libido, impotence
	Monoamine oxidase inhibitors (MAO) (Nardil)	Impotence, ejaculation, priapism, sexual dysfunction
Antipsychotic	Neuroleptic[d]	Libido
Mood disorders	Lithium	Libido
Weight control	Amphetamines	Sexual dysfunction
	Mazindol (Sanorex)	Sexual dysfunction

[a]Priapism: persistent erection of the penis due to disease rather than sexual desire; impotence: erection is either absent, or cannot be maintained; libido: sexual desire low or absent; ejaculation: absent or premature; sexual dysfunction: general term covering all sexual problems: female low arousal, male difficulty in reaching orgasm, decreased orgasmic pleasure, female or male dyspareunia (pain during intercourse).
[b]Representative brand name.
[c]See Table 10.1 for specific drug name.
[d]See Table 10.3 for specific drug name.

Non-COPD Drugs Some non-COPD medications that can make erections more difficult to achieve, or decrease desire to start with, are prescribed fairly frequently for COPD patients as well as others. These include some of the antihypertension drugs, some cardiac medications, antiulcer drugs, and the psychoactive mood-altering medications.

Alcohol Although not strictly a medication, alcohol's pronounced loosening up effects are sometime relied upon to help people relax and get "in the mood." The problem is that too much—and this amount, which varies with the individual, can be reached well before the sensation of having drunk too much—can actually lower sexual desire and prevent erection and orgasm.

Extending Your Limits

We presented our general arguments for adopting a routine of daily exercise in Chapter 13. We emphasized the importance of regular exercise for helping maintain general strength, flexibility, and endurance, and for improving your mental alertness and self-esteem. All these positive changes also contribute to stronger sexual feelings. And your improved endurance will aid you in carrying them out.

Because sex is strenuous exercise, patients should expect an increase in heart and breathing rates even if they're physically fit. *But if heavy breathing turns into dyspnea, don't panic, and don't give up.* First, stop and give yourself time to recover. Then, handle it the same way you do your regular exercise.

Medication to Help Breathing

If an inhaled bronchodilator usually helps you during exercise, it should also improve your breathing during sex. When dyspnea is only an occasional problem during sex, use your bronchodilator at those times to bring your breathing under control. But if it's a regular occurrence, make your bronchodilator routine. In essence, it's exercise premedication. Before sex, use albuterol/salbutamol. Then keep your MDI on your night table to make it as convenient as possible if you need it again.

The patient on medication every four hours should find it fairly easy to schedule the last dose at bedtime. Otherwise, use it when you think you might need it. Just remember that one dose gives you about four hours of protection. If you and your partner are both feeling sexy again at a point that would take you beyond this protective range, use your inhaler again.

If you are on supplemental oxygen, your physician has probably advised you to increase your flow rate when you exercise. So extend this principle to sexual exercise, and increase your flow rate before you get started.

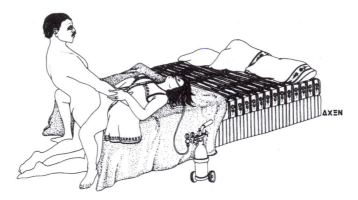

Figure 17.1 The lovemaking position considered least tiring for a female patient.

Avoid Fatigue

Don't forget that fatigue can put a damper on sexual relations. If this is a particular problem of yours, try to set up your schedules so that lovemaking can usually be when you are both well rested.

Conserve Your Energy

Another aspect to consider is the sexual position(s) you use. Since positions that are less strenuous and more comfortable ease the effort we put out, switching to one requiring less work can make a big difference. Patients who cannot tolerate any real weight on their chest also need to work with their partner and find some enjoyable substitutions. All of our suggestions—and don't be afraid to invent your own—can be used with supplemental oxygen.

1. Partners lying on their sides face-to-face allows free breathing for both.
2. Partners lying on their sides back-to-front, with the man entering from behind, has the same advantage.
3. In a variant of this, the woman kneels on the floor at bedside with her upper body flat on the bed so her chest is supported and free of pressure from the man's weight.
4. The man on the bottom with the woman sitting on top is very easy for male patients, since the woman provides most of the energy.
5. Perhaps the easiest position for a female patient (Figure 17.1) has her seated at the edge of the bed, feet on the floor, with her upper body comfortably semi-reclining on pillows. Her partner kneels on the floor in front of her. This position also makes oral sex very easy to add or substitute.

You may find that building a repertoire around petting, stroking, massaging, mutual masturbation, and oral sex works best for you. For some patients in this category, it means engaging in sexual behaviors they have spent many years regarding as inappropriate. Try keeping your focus on what you are trying to win back from COPD. These behaviors are legitimate, energy-conserving, and satisfying avenues to pleasure and intimacy. Don't let baseless old taboos deprive you of victory.

Summary

- [ ] Partners must be open-minded and *keep communication going*.
- [ ] Education is needed about: your disease; normal age-related changes; your medication(s)—how they can hurt and/or help sex for you; ways to help sex become satisfying again.
- [ ] Seek counseling for continuing problems.

18

COPD and Successful Travel

We are a mobile society. Both business and pleasure travel are integral to the American lifestyle. And for many of us, an anticipated pleasure of getting older is extended time to travel and explore. The eventual "empty nest" will give us, too, the freedom to leave it.

But COPD has—needlessly—destroyed this dream for the great majority of patients. They now feel bound to home more tightly than ever by their diminished energy and endurance, by whatever degree of supplemental oxygen they need, and by their sense of fragility. They feel safest with what they know. This means home—certainly not some faraway place where who knows what will happen, and who knows what they will be able to do about it.

It's true that travel disrupts your routines, can require some increases in energy expenditure, and separates you from your reassuring medical support systems. But it's also true that successful travel away from home does wonders for your self-confidence—especially when you're successfully coping with a major chronic disease—while it broadens your horizons. And it's fun and relaxing. Who doesn't benefit, from "running away from it all" for a little while?

Most patients don't need to give up their dreams. The availability of portable oxygen sources—combined with sensible advance planning—permits all but the most severely ill COPD patients to enjoy distant travel (Figure 18.1). Oxygen is safe to carry. Despite many patients' fears, it won't explode or catch fire unless the actual supply tubing is directly ignited. *Planning* means knowing—*in advance*—what your potential trouble spots are, and making *advance* arrangements for preventing or handling things if the worst should come to pass. This chapter is devoted to successful planning.

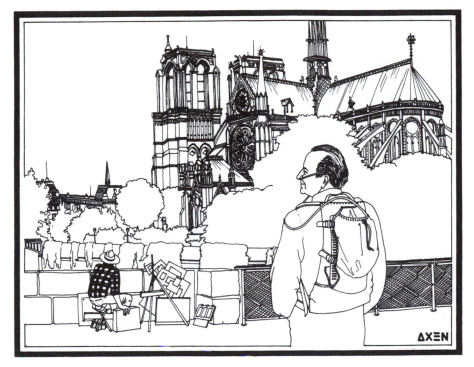

Figure 18.1   The presence of high capacity portable oxygen delivery systems gives oxygen-dependent COPD patients the freedom and comfort to travel. (Illustrated is the AirLift backpack designed to accommodate a liquid oxygen dispenser.)

Your Medical Needs Away from Home

Medication

Well before your departure date, work out a medication plan with your doctor. You need to prepare for two possibilities. Developing a respiratory infection will require an antibiotic on hand, and knowledge of the appropriate schedule for taking it. Know, also, when to increase your bronchodilator dosage, and by how much. You will need to do this, for example, if a pollution alert is forecast or if you will be at a gathering where many people will be smoking (a niece's wedding, perhaps).

But the best planning won't help if you don't have your medication with you. *Carry enough to cover your entire trip.* This includes your routine medication(s) as well as anything your doctor recommends for emergencies. Fill your prescriptions for emergency supplies—for example, steroids, antibiotics, cough medicine—right away, and keep them at hand throughout your trip. *Keep a full duplicate supply* of routine and emergency medications in your suitcase, with your name, type of medication, and your dosage and schedule information written on each container.

Medical Help

Go over your itinerary with your doctor to get recommendations of doctors, clinics, and hospitals where you will be. You can supplement this list by getting in touch with the American Lung Association, local Lung Associations in your destination cities, and the National Jewish Medical and Research Center's Lung-Line, 800-222-LUNG. They can also give you information on the spot if you run into unexpected problems. For travelers who venture outside the United States, contact the nearest United States government office if such trouble develops. This means our embassy if you are in a capital city, and our consulate if you aren't. These offices normally maintain a list of English-speaking physicians and hospitals.

Oxygen Supplies

If you need continuous oxygen, set up your supply network *before you leave*. Suppliers for liquid or tank oxygen are found in most large U.S. cities. Locate dealers' names both along your route and at your destination(s). Your home supplier should be able to help you find them. If not, call local Lung Associations or see if the local telephone information operators can help you.

Outside the United States, oxygen is less easily available. That makes it particularly important for foreign travelers to make sure they will have a supply at their destination(s). Most countries maintain an embassy in Washington D.C., and a consulate in Manhattan. These offices may have information on the feasibility of getting oxygen.

Several groups have come into existence since the first edition of this book that are devoted to helping travelers who must rely on supplemental oxygen. These groups, their services, and the means for contacting them are described in the final paragraph of Chapter 12 on page 178.

Insurance

Getting your medical insurance in order is also part of your medical needs. Find out if your policy covers you on your planned trip. If your insurer doesn't cover subscribers traveling outside the United States, for example, you can get a temporary policy to cover any medical expenses that arise during such a trip. But look around carefully. Many insurers won't cover a preexisting condition. Your travel agent should have the necessary information.

Don't neglect flight-cancellation and trip-interruption insurance. Think optimistically, but plan for the worst so you won't suffer unduly if it comes to pass. Vacations are more and more expensive these days. Some airlines and many charter companies won't refund your money if you cancel or interrupt your trip, no matter how serious and verifiable the reason. The relatively little you pay for such insurance is amply worth the peace of mind it buys you. Again, check with your travel agent for details.

Documents to Keep with You

Carrying your doctor's summary of the medication you have with you will facilitate your passage through Customs outside the United States—and through the occasional domestic airport that is particularly stringent in checking luggage. Having this summary include information on your disease—such as your history, test results, characteristic blood gases, and so on—can be of great help if a medical emergency arises.

Where to Go; When to Travel

For a trip not dictated by work, give some thought to your destination. COPD invokes three criteria of concern: altitude, temperature, and allergens.

Altitude

The higher up you go, the less oxygen is in the air. The air in "mile-high" cities—Denver and Mexico City, for example—has 20% less oxygen than sea-level cities such as Paris, London, and New York. If you have doubts about how you'll do in a high-altitude environment, ask your doctor to order a high-altitude simulation study for you. This test will determine how breathing oxygen-poor air affects you.

Climate

COPD patients tolerate warm climates better than cold ones. But temperatures over 90°F are considered extreme heat, and should also be avoided.

Allergens

If you have an allergy with a known cause, find out if this allergen is present in the area you want to visit. If it is, don't go. If you are allergic to dust and mold, for example: don't stay at old inns and hotels no matter how charming they are; avoid anything in lake and seashore areas that isn't newly built; don't visit heavily forested areas after rainy periods or once the leaves have fallen.

Going by Car

The family car is the most popular way to travel in the United States. It offers the traveler a great deal of independence, particularly if that traveler has to carry along an oxygen source. Both reservoirs and portable units are fairly easy to transport by car and refill from suppliers along the way. Remember to plan ahead and know which suppliers can, in fact, refill your particular unit. Some of the newer oxygen concentrators are actually small enough to put in the trunk of a large car.

Highway pollution can be a disadvantage of car travel. But you can minimize your exposure by: (1) keeping the air conditioner on and windows closed; (2) traveling only during periods of lighter traffic, always avoiding rush hours; (3) using back roads instead of heavily traveled highways whenever you can (and it's also far more pleasant).

If you don't do well at higher altitudes, you need to be aware of the altitudes you're driving through en route to your low-altitude destination. To remain an alert and responsive driver, you may have to increase your oxygen flow to compensate for reduced oxygen at higher altitudes. If you aren't on supplemental oxygen, try to avoid being at the wheel in high-altitude locales.

Going by Train or Bus

If a bus or a train will take you where you want to go, you may lose some freedom but you'll save in energy expenditure. The biggest advantage for oxygen users—on relatively short trips—is that train and bus lines do not restrict carrying a portable oxygen unit aboard. But remember that there are no transfilling facilities on trains and buses. So the crucial piece of advance information you need is the longest the trip could possibly take. If it won't outlast your oxygen supply, you're in good shape.

Airplane

Poor Cabin Air   Airplanes magically telescope distances and extend time. But the air they give you to breathe can also spell trouble if you have COPD. Except for the pilots' area, cabin air is typically underventilated. This means passengers breathe a significant volume of respiratory irritants over and over for the length of their trip.

Toxic fumes—including ozone, a major smog alert component—from the plane's engines pollute the air with respiratory irritants that are stated health threats in the National Academy of Sciences' August 1986 report on airplane cabins' poor air quality. The typical partial-strength air conditioning distributes it evenly throughout the air and it recycles to everyone. This recycled, inadequately cleaned air also spreads respiratory viruses efficiently and democratically throughout the cabin.

The American Association of Flight Attendants analyzed written complaints from 473 flight attendants who had individually contacted Congress about poor passenger-cabin air. The results: 268 cases of frequent respiratory irritation connected with flying, 11 cases of medically documented lung scarring or pneumonia, 49 cases of a bronchitis-like condition.

It isn't that airplanes *can't* clean their air of pollutants and infectious agents. They have catalytic converters to reduce ozone, and a fuel-powered air conditioning system to bring in fresh air. It's that they often *won't*. Airline companies cut fuel costs by having pilots reduce air conditioning use in passenger cabins. They also economize by infrequent maintenance of catalytic converters. This can happen because the FAA—the Federal Aviation Agency—doesn't regulate cabin air except for ozone levels—and even that regulation isn't backed up by enforcement provisions.

Also consider that the FAA's short-trip ozone limit—.25 parts per million—is much higher than the prevailing federal standard for protecting human health. And for New York State's Department of Environmental Conservation, that same level is the red flag to look out for a major smog alert. Because the FAA virtually ignores cabin air quality, passengers typically get as much fresh air as riders in an underground subway car—one-tenth the fresh air that pilots enjoy.

The airlines' response to the National Academy of Sciences' report has been to turn up the fans instead of the air conditioning. All that does is send the stale, recirculated air around a little faster. Major improvement seems a long way off.

So flying often means you risk catching a viral respiratory infection, which would develop in the few days after you land. A cold or flu can stress your meager respiratory reserves. Respiratory irritants you inhale on board worsen your symptoms—coughing, wheezing, shortness of breath—during the flight.

Precaution: Borrow a piece of advice from Mary O'Brien, M.D., a geriatric specialist who regularly adds elements of complementary medicine to the health care of seniors in her practice. She instructs *all* of her patients to take the herbal medicine *echinacea* whenever they are going to fly. The schedule is twice a day starting 3 days before the flight and continuing for 2 days after the flight, both going and returning. Echinacea is proven to stimulate the number and activity of macrophages, white blood cells that play an important role in subduing invading microbes. *HerbPharm's* "Super Echinacea" is an excellent brand for those who don't mind taking it in tincture (liquid) form. It's available in many health food stores. Among good brands for those who prefer swallowing capsules are *Enzymatic Therapy* and *Nature's Herbs*.

Minimizing Problems   For the flight itself, again, the key is to *plan in advance*. *Premedicate* when you are about to fly, using prescribed medication to minimize irritation. Use a spray bronchodilator 10 to 20 minutes before boarding. Those who must take medication via an electrically powered nebulizer can medicate shortly before leaving home if they live near the airport. If not, most airports have a first-aid room where the nebulizer can be used before boarding. But remember to schedule in the extra time your treatment takes. Don't forget to leave your nebulizer out of the suitcase and carry it with you! And get an explanatory note from your doctor to prevent delays at airport security metal detectors.

Keep These Tips in Mind

☐ Carry all your medication—not just your spray or nebulizer—with you. Needed medication can't help you from the baggage compartment.

☐ Talk to your doctor about Atrovent, a drug particularly effective in preventing bronchospasm from airway irritants.

☐ Consider a flu vaccination if you need to fly during flu season.

☐ Telling your flight attendant you have respiratory problems—and demanding full operation of the plane's air-conditioning system—sometimes gets results.

Oxygen   Airplane cabin pressure is not required to bring us any closer to sea level than 8,000 feet. This pressure gives you the same amount of oxygen you'd be breathing in Denver, Salt Lake City, Albuquerque—any of the "mile-high" cities.

What about COPD patients who need more? You would think that airplanes—because they always have oxygen on board in case the cabin suddenly depressurizes—would be ideal for these patients. Not so, we discovered.

First off, most airlines won't let you use your own oxygen supply, although they will let you check your empty reservoirs in the baggage compartment. Most airlines will agree to give you medicinal oxygen from their supply if you notify them well in advance and provide a doctor's prescription, but after that it gets complicated.

Phil Porte, Executive Director of NHOPA (National Home Oxygen Patients Association), describes a difficult, arbitrary situation in securing oxygen for air travel that he calls "gross and blatant discrimination." Of the roughly one million patients requiring 24-hour supplemental oxygen, an estimated 650,000–700,000 are able to fly as long as they have access to supplemental oxygen while in the air. Yet within the United States, not only are passengers prohibited by law from bringing their own oxygen system on board, but any airline—domestic or foreign—is permitted to deny boarding to anyone requiring oxygen. Although more U.S. airline carriers will now agree to provide oxygen compared to the state of affairs when our first edition was published, progress has moved at a snail's pace. The major domestic airlines all agree to provide oxygen, but Mr. Porte notes that this is limited to jet planes, has to be arranged from 48 to 72 hours in advance, and adds substantially to the ticket price. And we can see from Table 18.1 that the charge on foreign airlines ranges from no charge up to $1,500 for a standard round trip, and the advanced time required can be as much as a full month. There are no provisions for the emergency, last-minute travel that is sometimes unavoidable.

The information in Table 18.1 was gathered by people pretending to be COPD patients who called the listed airlines. According to Mr. Porte, though, the reality encountered once you are actually aboard can be distressingly different from the arrangements you thought you had made. "Just because the airlines acknowledge that you are coming and that they will have oxygen available—there is no binding agreement." He describes experiences that patients have reported all too frequently. "Oftentimes airlines will provide empty tanks," he says. "They will often provide tanks that they do not know how to operate. The patient who says: 'I don't see a flow meter. Could you tell me what the rate is set at?' can often expect to be told: 'Well . . . it's turned on!' Some of the oxygen setups provided are mask-only," Mr. Porte adds. "In virtually every other country in the world, you would be able to board a plane and use your own portable oxygen system without any difficulty. The situation here is a national disgrace."

What Mr. Porte hopes eventually to see is adoption of laws and regulations requiring airlines either to provide supplemental oxygen to those who need it, or to permit passengers to bring their own FAA-approved system on board. Despite today's new technologies, and further advances on the near horizon, FAA regulations are still archaically tied to the state of knowledge that existed back in the 1970s. "There are certainly legitimate safety and security concerns, but when you think of the money being spent now to put defibrillators on every plane," he observes, "we

Table 18.1 COMMERCIAL CARRIERS SAMPLED

Carrier	Permits O_2	Total Telephone Time, Min.	No. of Calls Required	No. of People Spoken To	Advance Notice Required	M.D. Notification Needed	Added Charge for a Standard Trip[1]	Devices Available	Liter Flow Options	Rating Value[2]
International										
KLM Royal Dutch	Yes	10	1	1	1 wk	Yes	0	Simple mask, NC[3]	2 or 10	3
China Airlines	Yes	15	2	2	1 wk	Yes	0	NC	1–6	2
Emirates	Yes	10	1	2	72 h	Yes	0	NC	2	3
Air Afrique	Yes	10	1	2	1 wk	Yes	$64	NC	2–4	2
BWIA	Yes	8	1	1	1 wk	Yes	$80	NC	2, 4, 6	2
Qantas	Yes	5	2	2	72 h	Yes	$100	Venti-mask, simple mask, NC	1–15	1
Air Ontario	Yes	8	1	1	48 h	Yes	$120	NC	1 or 4	3
British Airways	Yes	15	1	1	48 h	Yes	$150	NC	2 or 4	4
Lufthansa	Yes	20	1	1	72 h	Yes	$150	NC	2–8	2
JAL (Japan Airlines)	Yes	6	1	1	1 mo	Yes	$250	NC	2	4
Canadian Airlines International	Yes	9	2	2	48 h	Yes	$260	NC	2–4	4
Mexicana	Yes	8	1	1	72 h	Yes	0	NC	Any	3
Swissair	Yes	5	1	1	1 wk	Yes	$274	NC	2–6	4
Singapore	Yes	4	1	1	2 wk	Yes	$1,100	NC	2–4	4
Alitalia	Yes	12	1	2	72 h	Yes	$1,500	NC	6	4
Aerolineas Argentinas	No	1	1	1	—	—	—	—	—	5

Airline									
Finnair	No	1	1	1	—	—	—	—	—	5
Korean Air	No	3	1	1	—	—	—	—	—	5
Philippine Air	No	2	1	1	—	—	—	—	—	5
Saudi Arabian	Yes	6	2	3	72 h	Yes	0	NC	2–4	2
Scandinavian	Yes	5	1	1	3–4 wk	Yes	0	NC	2–4	4
South African Express	Yes	6	2	2	3–4 wk	Yes	0	NC	2–4	4
U.S.-Based										
American West	No	10	2	2	—	—	—	—	—	5
Delta	Yes	18	2	2	72 h	Yes	$100	NC	2–8	2
Midwest Express	No	5	1	1	—	—	—	—	—	5
United	Yes	15	2	2	48 h	Yes	$100	NC	2, 4, 6	3
American	Yes	10	2	2	48 h	Yes	$150	NC	2 or 4	4
TWA	Yes	7	2	2	48 h	Yes	$150	NC	2–8	4
Continental	Yes	16	1	2	48 h	Yes	$200	NC	2–4	3
US Airways	Yes	10	2	2	72 h	Yes	$120	Simple mask, NC	2, 4, 6	2
Northwest	Yes	15	1	2	48 h	Yes	$150	Simple mask, NC	2–8	3
Southwest	No	3	1	1	—	—	—	—	—	5
Skyway	No	3	1	1	—	—	—	—	—	5

[1] A standard trip is defined as a nonstop, round-trip 6-hour excursion requiring 2 liters/min.

[2] Rating—scored using a subjective 5-point ordinal scale (from *1 = best* to *5 = worst*)—integrated 4 elements: (1) ease of eliciting information, (2) ease of arranging for in-flight oxygen, (3) charge for in-flight oxygen, and (4) amount of advance notice required.

[3] NC = nasal cannula

(Reproduced with permission from Stoller JK, Hoisington E, Glen A. A comparative analysis of arranging in-flight oxygen aboard commercial air carriers. *Chest* 1999;115:991–995.)

should also be able to find a safe way of providing oxygen on board to those who need it."

He doesn't expect change to come quickly, though, because of what he sees as a two-pronged barrier. To begin with, he finds that the airlines do not understand oxygen, so their attempts to provide it are needlessly inadequate and unnecessarily expensive. In addition, his experience with the FAA has been extremely disillusioning. They talk a good line, but there is no action to back it up. Mr. Porte quotes as an example the notice published by the Department of Transportation in the August 20, 1997, *Federal Register.* "FAA, RSPA (Research and Special Programs Administration), and the Office of the Secretary are initiating a project, separate from this rule-making action, to explore whether safe alternatives exist for accommodating passenger needs in regard to the use of oxygen. This project could result in proposals to amend the relevant portions of . . ." The language is very specific, he points out: they *are initiating* a project, placing it squarely in the present tense. Yet whenever he has called the FAA, RSPA, or the Office of the Secretary, he cannot find a single staff person who works on this project. "What project?" is the only response he has ever had.

Mr. Porte urges patients to joint NHOPA to add their voices—and sometimes their letter-writing efforts—to the Association's advocacy efforts.

National Home Oxygen Patients Association
5454 Wisconsin Ave., Suite 1270
Chevy Chase, MD 20815
888-NHOPA44; fax: 310-718-2976; *homeoxygen@erols.com*
www.homeoxygen.org

Final Words

Get out your maps, make *all* your plans, and "Bon Voyage!"

19

Surgical Options

When this book was first published (in 1990), surgery was not a viable option for COPD patients. Since then, two procedures have become a reality for *appropriate* patients. Lung *transplantation*—the first, and more extreme, option to emerge—is now an approved, accepted procedure. The second—specifically for a subgroup of severely ill emphysema patients—is lung volume *reduction*. Although this procedure is still considered experimental because the final definitive study is in progress, these results will be a fine-tuning of our understanding of the definite benefits already published in a variety of small studies. For each procedure, this chapter will discuss what it consists of, what we know about benefits and side effects, what makes a good or poor candidate, and any other important relevant considerations.

Lung Transplantation

Lung transplantation involves replacing your diseased lungs with the healthy lungs of a person who very recently died. Depending on the severity of your disease, this can involve transplanting the entire lung (all five lobes) and heart together, or the entire lung by itself, or, most often, part of an entire lung that has been divided between two patients. Each one receives half of the lung—which doctors call a *single lung*—either the two-lobed left side or the three-lobed right side.

The very first lung transplant was attempted in 1963 by Dr. James Hardy at the hospital affiliated with the University of Mississippi Medical School. The patient was a 58-year-old convict, serving a life sentence, with terminal lung cancer who had volunteered for the experimental surgery. His new lungs kept him alive for almost 3 weeks, proof that this new procedure—once sufficiently improved—would work. Bringing it to this point took 20 years.

The first clinically successful single-lung transplant was done in 1983 by Dr. Joel Cooper in Toronto, Canada. At that point it became an option reserved for patients dying from interstitial fibrosis, a disease in which the lungs stiffen and prevent oxygen from passing easily into the blood. The first lung transplant for a COPD patient was in 1989. And since then, COPD patients—including the alpha$_1$-antitrypsin group—have become the rule rather than the exception. By 1995, COPD patients already represented almost half (47.5%) of the 1,932 lung transplants that had been done in the United States since that very first success in Toronto.

It is essential to understand, though, that the long-term survival statistics make lung transplantation a last heroic intervention. COPD patients receiving a single lung transplant have approximately a 90% chance of surviving the year following the surgery. But at the 5-year point, the 1995 survey showed only a little over one-third (37%) of the transplant patients still alive.

The Ideal Candidate

The worst medical picture—in the terminal stages of COPD, with a life expectancy of 12 to 24 months despite optimal medical care—is what qualifies a patient to be evaluated for a lung transplant. But because transplantable lungs are very scarce compared to the number of patients who need them, stringent eligibility criteria (Table 19.1) have been set to maximize the likelihood of a successful outcome. Medically, the ideal recipient does not have any other chronic diseases, is under 65 years old, and does not abuse drugs or alcohol. (No smoking for 6–12 months prior to listing is another important requirement.) In addition to that, the presence of strong social support—such as a close-knit family—is essential for helping the patient stick to the strict and complicated life-after-transplant medication regimen that can involve taking 60 pills a day.

In contrast, the poor candidate has one or more of the following characteristics: an additional chronic disease (such as insulin-dependent diabetes, significant heart disease, poor resistance to infection), age above 65, previous thoracic surgery, uses more than 15 mg of steroid drugs daily, or is actively psychotic or a drug abuser (which would impair adherence to the demanding medication regimen). Interestingly, by 1995, more than 57% of the approved candidates were women.

But even with strict criteria for determining eligibility, the number of people waiting for healthy lungs is still far greater than the number of organs available. This means that 70% of the eligible candidates have to wait for more than 1 year from the time they are first listed at the approximately 94 centers in the United States that do lung transplants. Sadly, some patients do not survive the wait.

Transplant Procedure

We'll limit this description to a single lung transplant, as that is by far the most common experience. It involves a large—big enough to pass the lung through—incision in the space between the fifth and sixth ribs. Whether the opening is made on the left or right side depends on which part of the entire lung is being replaced. During surgery the patient is on a respirator, and blood pressure and heart function are carefully monitored. The thin membrane covering the heart—called the *pericardium*— is slit open. The lung that is about to be replaced is separated from all of its "attachments"—the pulmonary artery (the large vessel carrying blood from the heart to the lungs for absorbing oxygen and shedding carbon dioxide), the veins that carry this blood back to the heart, and the airway attaching this lungs to the large bronchi. The lung itself is emptied of air and removed, and replaced with the healthy donor lung. The patient's pulmonary artery, the veins that return freshly oxygenated blood to the heart, and the connecting airway are sewn into place.

Once surgical recovery is over, the first step is a detailed and comprehensive education concerning how you must care for yourself—for the rest of your life as well as the immediate postsurgical period. The length of your hospital stay is impossible to predict because even without complications, the speed of recovery is a very individual matter. Immediately upon discharge from the hospital, you are enrolled in a pulmonary

Table 19.1 REQUIREMENTS FOR LUNG TRANSPLANT SURGERY ELIGIBILITY

- □ End-stage COPD (primarily emphysema) with a life expectancy between 12 and 24 months
- □ Less than 65 years old
- □ Absence of other significant systemic disease (especially kidney or liver disease) or recent major cancer
- □ Medical compliancy and reliability
- □ Psychological stability, with no history of substance abuse
- □ Ambulatory with oxygen
- □ Adequate social support
- □ Adequate nutrition
- □ Oral steroids—less than 15mg/day

rehabilitation program for at least one month. Rehabilitation will *substantially* improve your quality of life, and also provide for regular close medical supervision.

The Bad News

Let's get the less pleasant aspects out of the way before detailing the benefits that have made this procedure worthwhile for many of the patients who have undergone it. There are two time frames for a discussion of side effects. One is the short-term perspective of possible complications arising directly or indirectly from the surgery itself. Second is the lifelong consequences of living with an organ that your immune system knows does not belong to you.

The surgical procedure itself can cause bloating, nausea, and disappearance of intestinal activity, as well as cardiac arrhythmias, blood clots, and mild anemia. Patients who—for whatever reason—find the experience highly anxiety-producing may find that this increased stress level has raised their blood lipids and/or blood sugar and/or blood pressure. If steroids are used—to counter airway inflammation, among other things—they can cause osteoporosis and increase blood sugar. In many respects, though, this is the easiest part of the transplant experience.

As soon as your new lung is in place, your immune system identifies it as a foreign object because it lacks the unique molecular fingerprint carried by all of your own cells. And your immune system is programmed to reject anything lacking your signature fingerprint. When it comes to bacteria, viruses, and fungi, this powerful immune surveillance and protection keeps us healthy. But for a life-sustaining organ transplant to succeed, your doctor has to prevent the massive rejection response that will otherwise make you exceedingly sick—and destroy the new lung. (The technical term for an acute rejection episode is *graft vs. host disease,* or GVH.) Controlling the immune response requires a lifelong daily regimen of immunosuppressive drugs (costing more than $3,000/month) that starts right before surgery. *Cyclosporine A* has been the cornerstone for a number of years, although the new drug *tacrolimus* (called FK506 before it was fully approved) is increasingly replacing it. They work in the same way and many of their side effects appear to be similar, but some patients feel much better on tacrolimus than on cyclosporine A.

Although these drugs have made transplant surgery a reality, they unfortunately create problems of their own when used long-term. This includes kidney and neural damage, high blood sugar, and GI (gastrointestinal) disturbances, and eventual high blood pressure from the kidney damage. Some people suffer from migraine-like headaches. In addition, immunosuppression leaves you permanently vulnerable to infections, and treating them requires aggressive treatment with antimicrobial and anti-fungal drugs. Despite aggressive infection-fighting treatment, though, infection is the primary cause of deaths in the first three months after surgery. And an infection also runs the risk of sparking a rejection episode.

For those who survive this early period, 30% eventually do succumb to infection and another 30% die because the transplanted lung deteriorates. This condition—technically called *obliterative bronchiolitis (OB)* or *bronchiolitis obliterans syndrome (BOS)*—involves a generalized, progressive obstructive airway dysfunction. We do not know why this happens, but it eventually occurs—although not always fatally—in about one-half of all lung transplant patients. This condition can appear as early as the second postsurgery month but usually develops between 6 months and 2 years later, and is fatal to somewhere between one-third and one-half of the patients it happens to.

The *Good* News

Despite the relatively poor long-term prognosis for lung transplant recipients, it is very important to remember two things. One is that the very recent survival statistics are actually much better than the averages we just quoted from the overview in the 1995 survey, because the past 10 years have witnessed substantial improvement in early-period survival. The other is that a successful lung transplant results in major benefits, even if they do not last as long as we want them to. Patients experience improved physical capabilities, they feel healthier and reconnected with their lives and friends, and they feel a sense of value and daily purpose. Although we lack general statistics as to how the side effects of immunosuppression may modify the surgery's otherwise positive impact on quality of life, it is instructive to read Preston Golder's comments at the end of this chapter. Preston—an alpha$_1$-antitrypsin patient who underwent a successful lung transplant in February 1993—clearly speaks to the potential for a highly positive balance when all of these elements are put together.

And progress is on the horizon in several areas. Patients whose transplanted lung does not develop OB are being examined very carefully for clues, so that scientists can search for ways to create these same helpful conditions in all (or most) patients. Scientists are also working at full speed to find nondestructive—or substantially less destructive—ways to neutralize the body's natural rejection response. New drugs are in the wings. Particularly exciting is work at the Emory University School of Medicine in which scientists there have found a way to reprogram the transplant-directed immune response during the first few days after surgery. The immune system never "learns" during this critical period that the new organ lacks your molecular signature, so it remains fooled forever—and no immunosuppressive drugs are needed! Current experiments involve transplants in dogs, and it is only a question of time until this new technique will be adapted to people. And to improve infection control until we can narrow immunosuppressive action specifically to the rejection response, the search is on for methods to diagnose common infections *before* symptoms develop, so they can be treated before they are established.

This kind of progress in transplant acceptance may eventually permit animal lungs to be used. *Xenotransplantation*—the term for grafting an organ from one species to another—would make today's long waiting lists a thing of the past. The most likely animal source is the pig. Not only are its lungs the right size, but the epithelial tissues of humans and pigs—whether it is external (skin) or internal (lungs and digestive tract)—are very similar.

Another type of good news is the Second Wind Lung Transplant Association, the patient support and advocacy organization for patients—and their family/friends/significant others—at all stages in this process: considering undergoing a lung transplant procedure, preparing for one, recovering from it, and living with a lung transplant in the long term. They provide information and education, local support groups, organized activities, and helpful products. The organization also maintains a chatroom on-line that operates for regularly scheduled one-hour sessions.

Second Wind Lung Transplant Association
300 South Duncan Avenue, Suite 227
Clearwater, FL 33755-6457
888-222-2690 or 727-442-0892
secondwind@netzero.net; www.2ndWind.org

Lung Volume Reduction Surgery

Until quite recently, lung transplantation was the sole—and not very reliable—hope for emphysema patients who had progressed to the final stage of their disease. Happily, Dr. Joel Cooper then turned his efforts to an intriguing surgical procedure called *lung volume reduction,* (LVRS) which involves removing 20–30% of the lungs. Despite the high mortality when Dr. Otto Branigan had introduced it in the 1950s, there were highly positive aspects that Dr. Cooper found extremely encouraging—and he went to work to iron out the problems. His initial success was reported in 1995, and since then he has continued to refine his technique.

Although still officially considered "experimental," Dr. Cooper has provided a viable—and perhaps preferable—surgical alternative for selected COPD patients. It is especially appropriate for older people whose age alone would exclude them from a lung transplant.

Ironically, Dr. Cooper's early highly favorable results created problems of another kind. Because a large pool of emphysema patients—about 2 million Americans—potentially stood to benefit from this procedure, there was a tendency for surgeons (not all of them qualified) to rush into performing it before enough patients had been followed long enough to document long-term advantages and disadvantages. An outcry for caution by some segments of the health care community, including the Agency for Health Care Policy and Research, led Medicare to deny reimbursement for the procedure. In response, the Health Care Financing Administration—the bureaucracy governing Medicare—joined with the National Heart, Lung, and Blood Institute (NHLBI) of the National Institutes of Health to fund a long-term multicenter (see Appendix) trial, which is now in progress, to assess the value of this new procedure. Although the trial is not yet finished, enough interim information has become available to give us confidence that lung volume reduction will be medically accepted as an effective intervention in end-stage emphysema. (See comments and criticisms concerning aspects of this national trial in Chapter 21.)

Current Observations on Effectiveness

Everything published so far indicates overwhelmingly that it works. But how well it works, for how long, and for how many people are still open questions. The current perspective on LVRS was excellently summed up by Richard Casaburi, M.D., Ph.D.—president of the Pulmonary Education and Research Foundation (PERF)—in PERF's April 2000 *Second Wind* newsletter.

How long do the benefits last? This is really the $64,000 question. If lung function declined to pre-surgery levels in, say, one year, we would likely judge the surgery to be not worth the risk and expense. If, on the other hand, benefits last 7 or 10 years, the procedure would be an unequivocal success. The true answer appears to lie somewhere in between. A recent small study demonstrated that, 4 years after surgery, 25% of the patients retained appreciable improvements over pre-surgery lung function.

Is survival improved? Again, no clear answer. A recent indirect analysis indicated that a modest survival benefit might be obtained by those undergoing LVRS.

Does the need for supplemental oxygen decrease? Many of us were surprised by early reports showing that the majority of oxygen-dependent patients no longer required oxygen (or required it only during exercise) after LVRS. What is now clear is that, for the majority of patients, this is only a temporary reprieve; within two years or so the majority will need supplemental oxygen again.

It is my educated guess that, eventually, LVRS will be proven to be an effective palliative measure for a select group of patients.

In any case, statistics don't convey patients' observations on the personal impact of this surgery. The great proportion of people who have undergone this procedure, for example, report a much diminished sense of breathlessness and a dramatically improved quality of life. Because research statistics tend to be extremely impersonal, at the end of this chapter we have included Barbara Allen's typical account of the powerful changes in her life before and after.

We still must keep in mind that the newness of this procedure—having come into use only in 1995—makes it impossible at this point to have any *long-term* effectiveness data. Although there is certainly no reason to anticipate surgery-related problems cropping up down the road, we need additional time before we can officially document the state of affairs 6 or 7 years down the line. And although we know what constitutes the ideal patient, we don't yet know how far we can deviate from this profile and still anticipate good results. All of this will emerge over time.

The large, long-term NIH study will also clarify the full range of benefits because it differs in two important ways from the typical small evaluations that currently make up the literature. Because relatively few patients will be lost to follow-up, we can be confident that the results reflect the range of possible outcomes instead of just those patients who cooperate and stay in touch. And the NIH data will be presented in much greater detail, giving the range of individual responses rather than just data averages—which can hide negative outcomes. (For example, if 10 patients improve by 100% and 10 patients don't improve at all, the average implies that all patients improved by about 50%.)

But balanced against these uncertainties—in addition to the persuasive data already published and the numerous personal testimonials we have heard—lung volume reduction makes basic physiologic good sense.

Lung Volume Reduction Gives You Room to Breathe

Starting with a summary of Chapter 2's explanation of what happens to the lungs in emphysema will make this explanation very clear. Gradual destruction of more and more of the tiny, stretchy, resilient air sac walls increasingly robs the lungs of elasticity, and thus the power and pressure that elastic recoil normally generates to move a healthy amount of air in and out of the lungs. Not enough stale air is pushed out of the lungs, and the general flow of air in and out of the airways encounters a lot more resistance. These two airflow barriers substantially limit the amount of air you are able to exhale, leaving your lungs constantly hyperinflated. This continuous hyperinflation puts your chest wall and respiratory muscles—the respiratory machinery—at a profound mechanical disadvantage, which adds a lot to the muscular work of breathing. Because muscle work requires oxygen, this greater effort uses up a lot more oxygen—which you really don't have to spare.

Exertion magnifies all of this. You breathe faster, which shortens expiration times and retains even more stale air in your lungs, leading to greater hyperinflation and thus leading to lungs with very little room for more expansion. Because expansion is what pulls fresh air in, little expansion means even less fresh air than usual (when you need even more), and much of what little does enter the airways is blocked by the volumes of stale air trapped in the air sacs.

And there are additional respiratory stresses during exercise. Dead space ventilation increases, leading to an even smaller proportion of useful ventilation, which interferes with normal gas exchange and creates even higher carbon dioxide and lower oxygen levels. Blood moving through pulmonary vessels encounters more resistance than usual. And this entire list of dysfunctional elements each contributes to reducing the amount of oxygen delivered to muscles throughout the body, leading to early lactic acid production. A consequence of inadequate oxygen for the muscles—intensified by the rising lactic acid levels—is the unbearable sensation of being suffocatingly short of breath during exercise. So emphysema patients feel they have reached their maximum physical limit despite the capacity to go a lot further—and quit before they need to.

What does lung volume reduction surgery accomplish by removing dysfunctional tissue that amounts to 20% to 30% of the lungs? The consequences benefit the lungs, the cardiovascular system, and the respiratory muscles.

In the lungs, getting rid of this amount of stretched out, hyperinflated, dysfunctional lung tissue basically gives the remaining—and healthier—lung tissue room to breathe. After surgery, lung function tests show that a significant amount of vital capacity has been regained. The major result is improved elastic recoil, leading to better expiratory pressure as well as less airway resistance overall, leading to less hyperinflation and airways that remain open, leading to still more effective expiration, less air trapped, and further reduction of hyperinflation. In addition, removing highly overstretched lung tissue permits healthy alveoli that were compressed by this diseased tissue and by hyperinflation to reinflate, leading to better ventilation and improved gas exchange throughout the remaining lung.

In the cardiovascular system, the right side of the heart—the side that pumps blood through the lungs—works with greater efficiency because the blood is flowing far more easily. The better elastic recoil has helped blood vessels outside the alveoli expand, and capillaries that had been compressed within crushed—and now reopened—alveoli permit blood to flow through them once again. And all of this means that the right side of the heart is not working as hard.

The smaller area now occupied by the lungs allows the respiratory muscles—the diaphragm and the muscles between the ribs—to return to a longer, more effective resting length much closer to their normal configuration. Because they don't have to work as hard as they had been, they use much less oxygen.

All of the various benefits combine to improve exercise capacity. Testing a patient at the same level of effort he or she reached before surgery shows that airflow is clearly improved, hyperinflation is minimized, and the respiratory rate is slower, so significantly more air is taken in on each breath. And perhaps even more importantly, dyspnea—that unbearable, suffocating sense of breathlessness—is dramatically minimized. Because this allows patients to be far more active again, a major potential benefit is that patients who want to can exercise and improve their cardiovascular aerobic fitness and overall muscle strength. Once arm and leg muscles can do far more work using a great deal less oxygen, the heart doesn't have to work nearly as hard to supply them with the fuel they need. And greater aerobic fitness lessens dyspnea even further. One of the studies attempting to quantify this improvement in the laboratory found that by 3 months after lung reduction surgery, exercising patients' thigh muscles had increased significantly in bulk and they also improved substantially in the 6-minute walk test.

Who Will Benefit from This Surgery?

Although it is clear that lung reduction is not for everyone, for the time being what defines the *right* patient continues to become more flexible. Reacting to this temporary lack of full clarity and the new and still-evolving nature of the procedure itself, surgeons for now tend to be fairly conservative in selecting patients. (As the procedure becomes more routine, and as both surgical techniques and postoperative care improve, the envelope will be pushed to admit sicker and sicker patients.) Although different hospitals and surgeons currently have somewhat differing criteria for selecting/excluding patients, there are common factors (listed in Table 19.2).

Patients meeting all of these criteria then have a CAT scan. The CAT scan of an appropriate candidate will reveal (1) a combination of diseased and healthy lung areas (called *heterogeneous* as opposed to *homogeneous emphysema*) that are (2) distributed so that a large enough amount of diseased tissue can be removed without sacrificing healthy lung tissue. Most often, diseased tissue is removed from both sides of the lungs. The occasional patient with disease predominantly in one lobe, or with some unusual limiting anatomical factor, will be given a single-sided reduction.

Preparing for Surgery: Pulmonary Rehabilitation—Round 1

Being approved for lung volume reduction surgery is *not* the final presurgical step. Now—to maximize your potential for a smooth recovery and the greatest gain from your upcoming surgery—you have to get into shape through participation in a pulmonary rehabilitation program. A lot of readers will be puzzled at this point: rehabilitation has such an obvious and essential role after surgery, but why do it now—when what you need is the surgery, and you're going to do pulmonary rehab afterward anyway? Even though the presurgical state of your lungs seriously limits what pulmonary rehabilitation will achieve, much less than it will after surgery, there is still *significant* progress to be made. *And that progress will greatly improve your surgical outcome.* It's a basic surgical fact that the less debilitated you are when surgery—any surgery—takes place, the better you will respond and the less the likelihood of complications both in the operating room and during the recovery period. So every lung volume reduction program has followed Dr. Cooper's lead and made presurgical pulmonary rehabilitation an *essential* requirement. (It's also helpful to remember that the more you gain during this preliminary rehab phase, the further ahead you will start rehab after surgery.)

Although individual program details differ, there is a general format. The 4 to 6 weeks before surgery involve supervised resistive and aerobic exercise Monday through Friday. (And during the entire program—as you will also find after surgery—optimal pulmonary hygiene is stressed.) During resistive exercises to strengthen the arms and legs, patients are on supplemental oxygen to keep their blood oxygen saturation above 90%. Arm endurance is improved with an upper body ergometer (like an exercise bicycle for the arms) for 5 to 10 minutes per session, ideally working to

Table 19.2   SELECTING PATIENTS FOR LUNG VOLUME REDUCTION SURGERY

Eligible

All of these factors must be present *to qualify* for surgery.

Abnormal test results show air flow limitation *and* air trapping:

    a. FEV_1 of only 15%–40% of normal shows severely limited air flow

    b. FRC or TLC more than 20% above normal suggests air trapping

    c. A difference of more than 15% between TLC measured in the plethysmograph vs. measured by gas dilution confirms air trapping

    d. X-ray evidence of severe emphysema shows substantial hyperinflation

Evidence of severe impairment despite optimal medical management

Impaired quality of life

Less than 75 years old

Abstains from smoking

Some centers add blood gas criteria: a carbon dioxide tension of 50 mmHg or less and an oxygen tension above 40 mmHg while breathing room air.

Ineligible

Any one of these factors *disqualifies* a patient.

Has continued smoking

Pulmonary function too impaired to withstand surgery:

    a. FEV_1 is less than 15% of normal

    b. PO_2 is less than 40 mmHg when breathing room air

    c. CO_2 is higher than 50 mmHg

Some form of severe cardiovascular disease exists:

    a. advanced coronary artery disease

    b. pulmonary hypertension (pressure greater than 50 mmHg)

Severe debilitation, with total body weight less than 70% of ideal

Any pulmonary disease expected to limit survival

Psychosocial dysfunction

maintain your heart rate at 75–85% of the maximum predicted for your age. A general endurance program is mapped out based on how far you can walk in 6 minutes on your very first day. If you completed more than 500 feet, you will start treadmill walking right away. Your initial speed will be slow enough so that you can walk for 30 minutes and still keep your oxygen saturation above 90% (with supplemental oxygen at 6–8 liters/min). As you become more fit, treadmill speed and/or inclination are gradually increased to push your exercising heart rate into the same range that we described for upper body ergometer work. If you walked less than 500 feet during your initial test, you begin on an exercise bicycle with a goal of 30 minutes of continuous cycling. You switch to the treadmill after 7 to 10 days, working in the sequence described above. And when you have achieved the fitness goals established by the specialists guiding and monitoring you, surgery is scheduled.

The Surgery

During surgery, you will be on a respirator and your cardiac function will be monitored very closely. Of the several techniques for gaining access to the lungs, the traditional—and more invasive—approaches involve either splitting open the breast bone or, more rarely, cutting between two ribs. The choice depends on the individual patient. For a patient with an abnormal breast bone, for example, entering between the ribs would be preferable. A newer, less invasive technique is based on video-assisted thoracoscopic surgery—or VATS for short—in which entry is through a minimal incision and the lung is viewed on a TV screen via a fiberoptically transmitted image. Although VATS seems physically less traumatic because it is less invasive, splitting the breast bone gives the surgeon better visibility and the more invasive approaches are used more often because of this. Yet comparing results indicates no substantial differences in outcome between these different approaches.

After surgical entry—by whichever technique—the diseased lung tissue slated for removal is cut away with a scalpel. Until special tools were developed, this step was where the problems began. When a portion of the lung has been cut, sealing that open border is extremely difficult under the best of circumstances. Imagine slicing a very soft and flexible sponge and then trying to seal off completely all of the myriad and minuscule nooks and crannies. And in emphysema even the healthier lung tissue has become tissue-papery, and the diminished elasticity interferes with retracting around the surgical staples used to bind the cut edges. Before a special sealant material was developed, the tiny holes usually remaining around many of the staples allowed air to leak out and the lungs could not reinflate. What made lung reduction possible in emphysema patients was the innovative use of membrane sections taken from cows (*bovine pericardial strips*) to seal these staple holes. Despite this, however, air leaks develop in some patients—and this accounts for the majority of postsurgical complications (see Table 19.3).

Table 19.3 COMPLICATIONS THAT CAN FOLLOW LUNG VOLUME REDUCTION SURGERY, FROM MOST TO LEAST COMMON

Air leak lasting from 7 to 14 days

Air leak lasting more than 14 days

Cardiac arrhythmia

Temporary neurological effects

Need to be intubated for short-term respirator support

Pneumonia

Gastrointestinal disturbances

Need tracheostomy for extended respirator support

Infection

Surgical wound healing problems

A more experimental technique—intended to reduce complications—has been used by a small number of surgeons. They use VATS to reach the lungs and then a laser to slice off the diseased tissue. The laser creates an unusually clean cut with much less bleeding than a scalpel can achieve. Despite the rationale behind it, as presently performed VATS plus laser is not nearly as effective as use of the traditional scalpel.

Who Should Perform This Surgery

At the writing of this book—5 years after the reintroduction of the procedure—it is still considered experimental, and thus only a relatively few medical centers are performing it. Once the NIH study is completed and published and lung reduction surgery becomes established, though, the estimated 50,000–100,000 patients a year who will be approved candidates will transform it into a lucrative and widespread procedure. The question then will be—how to choose where to go for this surgery?

This decision involves several factors. In choosing your hospital and the pulmonary surgeon there who will do it, the *most* important criterion is *experience*—having already done this procedure on a large number of patients. As with any complex skill, the more often a hospital and surgeon perform a procedure, the better they get at the procedure itself and the fewer the postsurgical complications. (As an example, after a large New York City hospital first introduced lung reduction surgery a few years ago, the mortality rate for their first 50 patients was about 12%. For the next 50 patients, it was down to 2%.)

Next come the advantages offered by a larger hospital, whether university-affiliated or a municipal hospital center. Lung reduction surgery requires intensive rehabilitation both before and after surgery, and larger medical facilities tend to be better staffed and equipped to provide this. And—as with other complex surgeries—because larger centers will be doing this procedure much more frequently than their smaller counterparts, they will often be willing to accept the marginal or potentially riskier patients that hospitals with less experience and support will automatically reject.

But if choosing a large medical center means leaving friends, family, and home behind, the choice may not be so clear-cut. The factors mentioned in the last paragraph must be weighed against the equally important benefits that come from this kind of support. There is also the reality that community hospitals often—though not always—provide more personal and responsive pre- and postsurgical care than large hospitals do. And data from a high-level community hospital in central Massachusetts suggest that—at a *good* local hospital—this kind of surgery can be performed as safely, and with similar outcomes, as in larger institutions.

What Happens After Surgery: Recovery Plus Pulmonary Rehabilitation—Round 2

The 72 hours immediately after you leave the operating room are as important as the surgery itself. Assuming that all went well in the OR, you will most likely be breathing on your own. But remember that you went in with bad lungs, so don't be distressed or apprehensive if you wake up and discover that you are still attached to equipment helping you to breathe. This is not unusual, nor is it unusual to need some kind of assisted ventilation for several days. As with a great many types of surgery, there are any number of very temporary pulmonary inefficiencies that require an equally temporary assist to the lungs to maintain enough oxygen in the blood. And don't be apprehensive if you find yourself in the ICU for a few days before going to a regular room. Some patients need that extra care and monitoring right after surgery.

Whether you are in the ICU, a step-down unit (a temporary special-care room that falls between the ICU and a regular room), or a regular room, you will have several slender tubes coming out of your chest for at least the first 2 to 3 postsurgery days. They allow blood to drain, and they permit control of air pressure to restore the vacuum between your chest wall and lungs—temporarily disturbed when your chest wall and lungs were cut—that keeps your lungs inflated. If any air leaks resulted from the surgery, which is not uncommon, you may need these tubes for 1 to 2 weeks.

Pulmonary rehabilitation begins as soon as possible. This is geared to retraining your out-of-shape respiratory muscles and continuing the overall fitness training that you began preoperatively. (Some centers start patients on upper arm ergometry even while they are in the ICU.) In most cases, your physical therapist will have you up and walking the day after your surgery and will put you on an exercise bicycle—perhaps in your room—three days afterward. Your activities will expand in a program designed specifically for you, and continue until you leave the hospital.

Then you will probably enroll in a supervised outpatient physical therapy program for 1 to 2 months. This is a critical period for maximizing the potential of your lung volume reduction surgery. Quite simply, it is in your profound interest to continue exercising. At this point, you are still severely limited by the effects that your years of debilitating inactivity have had on your muscles and heart. The only way to get your heart and muscles to the point where they—and you—can take advantage of the substantial capabilities your lungs have regained is to continue exercising!! We cannot emphasize this strongly enough.

Continuing your exercise program once you are on your own is extremely hard for many people—the hardest part of the entire experience. *If the pulmonary and rehab staff have done their job, you will be taking home the clear message that exercise will be a central part of the rest of your life.*

In Their Own Words . . .

Preston Golder, who underwent a *lung transplant* 5 years before this interview, at age 48, was working as a bus driver for Santa Clara County in California when he was diagnosed with alpha$_1$-antitrypsin emphysema at age 43. He had consulted a doctor only because his co-workers had begun pointing out that the short walk across the bus yard would leave him breathless. He deteriorated rapidly, even for alpha$_1$-antitrypsin emphysema, and within 3 years was dependent on a wheelchair and oxygen. Not quite 2 years later he became a lung transplant candidate, and luckily he waited only 4 months for a lung to become available.

I was transplanted in February 1993 at Columbia-Presbyterian Hospital in New York City. I moved back to New York for my surgery because that's where I grew up, and my family and most of my friends—my support system—are there. The period after surgery was not easy. *Everything* hurt—even my mouth—and my eyes burned. My electrolytes were completely unbalanced. The equilibrium I had achieved with my lousy lungs was suddenly gone, and my body and I had to learn to live with my healthy new lungs! My leg muscles were so debilitated after 2 years in a wheelchair that I had to learn to walk again. And I had to learn to breathe again! When you have severe lung disease, you learn to get the maximum out of each breath. By the time you get your new lungs it's become your natural way of breathing—but now you're really overbreathing, and you tend to hyperventilate. Until I learned to control this, I would wake up in the middle of the night with panic attacks. But once I readjusted, for the most part I've lived a fairly normal life since the transplant.

The negative side has been that the medication [immunosuppressive medication—which forms part of the approximately 60 pills Preston must take every day] gives me severe migraines several times a month, occasionally so bad that I have to be hospitalized for painkilling medication. Because the immunosuppressive medication weakens my immune system, I can't fight off ordinary infections the way most people can. Some people on these drugs are real fanatics about protecting themselves from infections. In general I don't make a big a deal about it, but I learned the hard way—after getting sick three times—that I *do* have to be careful when I fly. Because planes usually recirculate stale air, which includes the germs breathed out by anyone who has a cold or flu, it's easy to catch something even if you have a normal immune system. And even worse for me, each time I got sick my immune system was stimulated enough to start rejecting my lungs. I was hospitalized for 2 weeks at a clip, and the drugs that saved my life also made me so sick while I was on them that I wished—briefly—I had died instead of being transplanted! Now I wear a hospital face mask when I fly. I get some strange looks—but I don't get sick! [Preston is also experiencing liver and kidney problems, side effects from the medications he has been on both before and after his transplant.] You've got to take the medications to stay alive, but they do damage. It's a trade-off.

But for those like me, there's no other alternative. After the transplant, the doctors told me that without it, I had had a week, maybe two, left to live. And now—I can *breathe* again! I can *run* up a flight of stairs again—and not even get winded! I would do it again without a doubt. You do trade one set of problems for another, but with healthy lungs and a positive outlook—you really can live a relatively normal life!

Barbara Allen underwent *lung volume reduction* surgery at age 42, not quite 2 years before this interview. She had been deteriorating steadily since her diagnosis with alpha$_1$-antitrypsin emphysema about 6 years earlier. Chronic esophageal reflux made eating a miserable experience, and she had dropped from 130 pounds to 98. She had become wheelchair-bound, and needed oxygen during exercise, whenever she would have an asthma attack, and when the air was bad. Cooking even the simplest meal was a major effort. Always a very active woman, playing golf, horseback riding, running around with her nieces and nephews, skiing and snow-mobiling with them, now these supreme pleasures—among many others—were only fading memories. Just being outside was more than her lungs could handle. Barbara was basically confined to the house, and waged a major battle—with family support—against depression, a significant problem for many advanced COPD patients.

I was being evaluated for a lung transplant at Columbia-Presbyterian Hospital. To my surprise, the doctors told me I might actually be a candidate for lung *reduction* because—unlike the typical alpha$_1$-antitrypsin patient, whose diseased lung tissue is usually spread all over the place—I actually had large sections of healthy lung at the top of each lobe. I decided to try lung reduction because, at that point, I didn't think anything could be worse than what I was already going through! [Barbara knows that because her emphysema is caused by an alpha$_1$-antitrypsin deficiency, she will need a lung transplant at some undetermined point in the future.]

So I went into a rehabilitation program before the surgery, and did my exercises at home on the off days. And I began to feel better just from that! It really strengthened me for surgery, and I think that had a lot to do with how well it went. I started rehab after surgery as soon as I could, and now I keep it up at home. It's the only time now that I still use oxygen. I have a treadmill in my living room that I use for anywhere from half an hour to a full hour every other day. On the alternate days I ride my exercise bicycle for half an hour. I also lift weights to strengthen my arms. When I go to South Carolina for the month of March to avoid the bad weather here in New York, I do aerobics to keep up my exercise. I still don't have quite one-fourth of a normal lung capacity, so if I miss even a few days I feel the difference right away. I was recently in Aruba for a week, with no treadmill—and no aerobics—and when I got back home, I could not go right back to my usual 2 mph pace!

One of my greatest joys since surgery has been *eating*! Reflux had been so awful for so many years—and after surgery it was gone. The very next day, I began eating real food for the first time in *years*! I can walk around the block now without stopping 100 times! I'm back out horseback riding—even when the wind is so strong it almost blows me off the horse! And I'm playing a little golf—not as well as years ago, but I'm *out* there! I can *walk* around a shopping mall instead of being pushed in a wheelchair! I can go to flea markets again! I've got my limitations, but I'm cooking again and doing other things at home I couldn't do for so long. I spend time in Aruba and South Carolina. I'm not running around with my nieces and nephews only because they're too old for that now! The surgery has given me back my life!

20

The Final Phase

The biological clock sooner or later runs out—even for the healthiest of us. People who must spend their waking moments confronting a disease that will never heal, and hopefully won't deteriorate too quickly, must be especially aware of that ticking in the background. Major issues arise for COPD patients—as for many others—when medicine and therapy can do no more. When the clock has run out, patients and their families need to know what these issues are, and have a sense about how they want to meet them.

Our society makes the inevitability of death very difficult to accept. The sadness of death's loss is human. The anguish we experience is much the mark of Western man. The Judeo-Christian foundation upon which our values and philosophy are built—including those that dominate the practice of medicine—regard death as our primary enemy rather than a natural, possibly desirable, transition. So when a patient at this transition point is in the hands of the medical establishment, he often becomes a battleground for the conflict between nature and the doctors caring for him. Patient and family become victims of this battle instead of getting the comfort and support they need.

This chapter is devoted to raising the problems and decisions you will eventually have to confront. Dealing with them effectively when the time comes means being prepared for them in advance. If your disease is still relatively mild, you may feel anxiety about reading this chapter now. Try to do it anyway. If you decide to postpone it, keep the book on an accessible shelf for that point when you will need it.

When Will That Point Be?

The Ninetieth Psalm advises that our clocks stop ticking at "three score and ten years, but if by reason of strength, they may be fourscore years."

Despite this ancient assurance, we can't predict anyone's life expectancy—healthy or not.

But your doctor can form a general impression about your COPD's rate of progression. His evaluation can help you make decisions about how you want to lead your life.

Of the many factors entering this equation, the two most important are the age at which your COPD was first diagnosed, and your FEV_1 (the volume of air you can blow forcefully out of your lungs in one second, described in Chapter 6) in relation to your age. Relative youth at diagnosis and a smaller FEV_1 both reflect a faster progressing disease.

Whatever the rate, most patients eventually reach the point where their remaining lung function isn't enough to maintain a good quality of life without using supplemental oxygen. You *may* finally reach the point where your life can't be maintained without a ventilator. *This is the final stage our chapter concerns, when "life" cannot continue without extreme measures whose value is coming more and more into question.*

Final Stage Care Is Moving from Hospital to Home

In-Hospital Care Under Severe Economic Pressure

The institutional response to the dizzying rise in health care costs over the last several decades—exacerbated by the desire for profits by private health care providers—has been: "Cut, cut, cut!"

The only way hospitals can cut costs—and stay in business—is by cutting the services they provide. This means that many medical decisions are now based on economic criteria as much as sound medical reasons. Doctors must bow to the "bottom liners" of their hospital's administration.

Another consequence of this politically pressured "cost-effective" approach to our health care is the institution of Diagnosis Related Groups—DRGs—by Medicare and private medical insurance companies in the mid-1980s. Administrators determined statistically how many days of hospital care a particular diagnosis requires. The hospital is reimbursed only for that number of days, no matter what.

Each company has its own set of figures, but the principle is the same. Medicare's DRG 88, for example, rules that a hospitalized COPD patient needs 6.3 days of inpatient care. If a particular COPD patient is discharged in 3 days, or actually needs 2 weeks of care to remove him from danger, the hospital will be reimbursed for 6.3 days. So hospitals are financially rewarded for short patient stays, and penalized for long ones.

This system puts subtle but real pressure on doctors to discharge many patients earlier—possibly to their detriment—following a hospital admission than they would have before DRGs were instituted.

It's true that before the advent of DRGs, hospitals chronically unable to fill their beds were tempted to hold on to patients longer than necessary. This is wrong. But we fault the existing system for heavily favoring economic belt tightening over people's health needs.

Outpatient and Home Care Haven't Been Penalized

Third-party repayment for both outpatient medical services and home care—at least for now—is not limited by DRG-like rules. So economic feasibility—plus the ready availability of home oxygen, intravenous antibiotics, and nutritional support—have reestablished the patient's home as the primary health care arena for the final stages of COPD.

The Team   *Successful* home care, though, is not a simple affair. It requires a team approach based on the family's willingness to support the patient, and the patient's willingness to cooperate. A doctor prescribes home care services and coordinates the team.

A professional nurse assesses and monitors the patient, directly supervises the team, and calls in other members when needed. These other members can be: a home health aide to help the patient with personal care; a homemaker to take care of housekeeping, food shopping, and meals; a physical therapist to do postural drainage, range-of-motion, and conditioning exercises. A respiratory therapist is sometimes used to help with mucus clearance, and instruction in using and cleaning respiratory support equipment. (Respiratory therapy is typically provided by the patient's DME dealer.) A social worker offers supportive counseling for both patient and family (see the discussion below), and is also a link with community support serves (for example, Meals on Wheels, transportation services, friendly visitor programs). The home health aide and the homemaker might be needed on a full-time basis. The others set up an appropriate schedule for visits.

Where you can turn for home care services depends on your community. Available agencies may include a branch of the Visiting Nurses Association, a public health nursing department, a hospital-based home care department, and/or private or nonprofit home health agencies. The National Association for Home Care—the organization of home health care agencies—is a valuable resource. They are located at 228 Seventh Street, Washington, DC 20002; 202-547-7424. Their pamphlet "How to Choose a Home Care Provider: A Consumer's Guide" contains a comprehensive education in a nutshell: what services are available, who provides them, how to locate, how to choose, how they bill, who pays, how to handle problems, what your rights are, etc. It also contains a list by state of all relevant government agencies with phone numbers. Their well-designed and helpful website (*www.nahc.org*) not only contains both highlight and full text versions of this pamphlet, but a detailed listing of hospice and home care agencies by city/state or zip code. If you still have difficulty finding or choosing a comprehensive home health provider agency, your hospital's Social Services Department and/or discharge planner should be able to help.

Respiratory Support Last but not least, respiratory support involves the necessary equipment and whatever arrangements are needed for servicing, oxygen delivery, and so on.

Mechanical ventilation for advanced COPD patients at home fills two different patient needs. Less frequent are the patients who can no longer breathe on their own. Reliable battery-powered ventilators make home care feasible for them, and even allow them some mobility.

The greatest number of patients benefit from just short periods of mechanical help. For some, this means temporary reliance on a respirator during a respiratory infection. Others need to give their exhausted respiratory muscles a periodic rest from the overwhelming effort their deteriorating respiratory system and oxygen level require. The idea is that periodic rests permit these muscles to recoup some strength.

A recent study of this kind of respirator use found an increase in respiratory muscle strength and exercise capacity, fewer and shorter hospital stays, and lower carbon dioxide levels. Although other studies have not been as positive, more work is needed for reliable results. The number of patients in all these studies was too small to draw strong conclusions from them.

When Death Is Finally Imminent

Even with the best treatment, death is inevitable. Unfortunately, Western civilization's view of death as an abomination often makes dying and death more difficult to deal with than need be for both patient and family. And when the patient is comatose, the family bears the most difficult burden. Beginning to recognize this, some hospital and religious organizations now offer home counseling to help patients and families approach death with more understanding and less anguish.

For the family, counseling educates them as to the stages the patient will go through as death occurs, how to know that death has actually occurred, and avoiding a last-minute panic that would subject the patient to "heroic measures"—intubation and mechanical ventilation—that would needlessly prolong his terminal state.

Many patients approaching death are terrified that they will experience agonizing suffocation as they struggle hopelessly to breathe. A counselor educates them, too, about the stages they will go through, which we describe in the next paragraph. Knowing the truth usually permits them to approach their death with a great deal of tranquility.

Death Without Medical Intervention

Without medical intervention (at home or in the hospital), the patient slips into a semistuporous state as his carbon dioxide level continues rising. At high carbon dioxide levels, his dyspnea becomes mild or completely disappears. He is resting comfortably at that point. Some patients periodically wake from this semiconscious state feeling refreshed. (Inexplicably, these episodes of recovery may recur over months or years before death actually occurs. Perhaps the mechanism for these temporary recovery periods involves the total muscular relaxation the carbon dioxide buildup produces.) Eventually this comfortable semistuporous state becomes continuous. Then the patient lapses into a coma. Death gently occurs when his oxygen level drops too low to sustain him even at this level any longer.

Death With Medical Intervention

Respirators, pacemakers, hemodialyzers, extracorporeal oxygenators—they can keep the patient's body alive well beyond the time his biological clock has stopped ticking. This use of hospital technology extends *physiological life*. Our Judeo-Christian heritage trains us—without our realizing it—to view death as our ultimate enemy. The medical community has taken this concept to its furthest extreme. The strong inclination among many doctors—and supported by many patients and families—is to prolong physiological life whenever possible, no matter how temporarily death is delayed.

There can be no argument against giving a patient additional years, or even months, of useful life. There are patients who can enjoy a happy and productive life—however long or short—tethered to their life-support systems. An example is one of the most brilliant minds of our time, Stephen Hawking, an acclaimed astrophysicist/philosopher and bestselling author. A crippling neurological disease paralyzed his respiratory muscles. Another is Baseball Hall of Famer Roy Campanella, the Brooklyn Dodgers' former star catcher, who broke his neck in an automobile accident and lived many years, at home, on a respirator. The actor Christopher Reeve—who has depended on a respirator ever since he broke his neck in a riding accident—leads an active life that includes advocacy for people with spinal cord injuries.

The question of appropriateness arises when death is delayed only at the cost of great suffering to the patient and his family. When life can only be sustained with massive technological intervention, the patient's medical care team and his family—and the patient, too, if he is conscious and competent—are faced with the critical questions: *When, if ever, is death preferable to a life of suffering? If it is, how is the issue to be resolved?*

Euthanasia

These questions address the concept of *euthanasia*. This exotic-sounding word comes from the ancient Greek roots *eu*, meaning "well," and *thanatos*, meaning "death." A faithful translation is "the good or gentle death." Today it is popularly translated as "mercy killing."

There are two types—or levels—of euthanasia. *Active euthanasia* involves committing an act to bring on death sooner than it would otherwise occur. *Passive euthanasia* is deciding to omit or end medical treatment that would prolong life.

Active Euthanasia

Active euthanasia is against the law in all "civilized" countries. But it is practiced openly in Holland, and secretly in the United States. Although the Dutch court punishes euthanasia with 12 years in prison, doctors who can meet "conflict of duty" criteria are not found guilty. "Conflict of duty" occurs when a patient's wish to die is deemed medically justifiable—"physical or mental pain is severe and without hope of relief"—and so outweighs any attempt to prolong his life.

The situation must meet these "conflict of duty" conditions: (1) Of his own free will, the patient clearly requested on several occasions to be killed. (2) All other options had either been unsuccessful, or refused by the patient. (3) The doctor consulted with another physician and kept a written record of their meeting.

This system has seemed to work in Holland. It is a country where society is more homogeneous than ours, everyone gets the same quality of medical care, and doctors have treated their patients for many years. Recently, a law allowing medically-assisted suicide was proposed in Holland to bring the law and medical practice into line with each other. As this book went to press, the Dutch government was on the verge of passing this law and making history.

Whether this kind of legalization can work here—in a melting-pot society with its many cultural and religious crosscurrents—is debatable. Change—if it comes—will start at the state level. Currently, California, Washington, Florida, and Hawaii are considering ways to legalize active euthanasia. In 1998, Oregon passed a law sanctioning a form of active euthanasia and in the first year 15 people took advantage of it. In response, the U.S. House of Representatives passed a measure that effectively blocks the Oregon statute.

Passive Euthanasia

A far more compelling issue is withholding or stopping life-sustaining therapy for a terminally ill patient. As long as it does not cause great suffering, passive euthanasia is much easier to contemplate—and carry out—because it does not involve killing another human being. It is finding increasing acceptance within the medical community.

In a recent poll of roughly 2,000 Colorado physicians, about one-half felt passive euthanasia was justified for some of their patients. And the American Medical Association found that 80% of their physicians favor passive euthanasia.

But even though the *concept* makes deep humane sense to many of us, there is still the problem of deciding when it should be applied. Dr. Gary L. Huber expressed the problem facing the family and physician of terminally ill patients in his introduction to a moving collection of editorials written in 1979 by four renowned pulmonary doctors. (The collection, "To Live and To Die," appeared in the *Archives of Internal Medicine*, vol. 139, pp. 916–921.) Dr. Gruber said:

> Perhaps medical technology has advanced more rapidly than . . . our capacity to employ it judiciously. Precisely the same mechanical devices and drugs that are used to manage respiratory failure can also be employed to maintain a state of *intolerable suffering from physical pain or mental anguish, beyond reasonable hope for recovery of normal human function* [emphasis is ours]. In other words, an indiscriminate application of technical and pharmacologic means to preserve a failing organ system may lose the perspective of quality of preservation of the patient as a whole human being.

The remaining discussion on passive euthanasia is based largely on these four eloquent editorials written by doctors who are confronted daily with these life-and-death decisions. Although written for other doctors, these soul-searching pieces clearly express the same spectrum of concerns and viewpoints that arise when patients and their families discuss passive euthanasia. And because they are couched in simple language, we have quoted them instead of putting them into our own words. (We have omitted the viewpoints of lawyers, medical ethicists, and the clergy because they tend to grapple with these issues in the abstract rather than from the bedside.)

The process of deciding how you want to respond to the reality of your imminent death applies equally to you and your family. You may want your family to make the decision with you. It may well be your family who must decide for you whether to continue or disconnect life support systems. Consequently, we indicate in italics where comments are applicable to family as well as patient.

In the Words of Dr. John J. Skillman

John J. Skillman, M.D., is with the Departments of Surgery at Harvard Medical School, and at Beth Israel Medical Center, both in Boston, Massachusetts. He is concerned about knowing when it is appropriate to let a patient die, and honoring one's duty in those circumstances with love and support.

Life begins at birth and extends in a continuum to death; or does it? Is there a point when it may be said that death is beginning? . . . There is a point when almost every physician and nurse of experience can say to himself or herself that the patient is beginning to die. . . .

The seriously ill patient with chronic lung disease represents an extremely difficult problem. As time goes on and the lung disease progresses, the patient's ability to ventilate himself without the aid of a machine nears an end. For such patients, the chronic lung disease has entered a terminal phase and the point of beginning death has been reached. They will require endotracheal intubation and artificial ventilation.

Even though the ventilator can be gradually removed, while keeping the patient comfortable with medication for pain and air hunger, the physician [*family*] may be unable to make this decision. What should be done now? Certainly the patient's wishes about discontinuation of therapy should be honored, even if they are different from wishes of the family. . . .

What is our obligation in such cases? I suggest it is one of caring for the human being in the broadest sense, not in a restricted or mechanical way. The physician [*family*] should learn to handle his guilt and frustration to avoid a withdrawal of emotional support and a dehumanization of the patient. I believe we need to use all of our love and human sensitivity to do the best that we can for these patients. Sometimes the very best we can do is avoid prolonging death by continuing treatments that may lead to a cruel, slow, and painful death. . . . When such a terminal point has been reached, when the likelihood of getting back to the previous minimal, dismal existence, without respirator, has disappeared, I do not support the continuation of ventilation. . . .

In the Words of Dr. Franklin H. Epstein

Franklin H. Epstein, M.D., is also with Harvard Medical School (Department of Medicine) and Beth Israel Medical Center. He is concerned with undue pressures that can lead to letting a patient die prematurely. He discusses his concept of dignified death in this context, and reminds doctors (and family) how fallible they can be.

Talk about a "dignified death" usually comes from onlookers, not from the patient. Most patients want to live. They need to have some hope of forestalling the inevitable end, and they need to feel that their physician is helping to keep hope alive. Dignity lies in their fight for life and in their struggle to maintain contact with humanity. Kindness, personal attention, and good nursing help to preserve a patient's dignity.

Euthanasia for elderly people whose bodily functions and control are failing primarily relieves the distress of the relatives, not that of the patient. Our obligation to assuage the pain of our patients is sometimes discussed as if it involved an equal obligation to minimize suffering for relatives, friends, and onlookers. In fact, much of the "suffering" of terminally ill patients . . . exists only in the imagination of shocked relatives, who are sickened and frightened by unfamiliar procedures and apparatus. The physician must remember that he has only one client—the patient. He is the advocate of the patient, not the family, nor the welfare agency, nor the kindly clergyman, squeamish at the sight of tracheostomy. . . .

Physicians are fallible. Their wisdom tends to be greatly exaggerated by the popular press and, too often, by physicians themselves. Patients have an enormous need to feel that their physicians can prognosticate with great accuracy, but the kindest, best-intentioned physician is often wrong. Moreover, a physician's prognosis tends to be weighted toward pessimism, because patients who do badly claim most of his time and attention and remain in his memory longer than those who do well.

In the Words of Dr. Gerald L. Baum

Gerald L. Baum, M.D., is retired from the Chaim Sheba Medical Center in Tel Aviv, Israel. He echoes Dr. Epstein's sentiments in his editorial *L'Chaim!* ("To Life!").

I wish to express my fervent and passionate commitment to life and to whatever I must do to protect and prolong it. As a physician I have always considered this my ethical and moral obligation in all situations. When the case before me is one . . . of end-stage chronic pulmonary failure, I feel uncomfortable with my commitment, but I still must act to preserve life. I have always assumed that my judgement is fallible, very fallible, and if this is true in ordinary situations, then why should my judgement be more precise in life-and-death situations? If I must make a mistake, let it be in the direction of life and not in the opposite direction. . . .

What I plead for in the situation of respiratory failure is humility on the part of the physican [*family*]. We should accept that we really are only slightly wiser than the apes in regard to the science of living and dying, and that we know very little about quality of life or the balance between a life of terror or a death of peace. When making an irrevocable decision for someone else, our actions should be guided by a notion of our fallibility and a surge of humility. If one accepts this philosophy as a guide, then there should be a rule to follow when the way is unclear, when the decision is difficult, or when the emotional pressures are overwhelming. I offer as that rule: *L'Chaim!*

In the Words of Dr. Thomas L. Petty

Thomas L. Petty, M.D., is with the Division of Pulmonary Diseases at the University of Colorado Medical Center in Denver, Colorado. He is one of this country's leading proponents of pulmonary rehabilitation to help patients live their lives to the fullest. In this spirit he coauthored *Enjoying Life with Emphysema* for patients and their families. In "Don't Just Do Something—Stand There," Dr. Petty formulates the four basic questions that help him make the life-or-death decision.

(1) Do I know the patient's underlying disease process and its course and prognosis? (2) Do I know the patient's quality of life in the context of his disease process? (3) Do I have anything more to offer the patient by resuscitative efforts designed to gain more time? (4) Do I wish to gain more time through resuscitative efforts to resolve these other questions?

If the first two questions are answered "Yes" and the second two are "No," he concludes:

When the patient's life is known to be miserable at best, and when the patient has indicated no wish to have his suffering extended by technological means—in short, when there is nothing to be gained by the additional hours, days or weeks one might achieve by supporting respiration and circulation—then intervention such as tracheal intubation, mechanical assistance, and cardiopulmonary support should be set aside. . . .

Central to the issue of passive euthanasia is the notion of quality of life.

Those who favor it assume that they are able to judge for the patient what is an acceptable quality, those who are against it feel that they cannot make that judgement for another. It appears obvious that only the patient can judge what is acceptable to him. The patient, therefore, should have the primary responsibility for making such a decision.

Dr. Petty revisited his 1979 editorial in *Chronic Obstructive Pulmonary Disease: Current Concepts*, a professional book he coedited in 1987. He modified question 4 and added question 5, both including the patient far more actively in the decision-making process. Question 4 became: "Do I wish for myself and on behalf of my patient to gain more time through resuscitative efforts to resolve these other questions?" Question 5: "Do I have a verbal or written contract with my patient about how I should handle situations when further medical care to sustain life is not appropriate?"

Deciding Your Fate

Hoping that others—your family, your doctor—will make the best decision for you at the crucial moment is asking them to grapple with an extraordinarily difficult issue under conditions of intense emotion and conflict. In the emergency room or intensive care unit, the instincts of the staff are to maintain life at all costs: you may be unconscious or unable to express yourself, your family may be emotionally distraught, and your physician typically is torn between the various ethical considerations imposed by his profession.

If the different parties disagree about what should be done, reaching a verdict takes time-consuming negotiations. Negotiation is often arbitrated by the hospital's ethics committee, where all parties express their feelings and the committee makes the final decision. *This is wrong. A committee should not—cannot—make this kind of decision.*

When a decision is needed, the outcome should be a matter of your personal conscience and morality. Some people find life an intolerable prison if they can do nothing—not even breathe—for themselves. Others find satisfactions that make these conditions acceptable. This personal judgment takes precedence over any ethical implications and legalities.

This Decision Is Your Legal Right

Fundamental legal principles uphold your right to make this decision privately with your doctor. The *U.S. Constitution*, for starters, guarantees your right to privacy. *Common law* guarantees your right to "bodily self-determination"—doing with your body as you see fit. Then there is the *principle of "informed consent,"* which gives you, the patient, the right to refuse or accept medical treatment once you understand its benefits and risks. (Remember the consent form you have to sign before surgery or special diagnostic procedures can legally be done?) Many medical ethics experts feel this right includes use of life-support systems, that the informed patient must be obeyed when he refuses—or requests—heroic measures to keep him alive. If how you live and how you die are to reflect your personal conscience and morality: *Don't leave the decision until the last moment. Make it in advance. Don't leave the decision up to someone else—especially a committee—if you can avoid it. It should be between you— or you and your family—and your doctor.*

If you are unsure, if you want someone to talk with who is without your family's emotions, without your doctor's possible professional bias, a counselor who helps patients come to terms with dying and death is the ideal person to help you reach an informed decision and communicate it to those who need to know.

Ideally, your decision should be in writing. And your doctor—whether you give him a written or verbal statement—should note it in your medical chart. But in the event that your doctor does not record your decision, it's wise to give a copy of your written statement to—or discuss it with—someone who will act for you in case your doctor is unavailable or you are unable to express yourself when that time comes. The person acting for you is called, in legal terms, your *surrogate*. In fact, some of those involved in the fight for patients' final rights advise patients to let *everyone*—children, spouse, doctor, friends—know about their decision, even if it's been written down in the "living will" we discuss in the next section. "It simply isn't enough to sign a living will," they counsel. "You have to go out of your way to be sure it's honored."

If you do not want to be kept alive on life support systems and you do not state this in writing, it's impossible to predict the hospital's response to your wishes stated verbally by your surrogate. If your doctor knows how you feel and accepts your decision, then it is highly likely that your wishes will prevail without difficulty. If your doctor prefers to keep you alive regardless of the circumstances, your surrogate may not be able to intervene with only a verbal statement. If your family is talking only with emergency room staff who have no prior history with you, the outcome can go either way.

The legalities can differ between states, and the unwritten rules can differ from one hospital to another and from doctor to doctor. If this aspect of your transition from life to death is important to you, then you need to learn in advance what you can expect from both your hospital and your doctor. The social work department in your hospital should be able to refer you to an appropriate person for this kind of discussion.

Living Will

Once you put your decision in writing, it becomes your *living will.* Such wills are now provided for by law in 38 states and the District of Columbia. The remaining states (except Michigan and South Dakota) have legal precedents that recognize this right.

Living will legislation states the patient's rights and the rules doctors must follow in carrying out their patients' wishes. **Caution:** Because not all states have written their legislation in the same language, one state's living will may not be accepted in another state. So if you make out a living will and then move to another state before the time has come to use it, find out whether you need to redo it or not. If you normally divide your year between homes in two different states, you may need two separate living wills.

If you want to make out a living will, your hospital's death and dying counseling service should be able to help you. If not, the organization *Choice in Dying* can supply you with information and documents at no cost. They provide the education—and the paperwork—needed to arrange for living wills, surrogate decisions, and so on; they publish a regular newsletter; and of course they have a website. Their National Office is at 1035 Thirtieth Street NW, Washington, DC 20007; phone: 202-338-9790; fax: 202-338-0242. Their Program Office is at 475 Riverside Drive, Room 1852, New York, NY 10115; phone: 212-870-2003; fax: 212-870-2040; *www.choices.org; cid@choices.org* for general inquiries; *services@choices.org* for membership and publications.

Health Care Power of Attorney

You can name a surrogate in your living will, but there is a stronger alternative. This alternative, which is recognized throughout the Untied States with the exception of the District of Columbia, is a *health care power of attorney.* "Power of attorney" means that the person you designate will have the legal authority to *make decisions for you* if you—at that time—cannot do so yourself. Executing a health care power of attorney protects you against the unforeseen: (1) the need for a decision arrives unexpectedly, yet you are unable to participate and you haven't yet written your living will; (2) you feel any meaningful decision must await the actual circumstances of that moment, yet you fear you may not be capable of a rational decision at that time.

The degree of decision-making power this position involves varies with the state. Twenty states currently permit a surrogate to issue the order ending or maintaining life-support treatment. But even in the weakest of cases, a health care power of attorney can't hurt, and might help.

For best protection, appoint two surrogates. Give each one the power to act alone. In case your primary surrogate is not available when the critical decisions have to be made, the designated alternate will be your stand-in.

A health care power of attorney should be drawn up by a lawyer, since it should be done to agree with your state's laws and court precedents.

Final Thoughts

Before ending this chapter, we want to put it into an appropriate perspective. We hope our attempt to deal honestly with the realities of COPD's final phase hasn't given you the notion that all COPD patients are at, or nearing, death's door. Over the last several decades, in fact, medicine has been able to push that door farther and farther into the future. Development of effective comprehensive pulmonary rehabilitation programs, the availability of home oxygen, and successful treatment of acute respiratory failure have significantly lengthened and improved the quality of life for COPD patients.

Most of you are living a decade longer than you would have just 20 years ago. With mortality typically staved off till the late 60s and early 70s, you now have an excellent shot at attaining your biblically allotted time on earth. And some of you will live to be much older than that.

But in addition to seeing COPD patients live well into old age, we want to see them live into their old age well. That is why we wrote this book. To the extent that it helps realize our hope, we have done our job.

21

Reflections: Taking the Measure

In our first edition we called this final chapter "Present and Future"—summing up the status quo, and trying our best to sense the winds of change. Now that we are at least a decade into this no longer uncharted future, we want to see how accurate we were.

Medical Optimism

In terms of treatment for COPD, we noted that patients found themselves in both the best of times and the worst of times. It was the best of times because—if you stopped smoking—medical knowledge of this disease could slow your rapid loss of lung function down to a normal rate of deterioration due to aging, giving you a satisfying and substantially longer life in return. Now, the evolution of technology has finally permitted lung volume reduction surgery to become a reality, and it appears to be a successful palliative measure in appropriate patients. In physical therapy, our greater understanding of the body's adaptation to exercise—especially the growing recognition of the value of weight training—has enhanced rehabilitation techniques.

We continue to be encouraged by the revolutionary breakthroughs allowing the missing enzyme in alpha$_1$-antitrypsin emphysema to be replaced by weekly injections of this essential protein. We had believed that by now scientists would have succeeded in incorporating the missing gene into patients' white blood cells, providing for their own natural production of the missing enzyme and making them normal. Perhaps we were a bit optimistic, but we still believe it is a question of time and the development of a more thorough understanding and a workable technology—it is simply that scientists did not yet know enough to be sufficiently aware of the complexities that still challenge us. And now on the horizon—with far more immediate application—is the possibility that a derivative of vitamin A may actually be able to restore lost lung tissue.

The future is likely to hold even greater miracles—probabilities that now sound like science fiction. We recently had dinner with a prominent geneticist who foresees a time when specific organs will be grown in test tubes to replace ailing ones. And on top of this, they will be custom-made—carrying each patient's unique immunologic fingerprint—allowing a healthy new organ to replace the diseased lungs with no need for immunosuppressive drugs and their harsh side effects. He also foresees the eventual capability to repair prenatally diagnosed genetic disorders—such as alpha$_1$-antitrypsin emphysema—in the unborn fetus.

So our sense that the continued development of science and technology would maintain this as the best of times for COPD patients has been borne out. Medical progress is unswerving in pointing to a brighter future for people with this serious chronic lung disease.

Economic Pressures Call the Shots in Health Care

But we had also predicted that the impact of this progress would be significantly blunted—"the worst of times"—because of economic pressures. And we erred, unable to imagine at that point the frightening extent to which economic pressures could interfere with optimal medical care.

Recently, the French farmer who led the demonstration that destroyed a McDonalds under construction in his town noted that the world had successfully faced and defeated the tyrannies of Fascism and then Communism, and that now we are contending with the tyranny of capitalism—that is, domination of the principle that *economics drives the system*. In the United States, this means that health issues concern the government only if: 1) they are likely to have a negative economic impact on the work force, and/or 2) they are a potential health threat to the power elite. Tuberculosis, for example, did not engender any government action as long as it was viewed as the wages of sin among the working class. Only once its negative effect on work productivity was realized, and the fact that its victims spanned all social classes, did the government enact public health measures and fund research. Similarly, HIV/AIDS measures received little federal funding while it was seen as a disease confined to promiscuous homosexuals, drug users, and the homeless. This remained the case until it was clear that AIDS has no social boundaries.

This brings us to the issue of national health insurance—the target of powerful opposition in the first half of this century from the American Medical Association, from industry, and from private insurance companies. The shameful result is that the United States is the only developed country without universal health care—leaving 44 million Americans out in the cold. The absence of a national health care system allowed private insurers to step in and create an industry—the health *management* organization. And here is the debilitating conflict of interest—they provide health care, the demands of which vary greatly with the individual patient, yet they insist on doing this at a highly respectable profit. These two goals are—on the large scale of such health care organizations—mutually exclusive. Since these large corporate entities can count on far more legal protection than can the individual patients they purport to exist for, we have seen a disheartening—and sometimes frightening—shift in the responsibility for health care decisions from physicians to administrators, and *their* strings are pulled by an establishment dedicated to earning substantial profit for its stockholders.

And perhaps the worst of it is that both private and governmental insurers are reluctant to pay for preventive medical care. Even though, as far as the COPD patient is concerned, prevention of exacerbation is *the* most effective form of therapy—and in general, regular preventive care is far less costly than the intensive treatments that advanced illness requires—insurers do not want to spend on early treatment now to guarantee savings later.

Although it is not our intention to politicize COPD, the essentially *unethical* nature of the system now providing health care in the United States makes this unavoidable. And because COPD patients tend to be older, and working hard simply to breathe, they are a vulnerable group. Far from the prototype of the squeaky wheel yelling to demand their rights, COPD patients concentrate on getting through their days—and nights—with enough air. They are easy prey.

Following is a summary of COPD health-related issues that we feel exemplify this blatant disregard of ethics. Although we have already detailed many of them in relevant chapters, there is virtue in bringing them together under a single spotlight. Perhaps it will help you find the anger and energy needed to turn up the volume on the squeaky wheel that advocacy groups like NHOPA and PERF have begun.

Although the National Institutes of Health clearly articulate their policy that participation in a program of exercise and breathing methods are part of the ". . . best known medical treatments for emphysema," there is no national policy authorizing Medicare reimbursement for pulmonary rehabilitation. It is left up to individual states, most of which do not recognize it. So it must be billed as "physical therapy," coverage is limited to 15 sessions, and the critical components of education and support groups are usually not covered at all. Place this in contrast to cardiac rehab patients—*who require essentially the same program*—for whom 36 sessions of comprehensive therapy are billed directly to Medicare as "cardiac rehabilitation."

Then there is the too frequent disgrace of inadequate and/or inappropriate oxygen provision to COPD patients, often flagrantly disregarding the physician's clearly written prescription. This effectively incarcerates these oxygen-requiring COPD patients in their homes—unless they can afford to pay for their oxygen—because the oxygen suppliers and HMOs place their profits ahead of the health and well-being of the patients they claim to serve.

Finally there is the federal government's handling of Medicare coverage for lung volume reduction surgery (LVRS). When the technology had developed to the point that this procedure became a reality for emphysema patients, and the benefits appeared to hold great promise, Medicare instituted coverage. Certain questions obviously required answers before a clear sense of its fundamental value could be determined: What are the benefits and risks compared with good medical therapy alone? How long do these benefits last? Does the procedure benefit some patients more than others? But we knew that these answers would emerge *in the course of our clinical experience.* Given enough time, we would know with confidence how representative or not the early success stories were.

Instead of allowing this time for natural evolution of knowledge, the federal government stepped in and required a long-term randomized controlled clinical trial (called NETT—the National Emphysema Treatment Trial) for answering these questions. And speaking through the National Institutes of Health and the Health Care Financing Administration (HCFA), the government decreed that Medicare will no longer cover LVRS until this trial is complete, and the data analyzed and deemed worthy. The many HMOs that take their lead from HCFA have followed suit, adding insult to injury.

This kind of study is not necessary or ethical, and we contend that it was put into effect because of reimbursement issues rather than legitimate scientific inquiry. Our government—at both federal and state levels—much prefers to invest in those segments of the population they see as productive and/or who do not tax existing resources. COPD patients—older people whose remaining years of economic productivity are few or nil, and whose annual medical cost have become fairly substantial—are unlikely to get high priority for existing funds. All too often, any excuse will do for denying support, or for taking it back once the economic bottom line is considered undesirable. A randomized clinical trial—meaning that volunteers are chosen randomly to be in the "experimental treatment" or "regular treatment" group—has meaning only when there is no way yet of knowing which treatment is actually best. With LVRS, however, we have data from as far back as the early 1990s indicating that this surgery provides significant palliative relief. So here we are with a government-sponsored clinical trial of a procedure that obviously provides benefit, yet half of the volunteers are being denied this treatment so that, in effect, we can get statistics to describe precisely how much benefit and how long it should last. But simply by observing our patients, and comparing these observations with the ample records that we have from the era before LVRS became available, we will reach these same conclusions—without denying treatment to half of the study participants, and without denying private treatment to all of those who cannot afford the $100,000 it currently costs to pay for it out of pocket.

How Can We Help Ourselves?

As far as health care insurance goes, even the institution of universal coverage will not eliminate a multilevel health care system. The wealthy will always get the most current and best available treatment, and those without substantial medical insurance will still be without support. Currently, the lowest rung of COPD patients are those who must rely on a municipal hospital clinic for their treatment. The clinic setting is unlikely to include any effort at rehabilitation—clinics simply cannot afford the needed time and personnel. But there is a system already in place that could help a great deal to narrow this gap. The U.S. government owns a large medical management organization. It is called the Veterans Administration: a network of 173 hospitals nationwide with approximately 51,000 beds; 391 outpatient, community, and outreach programs; 131 nursing home care units; and 39 domiciliaries. With the country's dramatically shrinking base of veterans—much smaller now than the VA system can easily handle—we suggest that the infrastructure needed to handle the medically uninsured is already in place. The one remaining step is to open it up to those in need.

On an individual level, we have two recommendations. One is to join the advocacy organizations that are marshalling their forces to make waves on your behalf. The more people they represent, the more letters that get written and the more phone calls that get made, the more powerful their voices will be. You'll find them listed in Chapter 12's discussion of the oxygen debacle, and in the Appendix.

And last but not least—*Hold on to your sense of humor!* This past decade of continued observation has confirmed our conclusion that the COPD patients who are success stories are those who do not take themselves too seriously. They *do* take their disease seriously—but not too seriously. Those who make it have not forgotten how to laugh.

Appendix

Additional Sources of Information

The Alpha1 Association
8120 Penn Ave. S., Suite 549
Minneapolis MN 55431-1326
800-521-3025 *or* 612-703-9979; *fax* 612-703-9977
A1NA@alpha1.org; www.alpha1.org

Considered to be the best-organized and most productive of all the patient support groups, they provide information, periodical publications, chat group opportunities, a support buddy network, great links, and more.

American College of Chest Physicians
911 Busse Highway
Park Ridge, IL 60068
www.chestnet.org
Professional society of chest physicians and surgeons that publishes *Chest.*

American Lung Association (ALA)
1740 Broadway
New York, NY 10019
212-315-8700
www.lungusa.org
The major national lung organization, the ALA publishes many pamphlets. Regional chapters exist in most areas.

American Thoracic Society (ATS)
1740 Broadway
New York, NY 10019
(212) 315-8700
www.thoracic.org
The medical section of the ALA. They publish the *American Review of Respiratory Diseases.*

National Heart, Lung, and Blood Institute
National Institutes of Health
Building 31, Room 4A21
9000 Rockville Pike
Bethesda, MD 20205
www.nhlbi.gov
The NHLBI is the major government sponsor of research in respiratory diseases.

National Jewish Medical and Research Center
1400 Jackson Street
Denver, CO 80206
www.njc.org
Large referral hospital for difficult COPD cases. They publish two quarterly newsletters: *New Directions* (for the lay public) and *Update* (for the physician). They also run Lung-Line, a free telephone information service, from 8:00 A.M. to 5:00 P.M. MST; 800-222-LUNG, or from inside Colorado, 303-398-1477.

Second Wind Lung Transplant Association
300 South Duncan Avenue, Suite 227
Clearwater, FL 33755-6457
888-222-2690 *or* 727-442-0892
secondwind@netzero.net; www.2ndWind.org
Although the focus is on pre- and post-transplant patients and their families, all patients with a chronic lung disease are welcome. This organization offers information, education, local support groups, organized activities, and products. They also maintain a chatroom on-line that operates for scheduled one-hour sessions.

Further Readings

Newsletters

Alpha$_1$News is published by the Alpha1 Association, 8120 Penn Ave. S., Suite 549, Minneapolis, MN 55431-1326.

The Pulmonary Paper—published by a group of health care professionals—is at P.O. Box 877, Ormond Beach, FL 32175, 800-950-3698, fax: 904-673-5044, *Belyea@aol.com.*

Respiratory News & Views is published by the Asthma/Emphysema Self-Help Group, 172 East 4th Street, #11F, New York, NY 10009, 212-777-0486, *respiratorynews@aol.com.*

Second Wind is published by the Pulmonary Education and Research Foundation (PERF), P.O. Box 1133 Lomita, CA 90717-5133, 310-539-8390, *perf@pacbell.net.*

Books for the Layperson

American Lung Association of Southwestern Pennsylvania Staff. *Self Help: Your Strategy for Living with COPD.* Bull Publishing Co., 1997.

Hubbard, K. and M. Williams, *To Air Is Human: A Manual for People with Chronic Lung Disease.* Pritchett and Hull Associates, 1999.

Jenkins, M. *Chronic Obstructive Pulmonary Disease: Practical Medical and Spiritual Guidelines for Daily Living with Emphysema, Chronic Bronchitis and Combination.* Hazelden Information Education, 1999.

The following books are out of print but may still be available. Two excellent on-line sources for locating hard-to-find books are *amazon.com* and *alibris.com.* Although Alibris is much easier to use and you get instant feedback, Amazon may be able to locate a book that Alibris doesn't have on hand.

Dewey, J. *Of Life and Breath.* Warner Books, 1986.

Petty, T. L., and L. M. Nett, *Enjoying Life with Emphysema.* (2nd ed.). Lea and Febiger, 1987.

Shayevitz, M. B., and B. R. Shayevitz, *Living Well with Emphysema and Bronchitis.* Doubleday, 1985.

Drug Information

Facts and Comparisons Drug Information. Updated monthly, and published by the Facts and Comparisons Division, J. B. Lippincott Co., 111 West Port Plaza, St. Louis, MO 63141.

Physicians' Desk Reference for Prescription Drugs. Published yearly by the Medical Economics Co., Oradell, NJ 07649.

United States Pharmacopeia Convention. One-page, easy-to-understand descriptions of medications; covers proper use, interaction with other drugs, side effects, how each drug works, and a list of generic types. For COPD these include:

adrenergic bronchodilator (aerosol inhalation)
adrenergic bronchodilator (oral/injection)
adrenocorticoids (aerosol)
adrenocorticoids (inhalation/oral)
xanthine (theophylline) bronchodilators (oral)

Medical Dictionary

Dorland's Illustrated Medical Dictionary. Philadelphia: W. B. Saunders. (We find it easier to use than Stedman's Medical Dictionary.)

Glossary

Words in **bold** type within a definition are also defined in the Glossary.

Accessory muscles of respiration   These muscles in the neck, shoulders, chest, and back help the main respiratory muscles during strenuous exercise and when it becomes difficult to breathe. Their contraction lifts the rib cage, making it larger.

Acinus   The acinus is the basic structural respiratory unit. Its structure combines the two final airway branchings (the tiniest **bronchioles**) with the alveoli they serve.

Adrenergic   Pertains to three related things: (1) the group of hormones—including *adrenaline*—produced by the inner segment of the adrenal glands, (2) the receptors on other organs that these hormones stimulate to achieve their effects, and (3) any drug that stimulates these same receptors. Adrenergic drugs dilate the airways.

Aerosol   A spray of fine particles that can be inhaled. Certain drugs available in liquid form can be taken this way. The aerosol is created with either a **nebulizer** or a **metered-dose inhaler**.

Allergy   A hypersensitive **immune system** response to a substance the person has been exposed to at least once before. People without this allergy are unaffected by the same substance. This response appears in one or more of the following ways: rash, hives, runny nose, itchy eyes, swelling, asthma.

Alpha$_1$-antitrypsin (AAT) or alpha$_1$-antiprotease (AAP)   The regulatory enzyme that prevents the **elastase** enzyme from digesting too much **elastin** protein in our lungs. Too little AAT can cause **emphysema.**

Alveolus   One of the millions of air sacs in the lungs, located at the ends of the narrowest airways. The *alveoli* (referring to more than one) are surrounded by **capillaries**. The exchange of **oxygen** and **carbon dioxide** occurs through the membrane separating the alveoli and capillaries. (See also **Acinus, Capillaries**.)

Arterial blood gases   The two gases carried in our blood are **oxygen** and **carbon dioxide**. The concentrations carried in our arterial blood—blood freshly oxygenated and cleansed of excess carbon diox-

306

ide by the lungs—are referred to as arterial blood gases. (See also **Hypoxemia, Hypoxia, Hypercapnia**.)

Atelectasis   Collapse of a small or large area of the lungs because all the gas in those **alveoli** has been absorbed and not replaced. It is encountered in severe **chronic bronchitis** when blocked airways prevent **oxygen** from entering.

Autonomic nervous system   This part of the central nervous system regulates the various organs in the body over which we have no voluntary control. Its two opposite-acting branches are the *sympathetic* and *parasympathetic nervous systems*. Stimulating the sympathetic branch causes the airways to dilate.

Beta-2 receptors   A type of receptor that is stimulated by **adrenergic** hormones. Activating beta-2 receptors causes bronchodilation.

Breath sounds   Sounds heard through the stethoscope as air moves in and out of the lungs. Certain breath sounds are characteristic of specific lung problems. Airway obstruction produces wheezing, the sound of turbulence caused as air is forced around **mucus** and through narrowed airways. A rale (or *rahl*) is the noise air makes as it bubbles through accumulated mucus.

Bronchi   The larger airways (meaning a diameter of more than 1/12 inch or 2 mm).

Bronchioles   The smaller airways, which branch off the **bronchi** and eventually end in the **alveoli**. The bronchioles get narrower each time they branch. The second narrowest airways are the *terminal* bronchioles. Each one ends in an **acinus** (see Figure 2.4): a *respiratory* (narrowest) bronchiole and the alveoli it serves.

Bronchoconstriction   Airway narrowing from one or more of the following causes: airway muscle contraction; swelling of the tissue lining the airways; excessive mucus clogging the airways.

Bronchoconstrictor   Any substance causing the airways to narrow.

Bronchodilator   Any substance that reverses bronchoconstriction.

Bulla   A large, air-containing space within the lungs created by the destruction and merging of neighboring **alveoli** that **emphysema** causes.

Capillaries   The smallest blood vessels, and the site of gas exchange throughout the body. In the lungs, capillary blood picks up **oxygen** from the **alveoli** while it discharges **carbon dioxide**. In other tissues, oxygen leaves the capillaries while they pick up carbon dioxide.

Carbon dioxide   Abbreviated CO_2, it is a waste product (the other being water) of energy metabolism. It is important in maintaining proper blood acidity, and is the major regulator of **ventilation.**

Chronic bronchitis   A **chronic obstructive pulmonary disease** in which chronic airway inflammation and **mucus** overproduction obstruct the airways, interfering with adequate **oxygen** supply and **carbon dioxide** removal.

Cilia   Microscopic hair-like structures on the cells lining the inner surface of the airways. They sweep particles out of the lungs after they are trapped in **mucus.** Inhaled cigarette smoke damages this sweeping mechanism. (See also **Sputum.**)

COPD (Chronic Obstructive Pulmonary Disease)   A group of lung diseases primarily affecting expiration, COPD commonly refers to **chronic bronchitis** and **emphysema**, but also includes asthma, bronchiectasis, and cystic fibrosis. (Sometimes called COAD, with *Airway* substituted for *Pulmonary*, or COLD, with *Lung* substituted.)

Cyanosis   The bluish tint appearing around the lips and under the fingernails when there is inadequate **oxygen** in the blood.

Diaphragm   The major inspiratory muscle. The larger, thin, dome-shaped muscle separates the chest and abdominal cavities.

Dyspnea   The subjective, highly unpleasant feeling of not being able to catch one's breath.

Edema   Excess fluid in the tissues, often from inflammation. In more severe COPD with accompanying heart failure, fluid accumulates in the lungs.

Elastase   The enzyme that digests the protein *elastin*, the lungs' primary structural elastic fiber that is so critical to its function. Normally, the **alpha$_1$-antitrypsin** regulatory enzyme ensures that elastase only destroys old elastin. With inadequate alpha$_1$-antitrypsin—from an inherited deficiency or from cigarette smoking—elastase also destroys healthy elastin fibers, initiating **emphysema.**

Elastin   See **Elastase**.

Emphysema   A **chronic obstructive pulmonary disease** that destroys **alveoli,** and so impairs **oxygen** and **carbon dioxide** exchange.

Expectorant   Any drug or other product (for example, garlic) that helps move and expel airway **mucus.**

FEV$_1$ (Forced Expiratory Volume in 1 Second)   The volume of air that can be forcefully expired from a maximum inspiration during the first second. This is a traditional test for evaluating how well the lungs are working. Airway obstruction reduces this volume, so it is always smaller in **COPD.**

FVC (Forced Vital Capacity)   The total amount of air that can be forcefully expired from a maximum inspiration. Whether or not it is reduced depends on **COPD** severity.

Generic drugs Drugs that are called by their common chemical name instead of a brand name. They are usually cheaper than their brand name counterparts.

Genetic Referring to the inheritance of biological traits.

Hypercapnia Abnormally high quantities of **carbon dioxide** in arterial blood.

Hyperventilation Breathing harder and faster than the body needs. Because it removes **carbon dioxide** from the blood much faster than normal, hyperventilation is technically defined as subnormal carbon dioxide in arterial blood.

Hypoventilation The opposite of **hyperventilation**, it is **ventilation** that cannot supply the body's metabolic demand for **oxygen** or remove enough **carbon dioxide**. It is technically defined as abnormally high carbon dioxide in arterial blood with subnormal oxygen content. (See also **Hypercapnia** and **Hypoxia**.)

Hypoxemia Inadequate **oxygen** in the blood.

Hypoxia A more general term for inadequate **oxygen**, it can be due to heart disease, lung disease, anemia, or high altitude (where there is not enough oxygen in the air). **Hypoxemia** and hypoxia are often used interchangeably.

Incidence The rate at which something occurs. For example, 6% of the American people have **COPD**. This term is often confused with **prevalence**.

Intravenous medication Medicine injected directly into a vein.

Lobule The cluster of **acini** branching off from a single terminal **bronchiole**. Viewed under the microscope, each lobule resembles a bunch of grapes (see Figure 2.4).

Metered-dose inhaler (MDI) A hand-held device that uses medication in liquid form to dispense a fixed dosage via **aerosol**.

Mucus Sticky airway secretion, produced by mucous glands and goblet cells, that traps foreign debris to prevent lung damage. It is seriously overproduced in **chronic bronchitis**, obstructing the airways. (See also **Sputum**.)

Nebulizer A device that converts a liquid into a fine spray inhaled with a mask.

Oxygen Abbreviated O_2, it is the gas that allows energy to be released from the food we eat. *Metabolism* is the process by which this happens.

Parasympathetic nervous system See **Autonomic nervous system**.

Phlegm See **Sputum**.

Prevalence The number of disease cases existing in a specified population at a particular time. For example, 16 million Americans currently have **COPD**. This term is often confused with **incidence**.

Prophylactic Preventive. In **COPD**, for example, flu vaccination is prophylactic medication because it prevents a type of upper respiratory infection.

Pulmonary function tests A series of tests designed to evaluate the health of the lungs (see illustrations in Chapter 5). (See also **FEV₁** and **FVC**.)

Rale Also called *rahl*. See **Breath sounds**.

Respiratory tract The system of tubes passing air from the mouth and nose to the **alveoli** (see Figure 2.1). The upper respiratory tract runs from the mouth and nose to the end of the **trachea** (windpipe). The lower respiratory tract goes from the end of the trachea to the alveoli entry points. *Upper respiratory infections* and *lower respiratory infections* refer to this division.

Sign Something observed about a patient, such as the bluish tint around his lips from inadequate **oxygen**. This stands in contrast to a *symptom*, which is something the patient notices or complains about. **Dyspnea** is the **emphysema** patient's classic symptom.

Sputum Also called *phlegm*, this is material coughed up from the lungs. It contains mucus and cells from the airway lining, cellular debris, bacteria, etc.

Sympathetic nervous system See **Autonomic nervous system**.

Symptom See **sign**.

Systemic The entire body. An oral or injected drug is called systemic because it is distributed throughout the body. A systemic drug becomes diluted as it spreads through the body, while a locally administered drug—because it doesn't spread—remains full strength in the desired area. So when a certain concentration of a **bronchodilator** drug is needed in the airways, a systemic preparation must be used in a higher dosage—to allow for dilution—than a local preparation.

Trachea The main windpipe connecting the mouth and nose to the lungs. It begins just below the Adam's apple and ends where it divides into the main right and left **bronchi**.

Vaccine A substance usually derived from live disease organisms which, when injected into animals or people, protects them against developing that disease.

Ventilation The amount of air that moves in and out of the lungs. It is usually measured for a given time period and recorded in liters per minute (called *minute ventilation*).

Wheeze See **Breath sounds**.

Index

dust, 217
dyspnea
  in cardiovascular disease, 77
  in chronic bronchitis, 41, 62
  disability evaluations and, 240
  downward spiral of, 4–5
  in emphysema, 44–45, 62
  exertional, 44–45, 164, 185, 271,
    272
  and fear, 204, 207, 208
  and oxygen, 164
  recovering from, 185–86
  and sexual activity, 209, 242, 249

echinacea, 152–53, 257–58
edema, peripheral, 64
elastase, 24, 37–38, 40, 46, 48
elasticity (elastance), 22–24, 25, 38,
    271
elastin, 24, 37–38, 46, 47
electrocardiograms, 72
emotional impact of COPD
  anxiety, 142–44, 156–58, 204,
    207–210
  dealing with, 210–13
  death and dying issues, 285–86
  denial, 167, 206
  depression, 142, 143, 144, 158,
    204, 206
  on family, 208–209, 212, 292
  fear, 4–5, 204, 207–208, 209
  help for, 210–13
  mourning, 206–207
  oxygen therapy and, 167
emphysema
  airway obstruction in, 25, 29, 44,
    271
  alpha$_1$-antitrypsin deficiency, 8–9,
    21, 24, 36–38, 46–51, 71–72, 296
  alveoli in, 6, 20–22, 29, 32, 38, 70
  centrilobular (centriacinar), 22, 42
  chest X-ray in, 70
  chronic bronchitis with, 36, 40, 44
  coughing in, 61
  course of, 38–39, 44–45

dyspnea and, 44–45, 62
elasticity and, 23, 24, 271
experimental treatment for, 141–42
ipratropium bromide for, 116
lung volume reduction surgery for,
    263, 268–78, 279–81
panlobular (panacinar), 21, 42
predominating, 44–45
resistance and, 25
smoking and, 9, 36, 37–38, 46, 48
symptoms of, 44–45, 59, 61–64
energy-saving strategies, 225–29,
    250–51
environmental irritants, 216–21,
    255–57
ephedrine, 105
euthanasia, 287–93
exercise
  aerobic, 191, 195, 272
  breathing exercises, 86, 182–86
  emphysema and, 271–72
  heart rate during, 192–93, 197–98,
    199
  lung volume reduction surgery
    and, 272
  medication adjustments for,
    198–99
  muscle-strengthening, 196
  oxygen therapy and, 164, 165, 199
  programs, 191–97
  respiratory process and, 22–23, 25
  sexual activity and, 249
  for smoking cessation, 93
  surgery and, 84, 86
  tests, 73, 74, 193
expectorants, 105, 139–40, 151
expiration
  carbon dioxide and, 15
  in COPD, 25, 26, 29, 38
  elasticity and, 22–23
  muscles of, 17–19, 23, 25, 38
  pursed-lip, 183, 184, 185, 189, 225
  resistance and, 25, 28, 38
  surface tension and, 24
expiratory reserve volume, 65, 66